McLaughlin and K

Continuous Quality Improvement in Health Care

FIFTH EDITION

Julie K. Johnson, PhD, MSPH

Professor, Department of Surgery
Center for Healthcare Studies
Institute for Public Health and Medicine
Feinberg School of Medicine, Northwestern University
Chicago, Illinois

William A. Sollecito, DrPH

Clinical Professor, Public Health Leadership Program
UNC Gillings School of Global Public Health
University of North Carolina at Chapel Hill
Chapel Hill, North Carolina

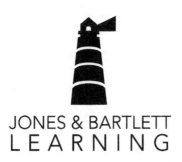

JONES & BARTLETT
LEARNING

World Headquarters
Jones & Bartlett Learning
5 Wall Street
Burlington, MA 01803
978-443-5000
info@jblearning.com
www.jblearning.com

Jones & Bartlett Learning books and products are available through most bookstores and online booksellers. To contact Jones & Bartlett Learning directly, call 800-832-0034, fax 978-443-8000, or visit our website, www.jblearning.com.

Substantial discounts on bulk quantities of Jones & Bartlett Learning publications are available to corporations, professional associations, and other qualified organizations. For details and specific discount information, contact the special sales department at Jones & Bartlett Learning via the above contact information or send an email to specialsales@jblearning.com.

Production Credits

VP, Product Management: David D. Cella
Director of Product Management: Michael Brown
Product Manager: Sophie Fleck Teague
Product Specialist: Carter McAlister
Production Manager: Carolyn Rogers Pershouse
Production Editor: Brooke Haley
Senior Marketing Manager: Susanne Walker
Manufacturing and Inventory Control Supervisor: Amy Bacus
Composition: codeMantra U.S. LLC

Cover Design: Scott Moden
Text Design: Kristin E. Parker
Director of Rights & Media: Joanna Gallant
Rights & Media Specialist: Merideth Tumasz
Media Development Editor: Shannon Sheehan
Cover Image (Title Page, Chapter Opener):
   © ALMAGAMI/Shutterstock
Printing and Binding: Command Robbinsville
Cover Printing: Command Robbinsville

Library of Congress Cataloging-in-Publication Data
Names: Sollecito, William A., author.
Title: Mclaughlin and Kaluzny's continuous quality improvement in health care /
William A. Sollecito, DRPH, UNC, Chapel Hill, Julie Johnson, PhD, MSPH,
Northwestern University Medical School, Chicago, Illinois.
Other titles: Continuous quality improvement in health care
Description: Fifth edition. | Burlington, Massachusetts: Jones & Bartlett Learning, [2019] |
Includes bibliographical references.
Identifiers: LCCN 2018029625 | ISBN 9781284126594 (paperback)
Subjects: LCSH: Medical care—United States—Quality control. | Total quality management—United States.
Classification: LCC RA399.A3 C66 2019 | DDC 362.10973—dc23
LC record available at https://lccn.loc.gov/2018029625

6048

Printed in the United States of America
24 23 22 21   10 9 8 7 6 5 4 3

To my home team—Paul, Harrison, Tore, and Elijah.

–JJ

To my family for their loving support always and especially to our newest addition, Mason, who represents the future, which is what this book is all about!

–WS

Contents

Contents

Acknowledgments

As we developed the fifth edition of *Continuous Quality Improvement in Health Care*, we were inspired once again by Drs. McLaughlin and Kaluzny. While we are very appreciative of their contribution of the Preface, their contribution has been so much greater through the years, as mentors and as colleagues.

We were also inspired by the thought provoking Foreword written by Dr. Paul Batalden where he outlined the model of CQI in improving quality, safety, and value and the model of coproduction in improving the "value of the health care service contribution to better health."

We have benefited greatly from the feedback of students who have provided insight and understanding of the importance of making this book a practical teaching tool that addresses the continuing challenges of improving quality and safety of health care in the future. We are most appreciative to our friends and colleagues around the globe who authored chapters. The coordination and integration of the contributing authors was a tremendous undertaking and we were privileged to work with excellent colleagues, who are truly expert practitioners of continuous quality improvement in health care.

The production of the book required a team effort at all levels and in multiple locations. We would first like to acknowledge the assistance and guidance of the editorial team at Jones & Bartlett Learning. In Chapel Hill, special appreciation goes to Dean Barbara Rimer, of the UNC Gillings School of Global Public Health, whose leadership inspires a learning environment that stimulates innovations and the motivation to pursue them. Deep appreciation is also given to the faculty and staff in the Public Health Leadership Program at the University of North Carolina and the Center for Healthcare Studies and Surgical Outcomes and Quality Improvement Center (SOQIC) at Northwestern University with whom we shared ideas that led to a better product. We especially thank Dr. Rohit Ramaswamy, who not only authored two chapters but also shared his wisdom about the current and future trends in CQI globally. Finally, we appreciate the feedback and guidance that we received from the readers of the *Fourth Edition*, which among other things led us to reduce the number of chapters in this edition, but also gave us the incentive to go into greater depth on some of the new topics, such as implementation science. While several chapters of the *Fourth Edition* have been eliminated, we would like to acknowledge several of the authors of those chapters here, as the concepts (listed below) were integrated into this edition's remaining chapters. They include:

- Vaughn Upshaw and David Steffen—the importance of the learning organization concepts in CQI
- Anna Schenck, Jill McArdle, and Robert Weiser—the use of Medicare data in CQI and the real-world example of the Clemson Nursing Home Case Study
- Curt McLaughlin and David Kibbe—the importance of health information technology and understanding the strengths and weaknesses of various data sources used in CQI

Once again, as with CQI itself, the production of this book truly required teamwork and we appreciate and acknowledge the vital role of all of our fellow team members, not the least of which includes our families.

Julie K. Johnson, Chicago, IL
William A. Sollecito, Chapel Hill, NC

Contributors

Paul Barach, MD, MPH
Clincal Professor
Wayne State University School of Medicine
Stavanger University Hospital, Stavanger,
Norway

Carol E. Breland, MPH, RRT, RCP-NPS
Research Recruitment Director
TraCS Institute
School of Medicine
University of North Carolina at Chapel Hill
Chapel Hill, North Carolina

Bruce J. Fried, PhD
Associate Professor
Department of Health Policy & Management
UNC Gillings School of Global
Public Health
University of North Carolina at Chapel Hill
Chapel Hill, North Carolina

David Greenfield, PhD
Professor and Director
Australian Institute of Health Service
Management
University of Tasmania
Sydney, Australia

Lisa R Hirschhorn, MD MPH
Professor, Medical Social Sciences and
Psychiatry and Behavioral Sciences
Member of Center for Prevention
Evaluation Implementation
Methodology (CEPIM)
Institute for Public Health and Medicine
Feinberg School of Medicine
Northwestern University
Chicago, Illinois

David Hardison, PhD
Vice President, Health Sciences
ConvergeHEALTH by Deloitte
Costa Mesa, California

Sara E. Massie, MPH
Senior Program Director
Population Health Improvement Partners
Morrisville, North Carolina

Mike Newton-Ward, MSW, MPH
Social Marketing Consultant
Adjunct Assistant Professor
Public Health Leadership Program
UNC Gillings School of Global Public Health
University of North Carolina at Chapel Hill
Chapel Hill, North Carolina

Marjorie Pawsey, AM, MBBS, FAAQHC
Senior Visiting Fellow
Australian Institute of Health Innovation
Macquarie University
Sydney, Australia

Edward Popovich, PhD
President
Sterling Enterprises International, Inc.
Adjunct Professor, Nova Southeastern
University College of Osteopathic Medicine
Satellite Beach, Florida

Rohit Ramaswamy, PhD, MPH, Grad. Dipl. (Bios)
Clinical Professor, Public Health Leadership
and Maternal and Child Health
Co-lead, MPH Global Health Concentration
UNC Gillings School of Global Public Health
University of North Carolina at Chapel Hill
Chapel Hill, North Carolina

Charlotte E. Randolph, BA
Research Assistant
UNC-RTI Evidence-Based
    Practice Center
Cecil G. Sheps Center for Health Services
    Research
University of North Carolina at
    Chapel Hill
Chapel Hill, North Carolina

Greg D. Randolph, MD, MPH
Executive Director
Population Health Improvement
    Partners
Morrisville, North Carolina
Professor, Department of Pediatrics
University of North Carolina School of
    Medicine
Adjunct Professor, Public Health
    Leadership Program
UNC Gillings School of Global
    Public Health
University of North Carolina at
    Chapel Hill
Chapel Hill, North Carolina

Hamish Robertson, PhD
Research Fellow
Centre for Health Services Management
Faculty of Health
University of Technology Sydney
Sydney, Australia

Joanne Travaglia, PhD
Professor and Director
Centre for Health Services Management
Faculty of Health
University of Technology Sydney
Sydney, Australia

Hal Wiggin, EdD
Adjunct Professor, Nova Southeastern
    University College of Osteopathic Medicine
Fort Lauderdale, Florida

Donna Woods, PhD
Associate Professor of Pediatrics
Center for Healthcare Studies
Institute for Public Health and Medicine
Feinberg School of Medicine and
Northwestern University
Chicago, Illinois

Preface

The first edition of *Continuous Quality Improvement in Health Care* was published in 1994. Continuous quality improvement in health care was in its infancy. Paul Batalden had kindly educated us, and others, on his philosophy and groundbreaking efforts at Hospital Corporation of America. The Joint Commission had recently launched the *Agenda for Change*. Within the larger health care community there was interest as well as skepticism as to whether manufacturing techniques that were popular and successful were applicable to health care. The obvious need was to explain the basics and provide documentation to illustrate its applicability to health care organizations. The *First Edition* provided the basics along with a series of cases to illustrate its relevance to health care. A key chapter was "Does TQM/CQI Really Work in Health Care?"

By the *Second Edition* in 1999, the issues of quality in health care had come of age with the publication of the IOM report *Crossing the Quality Chasm*. Many issues of implementation had become evident and a new key chapter was "CQI, Transformation and the 'Learning' Organization." At the same time the importance of such efforts was recognized by the health care version of the National Malcolm Baldrige Quality Award, whose standards were included in the text.

The *Third Edition* in 2006 emphasized measurement, especially outcomes measurement, as the use of CQI concepts expanded. It also paid attention to information technology that had the power to enhance implementation and to disseminate results more widely. At the same time the barriers to widespread adoption

of the knowledge produced were evident. The new cases on Intermountain Health Care and the American Board of Pediatrics efforts at organizational and professional learning were featured illustrations.

The *Fourth Edition* in 2013 was under the capable leadership of Bill Solliceto and Julie Johnson. Its publication aligned with the passage of the Affordable Care Act expanding the insurance coverage to 50 million people and the role of the CMS to assess different delivery models of care. It was a time of great expectations with emphasis on measurement and the movement of these efforts into a number of professional, governmental and international spheres. The CQI approach to quality and quality improvement had now achieved global prominence and led to the development of the companion volume, McLaughlin, Johnson, & Sollecito, *Implementing Continuous Quality Improvement in Health Care: A Global Casebook*.

As the *Fifth Edition* goes to press, basic elements of the ACA have been dismantled and, while quality improvement is a well-accepted management tool, issues of institutionalization, measurement, implementation and adaptation to environments remain challenging. One is tempted to conclude that not much has changed; major segments of the population are at risk of losing insurance coverage, interest in empirical evaluation of alternative care models and quality improvement efforts has slowed, and some evaluation studies on cost savings of quality improvement have not met expectations.

Over the past 25 years we have learned a lot about quality improvement, its implementation and the challenges and opportunities of quality and quality improvement as a core function in health care. What has changed is the context within which health care is provided that must be accommodated within future quality improvement processes. Many of these contextual changes were un imaginable 25 years ago; the sequencing of the genome and its implication for genomic medicine, the commercialization of health care, the consolidation of heath care organizations on a massive scale, and the introduction of new forms of provider organizations, (e.g., ACOs, Walmart, and Humana), the deprofessionalization of health care providers, the basic demographics of the population, and the types of care that will be needed in the years ahead.

With these changes have come new issues involving quality improvement:

- Will the addition of ever more quality and "value" measures turn attention away from an overall culture of improvement? Will people focus in on what is measured? That is already one reason why health care is great at increasing revenue, but not at reducing waste.

- Can we overcome the gaps between professional points of view? Or will we continue to have an attending specialist see the story boards in the his unit as "something the nurses are doing?"

- Will the institutionalization and professionalization of quality in ever large and more complex institutions be relegated to the quality officer/office rather than a fundamental responsibility of all personnel?

- Will health care management recognize that their departments and institutions are part of a larger system of care? A system of care characterized by handoffs that transcend organizational boundaries involving an array of organizations and providers with different professional and organizational cultures yet critical to providing an integrated seamless care continuum from prevention to end of life.

These are not abstract academic issues. These are real issues, involving real people, of which we are all at risk. We know what it is like to observe specialists exhibit mutual hostility at the bedside because one didn't comprehend why the other demanded a prompt weekend consult, or wonder how a case manager can expect an emotionally exhausted family, following an extended and traumatic hospital stay, to select from a list of long term care facilities without any guidance or insight about the facilities. These experiences change your perspective on quality, quality improvement and the role of management in implementing organizational structures and mechanisms to assure interdisciplinary collaboration and training hospital personnel to effectively manage the transition points in the care continuum.

As we enter an era of an aging population and precision medicine supported by genomics and big data, the quality of care at the front end will rapidly improve leaving the greater challenges and the greater payoffs to society in chronic and end-of-life care. What Deming, a pioneer in quality improvement, stated 50 years ago remains relevant today—that the problems are with the system and the system belongs to management. Our methods of quality improvement must encompass these larger, increasingly relevant systems.

Curtis P. McLaughlin, DBA
Arnold D. Kaluzny, PhD
Chapel Hill, North Carolina

Foreword

...questions
that have no right
to go away (Whyte, 2007).

This book invites two questions that may "have no right to go away" in our journey toward better health:

1. If we make improving quality, safety, and value an "enterprise-wide effort," what do we need to know and do?
2. If we make improving the "value of the health care service contribution to better health" our focus, what do we need to know and do?

▶ Enterprise-Wide Effort?

In response to this question, our attention has been directed at the ways and structures through which leaders lead organizations and the way(s) organizations and their people respond. In the last few decades, in addition to work "inside," we have been encouraged to look outside of the health care services sector to organization-wide efforts in automotive, computer, aerospace, and elsewhere, where great gains in quality, safety, and value have been made. We have learned a great deal about our own work: health care service as a system, process; system leadership; measurement of outcome; unwanted variation; system failure and unreliability; organization-wide contributions to better health; making improvement part of everyone's job; accountability for better performance and many other themes.

The *First Edition* of this book was published as we were deeply into these pursuits and learning (McLaughlin & Kaluzny, 1994). Several chapters in this edition of that book honor this question and help identify what might be known and done currently. Their content helps frame important contributions to leader development, selection, and performance assessment. In the short-term, following these chapters can offer today's leaders and organizations real substance in the performance of "leader and organization-wide work" for the improvement of health care service.

▶ Value of Health Care Service Contribution to Better Health?

This question invites focus on the words "service," "value," and "contribution." It suggests that we recognize that we are mainly in the business of making services, that we are invited to attend to the economic value of our efforts and that we acknowledge that our services are best thought of as a contribution to health.

Service

Victor Fuchs in his early review of the emerging service economy noted that making a service was different from making a product (Fuchs, 1968). Services always required the active participation, insight from two parties: the professional and the beneficiary. Vincent and Elinor Ostrom were the first to call that

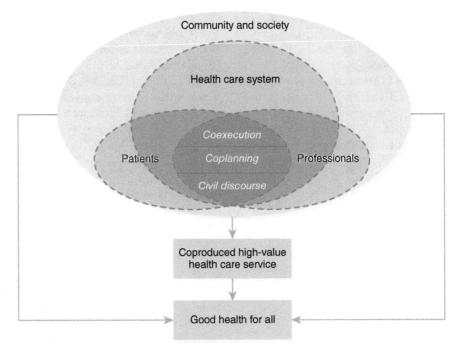

FIGURE 1 Conceptual Model of Health Care Services Coproduction

Reproduced from Batalden M. et al. *BMJ Qual Saf* 2016;25:509–517.

phenomenon "coproduction."[4] Building on the work of Lusch and Vargo (2014), Osborne, Radnor, and Nasi suggested that a "product-dominant logic" had overtaken a clearer view of the logic involved in making a service.[6] Building on these ideas of "service" and how "making a service" might be different from "making a product," Batalden and colleagues offered a description of the coproduction of health care service and a model for understanding and use, as illustrated in **FIGURE 1** (Batalden, Batalden, Margolis, et al., 2016).

The model invited attention to the interactions of patients and professionals. It suggested that a variety of interactions might be possible, ranging from "civil discourse" to "co-execution." It recognized that these interactions occurred partly within an openly bounded health care system and in the context of social and community systems. This

variety of interaction depended in part on the knowledge, skill, habits and willingness to be vulnerable as the parties engaged in the relationships and actions that characterized a health care service.

These insights formed the basis of a clearer idea of the interdependent work of two groups of people, some of whom might be named "patients" and some named as "professionals"—though in reality they each brought different expertise to their shared interactions.

If we really mean that health care services are "coproduced," new tools that enable visualization and design that reflect the contribution of patients and professionals will be helpful. The measurement of process and result will need to reflect both the implementation and effect of the professional's science-informed practice (Greenhalgh, 2018) and the methods of addressing and the degree of attainment of the patient's goal.

But not all health professional work seems to fit this service logic. Sometimes the health care work seems to better fit "making a product." Helping professionals know when to use which logic—service-making or product-making—will open new approaches to design, as well as professional education, development.

Value

Øystein Fjeldstad has suggested that multiple system architectures might be useful to create value in modern service-making. He includes the development of standardized responses to commonly occurring needs in linked processes (value chains), customized responses to particular needs (value shop), and flexible responses to emergent needs (value network) (Stabel & Fjeldstad, 1998; Fjeldstad, Snow, Miles, Lettl, 2012). Using this typology one can begin to imagine the opportunity to link them in ways that match need and system form. Much more development of these multiple ways of creating value seems likely.

Contribution

This word invites us to remember that a person's health is not easy to "outsource" to a professional. At best, the health professional's coproduced service makes a contribution to further another person's health. Recognizing that the shared work is a contribution to health, invites inquiry into patient need, patient assets, patient supports, patient knowledge & skill, patient's lived reality as part of the understanding for service coproduction design. A similar inventory of knowledge, skill, habits, capability and interest of professionals seems in order. Even the professional-patient relationship itself could be explored for its capability in contributing to the process of coproducing a service. Assessments of the role that other complementary resources & services, such as

social services must become even more clear and reliable as we use and integrate them with health care services for "improved outcomes" (Bradley & Taylor, 2015).

With this edition, the editors point to the future of the second question and have opened this space for readers (Chapter 14).

▶ In Summary

Both questions seem to have "patiently waited for us" in the poet's words (Whyte, 2007). They both invite strategic thinking and aligned professional action. Both recognize that "knowing" alone is not sufficient. Books like this can invite knowing and doing, but it is the reader who makes things happen. Enjoy the authors and editors' words in this book but enjoy their intent in the work of an informed, acting reader even more. Let me close with Mary Oliver's words (Oliver, 2005):

What I Have Learned So Far

Meditation is old and honorable, so why should I not sit, every morning of my life, on the hillside, looking into the shining world? Because, properly attended to, delight, as well as havoc, is suggestion. Can one be passionate about the just, the ideal, the sublime, and the holy, and yet commit to no labor in its cause? I don't think so.

All summations have a beginning, all effect has a story, all kindness begins with the sown seed. Thought buds toward radiance. The gospel of light is the crossroads of—indolence, or action.

Be ignited, or be gone.

Paul Batalden, MD
Active Emeritus Professor
The Dartmouth Institute for Health Policy
and Clinical Practice
St. Paul, MN 55108

▶ References

1. Whyte D. Sometimes. In Whyte D., *River Flow: New & Selected Poems: 1984-2007*. Langley, WA: Many Rivers Press, 2007.
2. McLaughlin C.P., Kaluzny A.D. (eds.), *Continuous Quality Improvement in Health Care: Theory, Implementation and Applications*. Gaithersburg, MD: Aspen Publishers, 1994.
3. Fuchs V. *The service economy*. New York, NY: National Bureau of Economic Research, 1968.
4. Ostrom V, Ostrom E. Public Goods and Public Choices. In Savas ES, ed., *Alternatives for Delivering Public Services: Toward Improved Performance*. Boulder, CO: Westview Press, 1977: Part 1: 7–44.
5. Lusch R.F., Vargo S.L. *Service-Dominant Logic: Premises, Perspectives, Possibilities*. Cambridge, UK: Cambridge Univ Press, 2014.
6. Osborne S.P., Radnor Z, Nasi G. A new theory for public service management? Toward a (public) service-dominant approach. *Am Rev Pub Adm* 2012;43: 135–158.
7. Batalden M, Batalden P, Margolis P, et al. The Coproduction of Healthcare Service. *BMJ Qual Saf* 2016; 25: 509–517.
8. Greenhalgh T. *How to implement evidence-based healthcare*. Hoboken, NJ: John Wiley & Sons, 2018.
9. Stabel C.B., Fjeldstad Ø.D. Configuring Value For Competitive Advantage: On Chains, Shops, And Networks. *Strat Mgmt J* 1998;19: 413–437.
10. Fjeldstad Ø.D., Snow C.C., Miles R.E., Lettl C. The Architecture of Collaboration. *Strat Mgmt J* 2012; 33: 734–750.
11. Bradley E.H., Taylor L.A. *The American Health Care Paradox: Why Spending More Is Getting Us Less*. New York, NY: Public Affairs Press, 2015.
12. Whyte D. Ibid.
13. Oliver M. What I Have Learned So Far. In Oliver M, *New and Selected Poems Vol. 2* Boston, MA: Beacon Press, 2005, p. 57.

CHAPTER 1

The Global Evolution of Continuous Quality Improvement: From Japanese Manufacturing to Global Health Services

William A. Sollecito and Julie K. Johnson

We are here to make another world.

—**W. Edwards Deming**

Continuous quality improvement (CQI) comes in a variety of shapes, colors, and sizes and has been referred to by many names. It is an example of the evolutionary process that started with industrial applications, primarily in Japan, and has now spread throughout the world, affecting many economic sectors, including health care. In this introductory chapter, we define CQI, trace its history and adaptation to health care, and consider its ongoing evolution. References to subsequent chapters and a previously published volume of case studies (McLaughlin, Johnson, & Sollecito,

2012) provide greater detail and illustrations of CQI approaches and successes as applied to health care.

Despite the evolution and significant progress in the adoption of CQI theory, methods, and applications, the need for greater efforts in quality improvement in health care continues unabated. For example, a major study from 2010 encompassing more than 2,300 admissions in 10 North Carolina hospitals demonstrated that much more needs be done to improve the quality and safety in U.S. hospitals, and it may have implications for health care globally. It found that "patient harms," including preventable medical errors and other patient safety measures, remained common with little evidence of improvement during the 6-year study period from 2002 to 2007 (Landrigan et al., 2010). In recent years, there has been substantial progress in the greater diffusion of CQI in health care in certain sectors. For example, there has been broader institutionalization of CQI in public health in the United States, much of which can be attributed to the broader application of accreditation requirements; this is described in Chapters 11 and 12. Great progress has also been seen in the broader adoption of CQI in resource-poor countries, as documented in Chapter 13. However, with greater complexity in health care comes greater challenges; for example, greater uses of technology bring benefits and risks, as described in Chapter 4, and more widespread applications of evidence-based interventions do not necessarily provide improved outcomes (Wandersman, Alia, Cook, Hsu, & Ramaswamy, 2016). As a result, the challenge of how to cross the quality chasm (Institute of Medicine [IOM], 2001) in health care clearly remains, and our goal in this text is to help to shed light on the scope of the problem and potential solutions.

▶ Definitions

Quality in Health Care

The exact definition of quality in health care varies somewhat for the various sectors of health care. The World Health Organization (WHO) provides a broad-based definition that encompasses global health care as:

> "the extent to which health care services provided to individuals and patient populations improve desired health outcomes. In order to achieve this, health care must be safe, effective, timely, efficient, equitable and people-centered."

Safe. Delivering health care that minimizes risks and harm to service users, including avoiding preventable injuries and reducing medical errors.

Effective. Providing services based on scientific knowledge and evidence-based guidelines.

Timely. Reducing delays in providing and receiving health care.

Efficient. Delivering health care in a manner that maximizes resource use and avoids waste.

Equitable. Delivering health care that does not differ in quality according to personal characteristics such as gender, race, ethnicity, geographical location, or socioeconomic status.

People-centered. Providing care that takes into account the preferences and aspirations of individual service users and the culture of their community (World Health Organization, 2017).

Quality Assurance

Quality assurance (QA) is closely related to, and sometimes confused with, CQI. QA focuses on conformance quality, which is defined as "conforming to specifications; having a product or service that meets predefined standards" (McLaughlin & Kaluzny, 2006, p. 37). QA is sometimes the primary goal of accreditation processes, for example in the 1980s and 90s hospital accreditation by the Joint Commission on Accreditation of Health Care Organizations (JCAHO) now known as The Joint Commission (TJC) was primarily focused on meeting predefined standards (i.e., QA). More recently, especially in public health, accreditation is intended to promote CQI (see Chapters 11 and 12). QA is sometimes included in broader CQI initiatives as a way of defining baseline care, as an interim goal or as part of the process definition, but CQI is much broader in its goals than QA.

A related concept that should be mentioned briefly is quality control (QC), which was widely used in the early development of procedures to ensure industrial product quality. Various definitions can be found for this term (Spath & Kelly, 2017), and in some cases, QC is confused with QA. It is our experience that QC is synonymous with inspection of products or other process outputs with the goal of determining which products should be rejected and/or reworked, often accompanied by counting the number of "defects." The role and weaknesses of inspection (in comparison to CQI) are further discussed by Ross (2014) as part of the evolutionary development of CQI.

Continuous Quality Improvement (CQI)

A succinct but accurate definition of CQI in health care is: "the combined efforts of everyone—health care professionals, patients and their families, researchers, payers, planners and educators—to make changes that will lead to better patient outcomes (health), better system performance (care) and better professional development (learning)" (Batalden & Davidoff, 2007, p. 2).

To expand on that definition, for example to include public health, and describe how this term has led to a broad movement, we provide a bit of history. What was originally called *total quality management* (TQM) in the manufacturing industry evolved into CQI as it was applied to health care administrative and clinical processes. Over time, the term continued to evolve, and now the same concepts and activities are referred to as *quality improvement* or *quality management,* or even sometimes simply as *improvement,* as in the Model for Improvement (Langley et al., 2009). Except when we refer to specific historical examples, the terms CQI and QI will be used primarily throughout this text.

In health care, a broader definition of CQI and its components is this: *CQI is a structured organizational process for involving personnel in planning and executing a continuous flow of improvements to provide quality health care that meets or exceeds expectations.*

CQI usually involves a common set of characteristics, which include the following:

- A link to key elements of the organization's strategic plan
- A quality council made up of the institution's top leadership
- Training programs for personnel
- Mechanisms for selecting improvement opportunities
- Formation of process improvement teams
- Staff support for process analysis and redesign
- Personnel policies that motivate and support staff participation in process improvement
- Application of the most current and rigorous techniques of the scientific method and statistical process control

Institutional Improvement

Under its various labels, CQI is both an approach or perspective and a set of activities applied at various times to one or more of the four broad types of performance improvement initiatives undertaken within a given institution:

1. Localized improvement efforts
2. Organizational learning
3. Process reengineering
4. Evidence-based practice and management

Localized improvement occurs when an ad hoc team is developed to look at a specific process problem or opportunity. *Organizational learning* occurs when this process is documented and results in the development of policies and procedures, which are then implemented. Examples include the development of protocols, procedures, clinical pathways, and so on. *Process reengineering* occurs when a major investment blends internal and external resources to make changes, often including the development of information systems, which radically impact key organizational processes. *Evidence-based practice and management* involve the selection of best health and management practices; these are determined by examination of the professional literature and consideration of internal experience, and more recently, especially in public health, accreditation requirements. The lines of demarcation between these four initiatives are not clear because performance improvement can occur across a continuum of project size, impact, content, external consultant involvement, and departure from existing norms.

Societal Learning

In recent years, the emphasis on quality has increased at the societal level. The Institute of Medicine (IOM) (now called the U.S. National Academy of Medicine) has issued a number of reports critical of the quality of care and the variability of both quality and cost across the country (IOM, 2000, 2001). This concern has increased with mounting evidence of the societal cost of poor-quality care in both lives and dollars (Brennan et al., 2004). It builds on the pioneering work of Phillip Crosby (1979), who provided a focus on the role of cost in quality initiatives that is quite relevant today. Crosby's writings emphasize developing an estimate of the *cost of nonconformance*, also called the *cost of quality*. Developing this estimate involves identifying and assigning values to all of the unnecessary costs associated with waste and wasted effort when work is not done correctly the first time. This includes the costs of identifying errors, correcting them, and making up for the customer dissatisfaction that results. Estimates of the cost of poor quality range from 20–40% of the total costs of the industry, a range widely accepted by hospital administrators and other health care experts.

This view leads naturally to a broadening of the definition of quality by introducing the concept of *adding value*, in addition to ensuring the highest quality of care, implying greater accountability and a cost benefit to

enhance the decision-making and evaluation aspects of CQI initiatives. This concept has seen a resurgence in recent years as national health plans, for example in the United States and the United Kingdom, look to minimize cost and increase value while providing the highest quality of care. For example, several leading experts propose refocusing on quality and accountability simultaneously, noting that "improving the U.S. health care system requires simultaneous pursuit of three aims: improving the experience of care, improving the health of populations, and reducing per capita costs of health care" (Berwick, Nolan, & Whittington, 2008, p. 759). These same sentiments are echoed by Robert Brook of the RAND Corporation, who proposes that the future of CQI in health care requires a focus on the concept of *value*, with consideration of both cost and quality (Brook, 2010).

Most recently, a large-scale reinforcement of these concepts in the United States is found in the goals of the Affordable Care Act (ACA), which jointly emphasizes improvements to access, quality of care, and cost reduction. Although some progress can be attributed to the ACA for example, in regard to lowering hospital acquired infections and readmissions—achievement of its long-term goals is still a work in progress (Blumenthal, Abrams, & Nuzum, 2015; Somander, 2015). These concepts are discussed in greater detail throughout this book, particularly in the final chapter (Chapter 14). Concerns about linking quality and value are not limited to the United States; similar evidence and concerns have been reported from the United Kingdom, Canada, Australia, and New Zealand (Baker et al., 2004; Davis et al., 2002; Kable, Gibbard, & Spigelman, 2002). This emphasis has played out in studies, commissions, and reports as well as the efforts of regulatory organizations to institutionalize quality through their standards and certification processes. As you will see throughout this book, concern for quality and cost is a matter of public policy.

Professional Responsibility

Health care as a whole is often likened to a cottage industry with overtones of a medieval craft guild, with a bias toward treatment rather than prevention and a monopoly of access to and implementation of technical knowledge. This system reached its zenith in the mid-20th century and has been under pressure ever since (McLaughlin & Kaluzny, 2002; Rastegar, 2004; Schlesinger, 2002; Starr, 1982). It is reinforced by the concept of *professionalism*, by which service providers are assumed to have exclusive access to knowledge and competence and, therefore, take full responsibility for self-regulation and for quality. However, much of the public policy debate has centered on the weaknesses of the professional system in improving quality of care. Critics point to excessive professional autonomy; protectionist guild practices, such as secrecy, restricted entry, and scapegoating; lack of capital accumulation for modernization; and economic self-interest as major problems. As we will see, all of these issues impinge on the search for improved quality. However, we cannot ignore the role of professional development as a potential engine of quality improvement, despite the popular emphasis on institutional improvement and societal learning. This, too, will be addressed in subsequent chapters.

▶ ## Rationale and Distinguishing Characteristics

As health care organizations and professions develop their own performance improvement approaches, their management must lead them through a decision process in which activities are initiated, adapted, and then institutionalized. Organizations embark on CQI for a variety of reasons, including accreditation requirements, cost control, competition

for customers, and pressure from employers and payers. Linder (1991), for example, suggests that there are three basic CQI strategies: true process improvement, competitive advantage, and conformance to requirements. Some institutions genuinely desire to maximize their quality of care as defined in both technical and customer preference terms. Others wish simply to increase their share of the local health care market. Still others wish to do whatever is necessary to maintain their accreditation status with bodies such as TJC, National Committee on Quality Assurance (NCQA), and others, after which they will return to business as usual. As you might imagine, this book is written for the first group—those who truly wish to improve their processes and excel in the competitive health care market by giving their customers the quality care that they deserve.

Although CQI comes in a variety of forms and is initiated for a variety of reasons, it does have distinguishing characteristics and functions. These characteristics and functions are often defined as the essence of good management and leadership. They include: (1) understanding and adapting to the external environment; (2) empowering clinicians and managers to analyze and improve processes; (3) adopting a norm that the term *customer* includes both patients and providers and that customer preferences are important determinants of quality in the process; (4) developing a multidisciplinary approach that goes beyond conventional departmental and professional lines; (5) adopting a planned, articulated philosophy of ongoing change and adaptation; (6) setting up mechanisms to ensure implementation of best practices through planned organizational learning; (7) providing the motivation for a rational, data-based, cooperative approach to process analysis and change; and (8) developing a culture that promotes all of the above (see Chapter 2).

The most radical departure from past health care improvement efforts is a willingness to examine existing health care processes and rework these processes collaboratively using state-of-the-art scientific and administrative knowledge and relevant data-gathering and analysis methodologies. Many health care processes developed and expanded in a complex, political, and authoritarian environment, acquiring the patina of science. The application of data-based management and scientific principles to the clinical and administrative processes that produce patient care is what CQI is all about. Even with all the public concern about medical errors and patient safety, improvement cannot occur without both institutional will and professional leadership (Millenson, 2003).

CQI is simultaneously two things: a management philosophy and a management method. It is distinguished by the recognition that customer requirements are the key to customer quality and that customer requirements ultimately will change over time because of changes in evidence-based practices and associated changes in education, economics, technology, and culture. Such changes, in turn, require continuous improvements in the administrative and clinical methods that affect the quality of patient care and population health. This dynamic between changing expectations and continuous efforts to meet these expectations is captured in the Japanese word *kaizen*, translated as "continuous improvement" (Imai, 1986). Change is fundamental to the health care environment, and the organization's systems must have both the will and the way to master such change effectively.

Customer Focus

The use of the term *customer* presents a special challenge to many health professionals (Houpt, Gilkey, & Ehringhaus, 2015). For many, it is a term that runs contrary to the professional model of health services and the idea that "the doctor knows best." Some health professionals would prefer terms that connote the more dependent roles of *client* or *patient*. In some

cases, it is professional pride about caring for patients and their families that causes disdain for the term customer. In CQI terms, *customer* is a generic term referring to the end user of a group's output or product. The customer can be external or internal to the system—a patient, a payer, a colleague, or someone from another department. User satisfaction then becomes one ultimate test of process and product quality. Consequently, new efforts and new resources must be devoted to ascertaining what the customer wants through the use of consumer surveys, focus groups, interviews, and various other ways of gathering information on customer preferences, expectations, and perceived experiences. Chapter 4 addresses some of the issues surrounding current methods for "surveying" customers to measure satisfaction, and Chapter 7 discusses the role of the patient in quality and safety.

System Focus

CQI is further distinguished by its emphasis on avoiding personal blame. The focus is on managerial and professional processes associated with a specific outcome—that is, the entire production system. The initial assumption is that the process needs to be changed and the persons already involved in that process are needed to help identify how to approach a given problem or opportunity.

Therefore, CQI moves beyond the ideas of participative management and decentralized organizations. It is, however, participative in that it encourages the involvement of all personnel associated with a particular work process to provide relevant information and become part of the solution. CQI is also decentralized in that it places responsibility for ownership of each process in the hands of its implementers, those most directly involved with it. Yet this level of participation and decentralization does not absolve management of its fundamental responsibility; in fact, it places additional burdens on management. In situations where the problem is within the system (usually the case), management is responsible for change. CQI calls for significant amounts of managerial thought, oversight, flexibility, and responsibility.

CQI inherently increases the dignity of the employees involved because it not only recognizes the important role belonging to each member of the process improvement team, but it also involves them as partners and even leaders in the redesign of the process. In some cases, professionals can also serve as consultants to other teams as well as to management. Not surprisingly, organizations using CQI often experience improvements in morale (intrinsic motivation) and higher levels of engagement. When the level of quality is being measured, workers can rightly take pride in the quality of the work they are producing. The importance of motivation and engagement to CQI efforts is discussed in greater detail in Chapter 2.

Another important aspect of having a systems focus is the recognition that health care systems are dynamically complex and can include many organizations, both large (macro-) systems and small (micro-) systems (see Chapters 6 and 9). An important part of a systems focus is the understanding that improving quality and safety of complex systems requires systems thinking (see Chapter 2), a management discipline that "acknowledges the large number of parts in a system, the infinite number of ways in which the parts interact and the nature of the interactions" (Spath & Kelly, 2017, p. 44). See Ross (2014) for further description of the components of systems thinking.

Measurement and Decision Making

Another distinguishing feature of CQI is the rigorous belief in fact-based learning and decision making, captured by Deming's saying, "In God we trust. All others bring data." Facts do include perceptions, and decisions cannot all be delayed to await the results of scientifically correct, double-blind studies. However, everyone involved in CQI activities is expected to study the multiple causes of events and to explore a wide array of system-wide solutions. The primary purpose of data and measurement in CQI is learning—how to make system improvements and what the impact of each change that we have already made has had on the overall system. Measurement is not intended to be used for selection, reward, or punishment (Berwick, 1996). It is surprising and rewarding to see a team move away from the table-pounding "I'm right and you're stupid" position (with which so many meetings in health care start) by gathering data, both qualitative and quantitative data, to see what is actually happening and why. Multiple causation is assumed, and the search for answers starts with trying to identify the full set of factors contributing to less-than-optimal system performance.

The inherent barriers that accompany CQI implementation include the tension between the professionals' need for autonomy and control and the objectives of organizational learning and conformance to best practices. Organizations can also oversimplify their environment, as sometimes happens with clinical pathways. Seriously ill patients or patients with multiple chronic conditions do not fit the simple diagnoses often assumed when developing such pathways; a traditional disease-management approach may not suffice, and a broader chronic-care model that incorporates a personalized approach may be necessary (See Chapter 7). There may also be a related tendency to try to over control processes. Health care is not like manufacturing, and it is necessary to understand that patients (anatomy, physiology, psyche, and family setting), providers, and diagnostic categories are highly variable—and that variance reduction can only go so far. One must develop systems that properly handle the inherent variability (called *common-cause variability*) after unnecessary variability (called *special-cause variability*) has been removed (McLaughlin, 1996).

▶ Elements of CQI

Together with these distinguishing character-istics, CQI in health care is usually composed of a number of elements, including:

- Philosophical elements, which for the most part mirror the distinguishing char-acteristics cited previously
- Structural elements, which are usually associated with both industrial and pro-fessional quality improvement programs
- Health specific elements, which add the specialized knowledge of health care and public health to the generic CQI approach

Philosophical Elements

The philosophical elements are those aspects of CQI that, at a minimum, must be present in order to constitute a CQI effort. They include:

1. Strategic focus—Emphasis on having a vision/mission, values, and objec-tives that performance improvement processes are designed, prioritized, and implemented to support
2. Customer focus—Emphasis on both customer (patient, provider, payer) satisfaction and health out-comes as performance measures
3. Systems view—Emphasis on analy-sis of the whole system providing a service or influencing an outcome and practicing systems thinking
4. Data-driven (evidence-based) analysis—Emphasis on gathering and using objective data on system operation and system performance
5. Implementer involvement—Empha-sis on involving the owners of all components of the system in seek-ing a common understanding of its delivery process
6. Multiple causation—Emphasis on identifying the multiple root causes of a set of system phenomena

7. Solution identification—Emphasis on seeking a set of solutions that enhance overall system perfor-mance through simultaneous improvements in a number of nor-mally independent functions
8. Process optimization—Emphasis on optimizing a delivery process to meet customer needs regard-less of existing precedents and on implementing the system changes regardless of existing territories and fiefdoms
9. Continuing improvement—Empha-sis on continuing the systems analy-sis even when a satisfactory solution to the presenting problem is obtained
10. Organizational learning—Emphasis on organizational learning so that the capacity of the organization to generate process improvement and foster personal growth is enhanced

Structural Elements

Beyond the philosophical elements just cited, a number of useful structural elements can be used to structure, organize, and support the continuous improvement process. Almost all CQI initiatives make intensive use of these structural elements, which reflect the opera-tional aspects of CQI and include:

1. Process improvement teams—Emphasis on forming and empow-ering teams of employees to deal with existing problems and oppor-tunities (see Chapter 6)
2. CQI tools—Use of one or more of the CQI tools so frequently cited in the industrial and health-quality literature: flowcharts, checklists, cause-and-effect diagrams, fre-quency and Pareto charts, run charts, and control charts (see Chapter 4)

3. Parallel organization—Development of a separate management structure to set priorities for and monitor CQI strategy and implementation, usually referred to as a quality council
4. Organizational leadership—Leadership, at the top levels and throughout the organization, to make the process effective and foster its integration into the institutional fabric of the organization (see Chapter 2)
5. Statistical thinking and analysis—Use of statistics, including statistical process control, to identify common vs. special causes of variation in processes and practices (see Chapter 4)
6. Customer satisfaction measures—Understanding the importance of measuring customer satisfaction, but also the strengths and weaknesses of available sources of data and survey methodologies in current use (see Chapter 4)
7. Benchmarking—Use of benchmarking to identify best practices in related and unrelated settings to emulate as processes or use as performance targets
8. Redesign of processes from scratch—Making sure that the end product conforms to customer requirements by using techniques of quality function deployment and/or process reengineering

Health Care–Specific Elements

The use of CQI in health care is often described as a major management innovation, but it also resonates with past and ongoing efforts within the health services research community. The health care quality movement has its own history, with its own leadership and values that must be understood and respected. Thus, there are a number of additional approaches and

techniques in health care that health managers and professionals have successfully added to the philosophical and structural elements associated with CQI, including:

1. Epidemiological and clinical studies, coupled with insurance payment and medical records data, often referred to as the basis of evidence-based practice
2. Involvement of the medical staff governance process, including quality assurance, tissue committees, pharmacy and therapeutics committees, and peer review
3. Use of risk-adjusted outcome measures
4. Use of cost-effectiveness analysis
5. Use of quality assurance data and techniques and risk management data

▶ Evolution of the Quality Movement

If you would understand anything, observe its beginning and its development.

—Aristotle

To fully understand the foundation of the CQI approaches that have developed over the years and the reasons for their successful implementation, it is important to understand the underlying philosophies of the founders of this "movement" and the way in which these methodologies that have been adapted to health care evolved from industry. The application of quality-improvement techniques has reached unprecedented levels throughout the world and especially in health care. What started as a "business solution" to address major weaknesses, including a reputation for poor quality, that Japan faced in its manufacturing after World War II has spread beyond manufacturing to encompass both products and services. This proliferation includes multiple industries across the world and, most notably, all sectors of health care. W. Edwards Deming described what happened in Japan as a "miracle that started off with a concussion in 1950." This miracle was the beginning of an evolutionary process whereby the Japanese military was transformed after the war and given a new goal: the reconstruction of Japan. As a result, "Japanese quality and dependability turned upward in 1950 and by 1954 had captured markets the world over" (Deming, 1986, p. 486). Built upon the expertise of Japanese leaders from industry, science, and the military, and with the guidance of Deming, using his own ideas and those of his colleague, Walter Shewhart, this miracle would transform industry not only in Japan, but also in many other countries around the world.

Although Deming and Shewhart both had been advocating a statistical approach to quality for some time, the Japanese were the first to implement these ideas widely. In Japan, the use of these techniques quickly spread to both product and service organizations. Outside Japan, despite slow adoption at first, this movement spread to the United States and Europe in the 1960s and 1970s. But its large-scale adoption did not occur until the 1980s in manufacturing, most notably due to competition from the Japanese automobile industry. In fact, the U.S. industry was perceived to be in a state of crisis when these methods began to receive wider acceptance. As Deming surmised, this crisis was due to poor quality that could be traced primarily to the incorrect belief that quality and productivity were incompatible. Deming demonstrated the fallacy of this notion in his landmark book, *Out of the Crisis*, first published in 1982 (Deming, 1986), thus forming the basis of what is now known as continuous quality improvement.

From this foundation, CQI has evolved exponentially—over time, across the world, and from industrial manufacturing to the provision of services. The beginning of the quality revolution occurred in America in 1980, when Deming was featured on an NBC television documentary, "If Japan Can, Why Can't We?" and a later PBS program, "Quality or Else," both of which had a major impact on bringing quality issues into the U.S. public's awareness (AmStat News, 1993).

Over many years, Deming made enormous contributions to the development of CQI, but he is perhaps best known for the 14-point program of recommendations that he devised for management to improve quality (see BOX 1.1). His focus was always on processes (rather than organizational structures), on the ever-continuous cycle of improvement, and on the rigorous statistical analysis of objective data. Deming believed that management has the final responsibility for quality because employees work in the system and management deals with the system itself. He also felt that most quality problems are management-controlled rather than worker-controlled. These beliefs were the basis for his requirement that CQI be based on an organization-wide commitment, including the important role and example of senior leaders.

The quality evolution later crossed fields as diverse as computer science, education, and health care—and within health care, it has evolved to encompass multiple levels and segments of health care delivery. As discussed earlier, this evolution has taken many forms and names over the years, encompassing and subsuming quality control, quality assurance, quality management, and quality improvement. Like the field itself, its name has evolved from total quality management (TQM) to continuous quality improvement (CQI), or simply quality improvement (QI).

From TQM to CQI

The evolution from TQM to CQI was more than a simple change in terminology; it represents a fundamental change in how organizations have come to recognize the importance of ensuring that changes are improvements

BOX 1.1 Deming's 14-Point Program

1. Create and publish to all employees a statement of the aims and purposes of the company or other organization. The management must demonstrate constantly their commitment to this statement.
2. Learn the new philosophy, top management and everybody.
3. Understand the purpose of inspection, for improvement of processes and reduction of cost.
4. End the practice of awarding business on the basis of price tag alone.
5. Improve constantly and forever the system of production and service.
6. Institute training.
7. Teach and institute leadership.
8. Drive out fear. Create trust. Create a climate for innovation.
9. Optimize toward the aims and purposes of the company the efforts of teams, groups, staff areas.
10. Eliminate exhortations for the work force.
11. a. Eliminate numerical quotas for production. Instead, learn and institute methods for improvement.
    b. Eliminate management by objective.
12. Remove barriers that rob people of pride of workmanship.
13. Encourage education and self-improvement for everyone.
14. Take action to accomplish the transformation.

Reprinted from *The New Economics for Industry, Government, Education* by W. Edwards Deming by permission of MIT and W. Edwards Deming. Published by MIT, Center for Advanced Engineering Study, Cambridge, MA 02139. Copyright © 1993 by W. Edwards Demig.

and that the improvement processes are ongoing, requiring learning and involvement in the process at all levels, from the individual to the organization level. CQI has been directly linked to management and leadership competencies and philosophies that embrace change and innovation as the keys to a vision of value-driven growth. The fundamentals of TQM are based on the scientific management movement developed in the early 20th century. Emphasis was given to "management based on facts," but with management assumed to be the master of the facts. It was believed to be the responsibility of management to specify one correct method of work for all workers and to see that personnel executed that method to ensure quality. Gradually, that perspective has been influenced by the human relations perspective and by the recognition of the importance and ability of the people in the organization. **FIGURE 1.1** illustrates the wide range of leaders who were involved in the quality evolution, with an emphasis on health care.

Some of the most notable contemporaries of Deming and Shewhart who were major contributors to the history of TQM, and later CQI, include Armand Feigenbaum, Joseph Juran, and Philip Crosby. Their contributions have been widely documented in the literature, as well as through organizations that continue to promote their ideas, such as the Juran Institute. They are included, along with many others, in websites that profile these gurus of quality improvement and their individual ideas and techniques that form the basis of modern CQI.

Ongoing Evolution in Japan

While the quality concepts originally applied in Japan were evolving across other countries, they continued to develop and evolve within Japan as well, with numerous original contributions to CQI thinking, tools, and techniques, especially since the 1960s. The most famous of the Japanese experts are Genichi Taguchi and Kaoru Ishikawa.

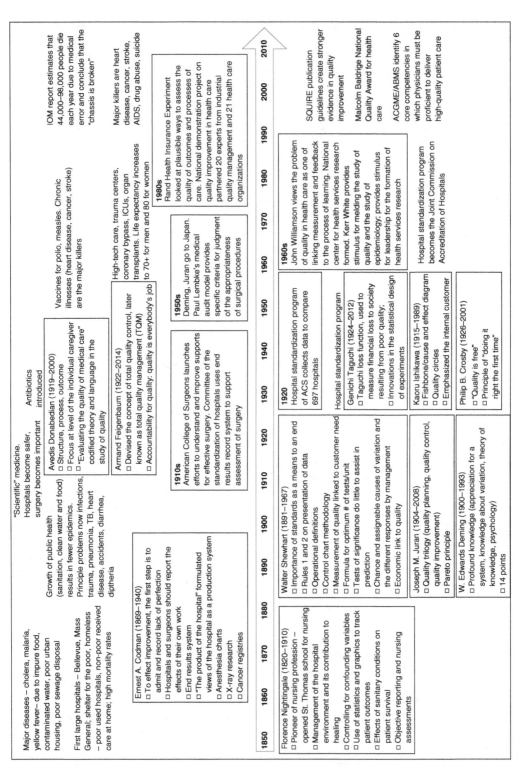

FIGURE 1.1 Some of the Evolutionary Context of Quality in Health Care

BOX 1.2 Recent Contributions of Japanese Quality Engineers

1. Total participation is required of all members of an organization (quality must be company-wide).
2. The next step of a process is its "customer," just as the preceding step is its "supplier."
3. Communicating with both customer and supplier is necessary (promoting feedback and creating channels of communication throughout the system).
4. Emphasis is placed on participative teams, starting with "quality circles."
5. Emphasis is placed on education and training.
6. Instituted the Deming Prize to recognize quality improvement.
7. Statistics are used rigorously.
8. Instituted "just in time" processes.

Taguchi was a Japanese quality expert who emphasized using statistical techniques developed for the design of experiments to quickly identify problematic variations in a service or product; he also advocated a focus on what he called a "robust" (forgiving) design. He emphasized evaluating quality from both an end-user and a process approach. Ishikawa is well known for developing one of the classic CQI tools, the fishbone (or Ishikawa) cause-and-effect diagram (see Chapter 4). Along with other Japanese quality engineers, Ishikawa also refined the application of the foundations of CQI and added the concepts described in **BOX 1.2**.

Cross-Disciplinary Thinking

More than a historical business trend or a movement, the growth of quality improvement represents an evolution of both the philosophies and processes that have been studied and improved over the years, through application, review, feedback, and then broader application. There has been a fair amount of scrutiny, and these approaches have not only stood the test of time but have evolved to address criticisms and have been adapted to meet specialized needs that are unique in some segments, especially in health care. This phenomenon has occurred naturally as a result of cross-disciplinary strategic thinking

processes, where learning occurs by focusing not on what makes industries and disciplines different from each other, but rather on what they share in common (Brown, 1999). A good example of this commonality is a focus on adding value to products and services for customers, be they automobile buyers, airline passengers, or hospital patients. This notion can be directly extended to quality improvement (see **FIGURE 1.2**) by noting that industries— for example, automobile manufacturing vs. health care—may differ in terms of specific mission, goals, and outcomes but may share strategies to add value, including the philosophy, process, and tools of CQI. As a result, the common strategic elements of CQI have been adopted from diverse industrial applications and then customized to meet the special needs of health care.

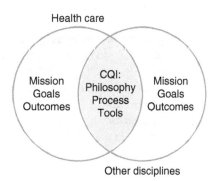

FIGURE 1.2 Cross-Disciplinary Strategic Thinking

Comparing Industrial and Health Care Quality

Cross-disciplinary learning between industry and health care was spurred during the 1990s and contributed to this evolutionary process. A comparison of quality from an industrial perspective vs. quality from a health care perspective reveals that the two are surprisingly similar and that both have strengths and weaknesses (Donabedian, 1993). The industrial model is limited in that it (1) does not address the complexities, including the dynamic character and professional and cultural norms, of the patient–practitioner relationship; (2) downplays the knowledge, skills, motivation, and legal/ethical obligations of the practitioner; (3) treats quality as free, ignoring quality–cost trade-offs; (4) gives more attention to supportive activities and less to clinical ones; and (5) provides less emphasis on influencing professional performance via "education, retraining, supervision, encouragement, and censure" (Donabedian, 1993, pp. 1–4). On the other hand, Donabedian suggested that the professional health care model can learn the following from the industrial model:

1. New appreciation of the fundamental soundness of health care quality traditions
2. The need for even greater attention to consumer requirements, values, and expectations
3. The need for greater attention to the design of systems and processes as a means of quality assurance
4. The need to extend the self-monitoring, self-governing tradition of physicians to others in the organization
5. The need for a greater role by management in assuring the quality of clinical care
6. The need to develop appropriate applications of statistical control methods to health care monitoring
7. The need for greater education and training in quality monitoring and assurance for all concerned (1993, pp. 1–4)

In reality, there is a continuum of CQI activities, with manufacturing at one end of the continuum and professional services at the other (Hart, 1993). The CQI approach should be modified in accordance with its position along this continuum. Manufacturing processes have linear flows, repetitive cycle steps, standardized inputs, high analyzability, and low worker discretion. Professional services, on the other hand, involve multiple nonstandardized and variable inputs, nonrepetitive operations, unpredictable demand peaks, and high worker discretion. Many organizations, including health care organizations, have processes at different points along that continuum that should be analyzed accordingly. The hospital, for example, has laboratory and support operations that are like a factory and has preventive, diagnostic, and treatment activities that are professional services. The objective of factory-like operations is to drive out variability to conform to requirements and to produce near-zero defects. At the other end, the objectives of disease prevention, diagnosis, and treatment are to do whatever it takes to produce improved health and satisfaction and maintain the loyalty of customers—including both patients (external customers) and employees (internal customers).

An important contrast between traditional industry and health care is evidence of the pace of quality improvement initiatives in health care relative to the traditional industries that spawned CQI methods globally. As described by a former director of the McKinsey Global Institute, William Lewis, "For most industry the benefits from the various quality movements have been quite large but … they are also largely in the past" with only incremental progress now being made, and he contrasts that development with health care, which is the "big exception" (Leonhardt, 2009, p. 11). So while health care has learned from manufacturing and commercial industry, its evolution in CQI has led to acceleration in comparison to the slowdown, and even reversal, seen in manufacturing and commercial industry; for example, consider the quality issues faced in 2010 by Toyota—a manufacturing pioneer from which some of these approaches have evolved (Crawley, 2010; Dawson & Takahashi, 2011). (It should be noted that reports in the commercial media in recent years indicate that these issues have been resolved by a return to best practices and greater customer focus [Rechtin, 2014].)

This evolution, or cross-disciplinary translation, continues within a variety of health care settings, as will be illustrated throughout this text, with some tools and techniques being especially good examples of cross disciplinary adoption. Probably the best example is the Plan, Do, Study, Act (PDSA) cycle originally developed by Shewhart (1931) for industry. (Although the PDSA cycle is often attributed to Deming, he attributes it to Shewhart [Deming, 1986].) It is especially amenable to widespread use in health care and continues to find new applications to meet an ever-widening range of clinical and programmatic problems (see FIGURE 1.3).

One very interesting example of the cross-disciplinary/industry phenomenon, which has been given much attention both in scientific journals and in popular media, is the adoption of surgical checklists to prevent errors. The checklist is a very simple but powerful project management and safety tool that has been used in various industries, but it is probably most well known for its effectiveness in the airline industry. A strong case has been made in scientific publications and in the popular media for greater adoption of checklists in surgery (Haynes et al., 2009) and other medical specialties (Gawande, 2009; Pronovost et al., 2006). Although its adoption in a wide range of settings has been seen in recent years, the effectiveness of this tool, used by itself, has been questioned by some (Bosk et al., 2009) and studied by many, with the goal of better understanding its role and improving its effectiveness (Avelling, McCulloch, & Dixon-Woods, 2013; de Vries et al., 2010; Wandersman et al., 2016). The use of checklists also provides a good illustration of some basic CQI principles that have broader implications. For example, checklist usage raises two key questions that are important in regard to a variety of CQI applications: (1) how much does the effectiveness of using checklists vary for different health care applications and settings? and (2) what is their specific role in improving health care safety and quality? One brief answer to these questions is that while the checklist is a simple tool, it is not a magic bullet—instead, it can be an effective means for helping ensure the application of other CQI principles in an overall

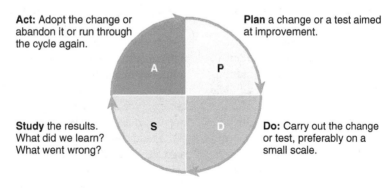

Act: Adopt the change or abandon it or run through the cycle again.

Plan a change or a test aimed at improvement.

Study the results. What did we learn? What went wrong?

Do: Carry out the change or test, preferably on a small scale.

FIGURE 1.3 Shewhart (PDSA) Cycle

program of quality assurance and improvement. For example, its use and effectiveness (or lack thereof) has broad implications about how health care teams communicate and share responsibilities; how leadership supports innovations and change—ultimately a cultural issue; and how to monitor and ensure compliance with CQI initiatives (Avelling, McCulloch, & Dixon-Woods, 2013; Dixon-Woods & Martin, 2016). Checklists provide an example of the importance of teamwork in CQI (see Chapter 6) and provide an example of a CQI tool (in Chapter 4) as well as an example of the broader issue of culture, leadership, and diffusion of CQI in health care (in Chapter 2). Checklists are also used as an example of the use of social marketing to increase compliance with CQI innovations and tools (in Chapter 8).

New approaches, refinements of older concepts, and different combinations of ideas are occurring almost daily in this ongoing evolutionary process. As more and more organizations adopt CQI, we are seeing increasing innovation and experimentation with CQI thinking and its applications. This is especially true of the health care arena, where virtually every organization has had to work hard to develop its own adaptation of CQI to the clinical process.

The Evolution Across Sectors of Health Care

The evolution in health care—which started in the most well-defined sector, hospitals—now includes all segments of the health care system and has become woven into the education of future practitioners, including not only administrators and physicians but also nurses, public health practitioners, and a wide array of other health professionals. It has spanned health care systems in many industrialized nations and now has become a way of meeting emerging crises, with widespread global health applications in resource-poor nations (see Chapter 13).

As illustrated in Figure 1.1, the health care evolution of CQI may be traced back to the work of Florence Nightingale, who pioneered the use of statistical methods to analyze variation and propose areas for improvement. As one of many quality improvement initiatives, Florence Nightingale used descriptive statistics to demonstrate the link between unsanitary conditions and needless deaths during the Crimean War (Cohen, 1984). The evolutionary context of quality in health care, described in Figure 1.1, has occurred at many different levels, spanning history and geography, and has included a broadening of applications and a sharpening of tools and techniques. Both within and outside health care, probably the most dramatic part of this evolution has been the wide dispersion of knowledge about how to use these techniques, first starting with a small group of expert consultants and later expanding to a broad range of practitioners with a common goal to make improvements in a diverse set of products and services. Coupled with that "practice" goal have been educational efforts to develop and disseminate quality-improvement competencies by teaching these methods to an ever-widening range of health care professionals. For example, these efforts have included recent initiatives in nursing, the primary profession of Florence Nightingale (Sherwood & Jones, 2013).

In parallel with this broadening health care evolution over time and space, the same improvement processes were being applied to CQI tools and techniques, leading to improvements and greater precision relative to the measurement of outcomes and processes. The improvement processes also spawned international private- and public-sector organizations, which can be thought of as "health care quality czars," that have applied and expanded these approaches. These organizations include the Institute for Healthcare Improvement (IHI) and both national and international regulatory agencies, such as the CMS in the United States, which, with the establishment of Quality Improvement Organizations (QIOs), uses data from the Medicare and Medicaid system to monitor quality of care and, more importantly, to define improvement strategies (Schenck, McArdle, & Weiser, 2013). Similarly, local, national, and international accreditation agencies, such as TJC in the United States and its global counterparts (e.g., Joint Commission International [JCI]), have mandated the need for quality improvement in large health care systems (see Chapter 12). Ultimately, this has led to the emergence of quality leaders, with recognized achievements via a health care organization's eligibility to receive awards such as the Malcolm Baldrige National Quality Award (Hertz, Reimann, & Bostwick, 1994; McLaughlin & Kaluzny, 2006).

Around the mid-1980s, CQI was applied in several health care settings. Most notable was the early work done by three physicians following the principles outlined by Deming: Paul Batalden at Hospital Corporation of America (HCA), Donald Berwick at Harvard Community Health Center and IHI, and Brent James at Intermountain Health Care. Examples of their work and ideas will be illustrated throughout this chapter and this book.

Armed with the ideas of these creative quality leaders who elaborated on techniques, such as the PDSA cycle that were drawn originally from the pioneers of quality improvement, an acceleration marked by more widespread applications has occurred throughout all sectors of health care in the 21st century. That acceleration was spurred greatly by "a wake-up call" describing the crisis that health care quality was facing entering the new millennium.

▶ The Big Bang—The Quality Chasm

Quality under the rubric of patient safety suddenly came to dominate the scene following the two significant IOM reports, *To Err Is Human* (IOM, 2000) and *Crossing the Quality Chasm* (IOM, 2001). Virtually all those concerns about cost and benefits and professional autonomy

seemed swamped by the documentation of unacceptably high rates of medical errors. The recognition that needless human suffering, loss of life, and wasted resources were related to unnecessary variability in treatment and the lack of implementation of known best practices galvanized professional groups, regulators, and payers into action. Suddenly, quality improvement was acknowledged to be a professional responsibility, a quality-of-care issue rather than a managerial tactic. Current investment and involvement levels are high as evidence has mounted that the variability in clinical processes and the lack of conformance to evidence-based best practices has cost the public dearly. Many of the actors identified previously are demanding accountability for patient safety and for achieving acceptable levels of clinical performance and outcomes achievement. Adverse events are now undergoing extreme scrutiny, and a broad range of quality indicators are being reported, followed, and compared by payers and regulators (see Chapter 10).

One important change that called even greater attention to the seriousness of medical errors was that, effective October 1, 2008, the Centers for Medicare and Medicaid Services (CMS) adopted a nonreimbursement policy for certain "never events," which are defined as serious, preventable hospital-acquired conditions. The rationale is that hospitals cannot bill CMS for adverse events and complications that are considered never events *because* they are preventable; the goal is to motivate hospitals to accelerate improvement of patient safety. A list of never events can be found at the Agency for Healthcare Research and Quality (AHRQ) website, and a summary of how this step came about is offered by Michaels et al. (2007).

Local and regional variability in health care has long been known to exist, but the translation of that variability into missed opportunities for improved outcomes has been slow in coming. With that veil of secrecy about medical errors lifted, the demands for action and professional responsiveness have become extensive. This sea-change goes well beyond concerns about malpractice insurance to issues of clinical governance, professional training, certification, and continuity of care.

For a while, financial questions seemed to have dissipated as the social costs took precedence. However, these cost issues have certainly been revisited and have grown in importance with the full implementation of the ACA in the United States and other health care reform initiatives in other locations around the world. Concerns about cost of care continue and need to be considered relative to CQI initiatives and the overall nature of the relationship of cost to quality and the role of value.

▶ From Industrialization to Personalization

Quality has been and continues to be a central issue in health care organizations and among health care providers. The classic works of Avedis Donabedian, Robert Brook, and Leonard Rosenfeld, to name a few, have made major contributions to the definition, measurement, and understanding of health care quality. However, the corporatization of health care in the United States (Starr, 1982) and other changes to the health care system have redefined, and will continue to redefine, how we manage quality. Given the increasing proportion of the gross national product allocated to health services and the redefinition of health care as an "economic good," health care organizations are influenced to a growing extent by organizations in the industrial sector. As part of this process, health care organizations have become "corporations," with expansion goals to create larger hospital systems. The long-held perception of health care as a cottage industry persisted into the 1960s and 1970s. In this view, health care was seen as a craft or art delivered by individual professionals who had learned by apprenticeship and who worked independently in a decentralized system. These practitioners tailored their craft

to each individual situation using processes that were neither recorded nor explicitly engineered, and they were personally accountable for the performance and financial outcomes of the care they provided.

The 1980s and 1990s witnessed a distinct change, which is often described as the "industrialization of health care" (Kongstvedt, 1997). This change affected almost all aspects of health care delivery, influencing how risks are allocated, how care is organized, and how professionals are motivated and incentivized. This industrialization process can be described utilizing the dynamic stability model of Boynton, Victor, and Pine (1993), which presents various industrial transformation strategies. These can be adapted to health care services to describe the transformation from craft to a more industrialized approach. For example, one strategy follows the traditional route of industrialization utilizing mass production to ensure high levels of process stability, as illustrated by the bundling of unique medical procedures into a few high-volume, specialized centers. However, most health care activities have followed an alternate route that is also described by this model, bypassing mass production due to the high variability in patient needs and using techniques of CQI and process reengineering.

The Victor & Boynton (1998) model for the organization suggests an appropriate path for organizational development and improvement. As presented in FIGURE 1.4, health care processes and product lines have begun to move from the craft stage to positions in all of the other three stages of that model. Each of the four stages requires its own approach to quality.

1. Craft requires that the individual improve with experience and use the tacit knowledge produced to develop a better individual reputation and group reputation. Craft activities can be leveraged to a limited extent by a community of cooperating and teaching crafts-persons.

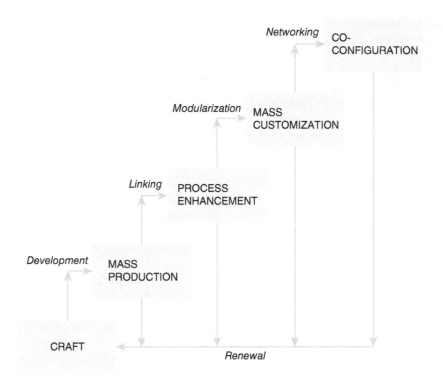

FIGURE 1.4 The Right Path Transformations Are Sequenced Along the Way

Reprinted with permission from Victorm B., and Boynton, A.C. (1998). *Invented Here: Maximizing Your Organization's Internal Growth and Profitability*. Boston: Harvard Business School Press.

2. Mass production requires the discipline that produces conformance quality in high volume at low cost. Critics sometimes refer to this approach using terms such as *industrialization* or the *deskilling* of the profession and occasionally mention Henry Ford's assembly lines as a negative model.

3. Process enhancement requires that processes be analyzed and modified to develop a best-practice approach using worker feedback and process-owning teams within the organization.

4. Mass customization requires that the organization takes that best practice, modularizes and supports it independently, and then uses those modules to build efficient, low-cost processes that are responsive to individual customer wants and needs.

Because health care is a complex, multi-product environment, various types of care can be found at each of the four stages, depending on the state of the technology and the strategy of the delivery unit. The correct place to be along that pathway depends on the current state of the technology. The revolution in health care organization is driven not only by economics, but also by the type of knowledge work that is being done. As described in Victor & Boynton (1998, p. 129):

Managers take the wrong path when they fail to account for the fact that (1) learning is always taking place, and (2) what learning is taking place depends on the kind of work one is doing. The learning system we describe along the right path requires that managers leverage the learning from previous forms of work. ... If managers attempt to transform without understanding the learning taking place ..., then transformation efforts will be at best slightly off the mark and at worst futile. In addition, if managers misunderstand what type of work (craft, mass production, process enhancement, or mass customization) is taking place in a given process or activity when transformation starts, then they may use the wrong transformation steps (development, linking, modularization, or renewal).

These authors, however, were referring to a single, commercial firm with a relatively limited line of goods and services. In health care, a single organization such as a hospital might contain examples of multiple stages due to the variety of its products. There is a recognition that complexity is ever-increasing;

for example, one hears complaints that some traditional definitions apply to patients with only one diagnosis, whereas most very sick patients, especially the elderly, have multiple diagnoses. Therefore, the prevailing quality and performance enhancement systems have to be prepared with much greater levels of variability—in patient problem constellations, anatomy, physiology, and preferences, as well as in provider potentials and preferences (McLaughlin, 1996). Furthermore, increased availability of genetic information will further fractionate many disease categories, making the definitions of disease even more complex. Among other ideas, this has led to the concept of personalization of medicine and an associated concept, individualization of care, which will be discussed in greater detail in the next section.

FIGURE 1.5 suggests how this has and will occur in health care. As scientific information about a health care process accumulates, it shifts from the craft stage to the process enhancement stage. After the process is codified and developed further, it may shift into the mass production mode if the approach is sufficiently cut and dried, the volume is high,

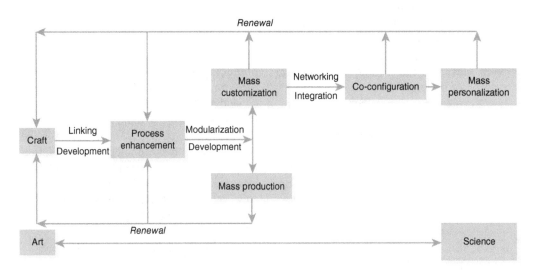

FIGURE 1.5 Revised Boynton & Victor Model for Health Care

and the patients will accept this impersonal mode of delivery. If there is still too much art or lack of science to justify codification, the enhanced process can be returned to the craft mode or moved into the mass customization and co-configuration pathway.

The craft mode contains multiple delivery alternatives. For example, if someone were to decide to commission an artist to make a custom work of art, that person has two ways to specify how it is to be controlled. The first is to say, "You are the artist. Do your thing, and I will pay whatever it costs." This is *fee-for-service indemnity*. The other is to say, "You can decide what to do, but here is all that I can afford to pay." This is *capitation*. In both cases, the grand design and the execution are still in the hands of the artist. However, that does not preclude the artist from learning by doing, obtaining suggestions from vendors of materials and equipment, or observing and collaborating with colleagues. Neither the artist nor the person commissioning the art commits to a single "best" way to do things, because neither is able to articulate or agree on the best way to reach the desired outcome.

The mass-customization pathway has long been thought of as the best way to produce satisfied health care customers at low or reasonable relative costs. The organization develops a series of modular approaches to prevention and treatment, highly articulated and well supported by information technology, so that they can be deployed efficiently in a variety of places and configurations to respond to customer needs. Clinical pathways represent one example of modularization. They represent best practices as known to the organization, and they are applied and configured by a configuror (the health care professional) to meet the needs of the individual patient. This requires an integrated information system that will give the health care professional, usually a generalist, access to specialized information and to full information about the patient's background, medical history, and status; the system will

also allow the health care professional to synchronize the implementation of the modules of service being delivered. In a sense, mass customization represents a process that simulates craft but is highly science based, coordinated, integrated with other process flows, and efficient. How does this differ from the well-run modern hospital or clinic? As described by Victor & Boynton (1998, pp. 12–13):

> The tightly linked process steps developed under process enhancement are now exploded, not into isolated parts, but into a dynamic web of interconnected modular units. Rather than the sequential assembly lines, ... work is now organized as a complex, reconfigurable product and service system.
>
> Modularization breaks up the work into units that are interchangeable on demand from the customer. And everything has to happen fast. ... Modularization transforms work by creating a dynamic, robust network of units.
>
> Within some of these units, ... there may still be active craft, mass production, or process enhancement work taking place, but all the possible interfaces among modules must be carefully designed so that they can rapidly, efficiently, and seamlessly regroup to meet customer needs.

Where does science come in? Victor and Boynton refer to architectural knowledge, a much deeper process understanding than that needed for earlier stages of their model. Also at a practical level, it takes hard science to legitimize the conformance by providers required to make such a system work.

The remaining stage of this model has been called "co-configuration"—a system in which the customer is linked into the network, and customer intelligence is accessed as readily as the providers' knowledge. In a futuristic sense, one should also be able to include the patient in the decision-making network to a high degree. The future has arrived in the form of what many authors call "mass personalization." It represents an even more intense involvement of customers in product and service delivery choices; in health care, patient-specific needs and wants are being more directly addressed.

Mass Personalization

Personalization is an evolutionary concept that is not only having an impact on how industries deliver products and services but also on how organizations are structured, such as in learning organizations. It is an example of a business application that continues to evolve within the business world and is now beginning to evolve at its own pace within health care. In business, this evolution is especially apparent in service industries, where the morphing of mass customization into mass personalization has been fueled by the rapid growth of technology, especially the Internet, search engines, and personal media, to bring each customer's wants and needs in direct contact with service providers.

This phase of evolution has happened quite rapidly, and its speed of growth is directly correlated with technological advances. "Two decades after its conception there is growing evidence that mass customization strategy is transforming into a mass personalization strategy" (Kumar, 2007, p. 533). It was not until 1987 that the term *mass customization* was first introduced; however, from 1987 to 2008, more than 1,100 articles on mass customization appeared in scholarly journals, with exponential growth in the 1990s (Kumar, 2007).

Personalization of products began in the 1950s, with affordability being the key component that led to its popularity and growth. As computer technologies have become more personalized, the concepts of mass customization and co-configuration have evolved into personalization, at an accelerated pace. As

Kumar explains, "Mass personalization strategy evolved from mass customization strategy as a result of strides in information and operational technologies" (2007, p. 536). Both strategies are in current use; while similar, they do have differences. As described by Tseng & Piller (2003, p. 7), who have written extensively on this trend:

Personalization must not be mixed up with customization. While customization relates to changing, assembling, or modifying product or service components according to customers' needs and desires, personalization involves intense communication and interaction between two parties, namely customer and supplier. Personalization in general is about selecting or filtering information objects for an individual by using information about that individual (the customer profile) and then negotiating the selection with the individual. ... From a technical point of view, automatic personalization or recommendation means matching meta-information of products or information objects against meta-information of customers (stored in the customer profile).

This leads to strategies that are directed at what Kumar calls "a market of one" (Kumar, 2007, p. 533).

Health Care Applications of Personalization

That mass personalization is directly applicable to CQI is quite obvious due to their common focus on adding value and customer satisfaction and their common reliance on data and technology. What is a bit surprising is that personalization can be applied directly to CQI in health care, and how rapidly this stage of evolution from business to health care is occurring. This concept is closely related to what Berwick calls "patient-centeredness," a consumerist view of quality of care, which he describes as involving "disruptive shifts in control and power out of the hands of those who give care and into the hands of those who receive it" (Berwick, 2009, p. 555).

At first glance, the importance and reliance on evidence-based practice as part of CQI in health care might seem contradictory to personalization; however, as noted by Sackett and many others, the steps in applying evidence-based practice include evaluating the best data available but also using individual clinical judgment and patient input, including patient preferences, in making final treatment decisions (Sackett, 1996; Satterfield et al., 2009). The current definition of health care personalization encompasses the concepts of individualized care and shared decision making, in addition to personalized medicine (Barratt, 2008; Pfaff et al., 2010; Robinson, Callister, Berry, & Dearing, 2008). In all forms, these concepts lead to greater focus on patient characteristics, needs, and preferences in decision making about their care, and they are all closely associated with the customer focus concepts that are central to CQI. With greater availability of information, via the Internet and other more traditional sources, patients and their families are playing a greater role in health care decision making and quality of care. Sources of data and information abound in numerous easily accessible formats. For example, for many years the AHRQ has provided information to encourage patient participation in their medical care and the quality of the medical care they receive; one example is the AHRQ website "Questions to Ask Your Doctor" (AHRQ, 2012). Similar resources have long been provided by other organizations to support patients with specialty needs; for example, the National Cancer Institute's Cancer Information Service was established in 1975 to help cancer patients find information

and treatment resources (NCI n.d.). What has contributed notably to the use of such information is that patients now have greater knowledge and access to technology, such as search engines to find medical information. This has led to input by patients and their families in their own health care decisions and in the quality of their care, which is discussed in greater detail in Chapter 7.

But the growth in health care personalization goes beyond patients having access to medical information; it relates directly to medical strategies and emerging science for providing higher quality, safer, more personalized treatments. This trend draws strength from a vision of personalized medicine primarily in terms of genomic medicine; it is a means of "focusing on the best ways to develop new therapies and optimize prescribing by steering patients to the right drug at the right dose at the right time" (Hamburg & Collins, 2010, p. 301). This vision includes partnerships among industry, academia, doctors, patients, and the public that will lead to a "national highway for personalized medicine." One of the earliest signs of success relates to identifying the optimal dosage and combination of treatments for cancer patients (Spector & Blackwell, 2009).

As in the business community, the personalization concept in health care has evolved to include broader components of health care, in part because of advances in research and technology. In medical care, this includes recent breakthroughs in genomics (Spector & Blackwell, 2009) but also tools provided by computer technology, including greater use of electronic medical records. Individualized treatment strategies are further extensions of these concepts, going beyond genomics to include patients' preferences and experiences in shared decision making with their providers, allowing greater patient participation in choice of drugs and dosages and administration; even more broadly, individualization leads to patients being more proactive in regard to prevention, screening, and early treatment, through greater use of information technology, electronic medical records, and decision-making tools, such as patient decision support technologies (Pfaff et al., 2010).

Health care personalization can be thought of more broadly as an extension of Wagner's (1996) chronic care model, which focuses on the individual rather than the condition. This approach is especially useful when individuals have multiple chronic conditions.

The evolutionary path of CQI within health care is an important catalyst to personalization that is reflective of broader societal trends spanning a wide range of businesses. These trends are reflected in the concept of customer relationship management (CRM). As described by Kumar (2007), "CRM is the philosophy, policy, and coordinating strategy connecting different players within an organization so as to coordinate their efforts in creating an overall valuable series of experiences, products, and services for the customer." Kumar notes that CRM also requires that the customer be integrated into all aspects of product and process design and that "customer driven innovation has become a key source of strategic advantage." This relates not only to health care personalization but also to the traditional focus on customers in CQI and on methods of gathering customer feedback. This is reflected in many ways including the greater use (and some abuse) of patient satisfaction surveys as a way of evaluating quality of care (see Chapter 4).

With new opportunities come new challenges. The greater amount of information available and the increased role of "untrained" patients and their families in care decisions present the challenge of knowing how to evaluate the quality and appropriateness of treatment options. This has led to some level of conflict as the two extremes of standardization vs. personalization strain the boundaries and definitions of evidence-based medicine, with both extremes striving to achieve the highest quality of care. There is an ongoing broad discussion throughout health care, locally

and globally, about how to balance these concepts (Pfaff et al., 2010; Robinson et al., 2008; Satterfield et al., 2009; Wandersman et al., 2016). What is clear is that these patient-centered concepts are here to stay and will lead to the next stages of the evolution in health care and, as with the previous stages, will continue to grow exponentially.

Likewise, referring back to Berwick's (2009) notion of "patient-centeredness," patients are playing—and should play—a greater role in health care quality improvement. These patient-centered trends have had an impact on quality improvement education for health care professionals. For example, they are being incorporated into nursing education (Sherwood & Jones, 2013). Day and Smith (2007, pp. 139–140) describe this need:

> Unfortunately there is wide variation in the quality of information provided by websites and no search engine screens for quality or accuracy. An important part of basic nursing education is helping students develop skills that enable them to evaluate web-based information, especially if that information is going to be passed on to a patient or family member or used as the basis for patient and family teaching.

Thus, as with other evolutionary stages in CQI, new challenges to quality management present themselves and will hopefully lead to new opportunities in an unending cycle of improvement.

▶ The Scientific Method of CQI

As CQI philosophies and processes have evolved within health care, a series of broad-based approaches have evolved and proven to be widely applicable across a range of health care settings. These can be thought of as umbrella approaches under which specific change methods can be applied. At the foundation of these is the scientific method and the historically proven PDSA cycle, which has been particularly successful in health care as frameworks within which a variety of improvement methods have been applied to measure and further initiate improvement strategies.

Walter Shewhart at Bell Laboratories, was the first to introduce the Plan, Do, Study, Act (PDSA) cycle, which was presented earlier in Figure 1.3. It should also be noted that over time, the abbreviation PDSA was changed by some to PDCA, the "S" for study being changed to "C" for check, as in *checking* what impact an improvement has made on the process being changed. Today the terms are used interchangeably, as we will do throughout this book. Either way, Shewhart's concept has become a very powerful and frequently used quality improvement methodology that has withstood the test of time.

Stated quite simply, PDSA cycles "provide a structure for iterative testing of changes to improve quality of systems. ... The pragmatic principles of PDSA cycles promote the use of a small scale iterative approach to test interventions, as this enables rapid assessment and provides flexibility to adapt the change according to feedback to ensure fit-for-purpose solutions are developed" (Taylor et al., 2014, pp. 290–291). The key features of any PDSA application are:

1. The use of repeated iterative cycles
2. Prediction-based test of change (developed in the plan stage)
3. Small-scale testing (build as confidence grows—adapting according to feedback and learning)
4. Use of data over time (to understand the impact of change)
5. Documentation (to support local learning and transferability to other settings) (Taylor et al., 2014, p. 293)

The two very successful and well-known applications of the PDCA/PDSA cycle that have evolved in health care are HCA's FOCUS–PDCA model (Batalden & Stoltz, 1993) and the Model for Improvement (Langley et al., 2009). These encompass two frameworks that have been developed to use in conjunction with PDCA/PDSA cycles. In addition to these two major PDSA applications, numerous other CQI initiatives have centered around this basic improvement cycle.

The broad applicability of the PDSA cycle in health care can be traced directly to its roots as it was applied by Deming. One of Deming's (1993) major premises was that management needs to undergo a transformation. In order to respond successfully to challenges to organizations and their environments, the way to accomplish that transformation, which must be deliberately learned and incorporated into management, is by pursuing what he called "profound knowledge." The key elements of his system of profound knowledge are (1) appreciation for a system, (2) knowledge about variation, (3) theory of knowledge, and (4) psychology.

The Deming process is especially useful in health care because professionals already have knowledge of the subject matter as well as a set of values and disciplines that fit the Deming philosophy. Training in Deming methods adds knowledge of how to build a new theory using insights about systems, variation, and psychology, and it focuses on the answers given to the set of basic questions that center around knowing what is to be accomplished. Furthermore, it applies a cyclical process of testing and learning from data whether the change being made is an improvement and what improvements are needed in the future (Batalden & Stoltz, 1993). A Deming approach, as adopted by the HCA in Nashville, Tennessee, is illustrated in FIGURE 1.6. It was referred to by the HCA as FOCUS–PDCA and provided the firm's health care workers with a common language and an orderly sequence for implementing the cycle

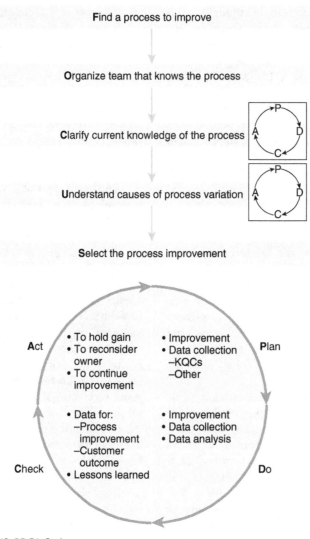

FIGURE 1.6 The FOCUS–PDCA Cycle

of continuous improvement. It focuses on the answers given to the following basic questions (Batalden & Stoltz, 1993):

1. What are we trying to accomplish?
2. How will we know when that change is an improvement?
3. What changes can we predict will make an improvement?
4. How shall we pilot test the predicted improvements?

5. What do we expect to learn from the test run?
6. As the data come in, what have we learned?
7. If we get positive results, how do we hold on to the gains?
8. If we get negative results, what needs to be done next?
9. When we review the experience, what can we learn about doing a better job in the future?

In parallel with the FOCUS–PDCA model was the introduction in 1992 of the Model for Improvement by Langley et al. (2009). It includes a PDSA cycle as its core approach, returning to the traditional "S," emphasizing the importance of *studying* what has been accomplished before making further changes (**FIGURE 1.7**). Careful study and reflection are points of emphasis made by Berwick (1996), who describes this model as "inductive learning—the growth of knowledge through making changes and then reflecting on the consequences of those changes."

Central to the Model for Improvement are three key questions:

1. What are we trying to accomplish?
2. How will we know that a change is an improvement?
3. What change can we make that will result in an improvement?

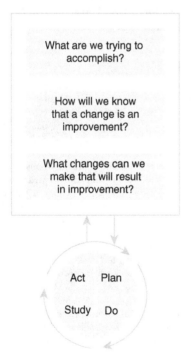

What are we trying to accomplish?

How will we know that a change is an improvement?

What changes can we make that will result in improvement?

Act   Plan

Study   Do

FIGURE 1.7 Model for Improvement

Reproduced from Langley, G.L., Nolan, K.M., Nolan, T.W., Norman, C.L. and Provost, L.P. (2009), The Improvement Guide: A Practical Approach to Enhancing Organizational Performance, 2nd ed., Jossey Bass, San Francisco.

The wide use of these approaches is due directly to the elegance and simplicity of the PDSA cycle. Likewise, the range of applications ties directly to the generalizability of the PDSA cycle. Recent applications have included public health (see Chapter 11), health care in resource-poor countries (see Chapter 13) and traditional medical care in industrialized settings, which are described throughout this book.

However, with the widespread use of PDSA, there have been some questions raised about how to assess validity and generalizability of specific applications before their results are transferred into clinical practice as new evidence-based methods (Speroff, James, Nelson, Headrick, & Brommels, 2004). These questions fall under the broad heading of how to apply critical appraisal criteria to PDSA, and other CQI initiatives, in a manner that is similar to appraisal of clinical research studies that are directed at efficacy and safety of new treatments or drugs. One approach to addressing these questions is to carefully review how well the key features of the PDSA methods (listed above) have been applied in a specific application; this approach is outlined by Taylor et al. (2014). Included in this approach is Berwick's emphasis on careful study of findings at the "S" stage of each cycle, before acting on those findings (Berwick, 1996).

A useful set of guidelines for strengthening PDSA applications as well as other CQI initiatives, and which parallel the recommendations of Taylor et al. (2014), are presented by Speroff et al. (2004, p. 36) and start with four core questions:

1. Is the quality improvement study pertinent and relevant?
2. Are the results valid?
3. Are appropriate criteria used to interpret the results?
4. Will the study help you with your practice or organization of care?

These authors also present detailed recommendations for how to address each of these four questions, including how to improve the causal inferences (internal validity) and generalizability (exernal validity) of PDSA studies (Speroff et al., 2004). Because of the simplicity and consequently the broad usage of PDSA, careful attention should be paid to the guidelines described above in order to ensure proper use and both internal and external validity of applications of the PDSA methodology.

Similar discussions have also been carried out recently in regard to improving the applicability of other well known CQI methods and specific results. Recommendations have been presented for greater emphasis on the fidelity of the applications and fuller understanstanding, and consideration of the context, in which project-specific results are obtained before broadly assuming the robustness of their findings. These recommendations help to explain why some CQI methods are not achieving the results that are expected and should be carried out before generalizing them to other settings, and we should always be cautious to not assume that a "magic bullet" has been found that will produce improvements in any situation, regardless of context (Dixon-Woods & Martin, 2016).

▶ Conclusions

The examples of how CQI has evolved in an exponential manner, especially since the advent of the new millennium, are many and varied. Whether this trend is due to greater customer awareness and demands, technology improvements, greater competition, or a combination of these factors, what is clear is that the trend is continuing on a global scale. While some traditional industries that had incorporated CQI are now "making only incremental progress" (Leonhardt, 2009) CQI in health care is leaping forward, using examples and lessons from outside as well as inside health care. National developments (e.g., the ACA in the United States) and international developments (e.g., applications of CQI in resource-poor

nations) have been both the result of and the source of global learning. This cycle of learning has led to innovations and paradigm shifts that will ensure further evolution in the future. The institutionalization of CQI in public health, which represents an extension of what has been learned in medical and hospital care, continues to grow due to various influences that mirror other health care sectors, such as national and local accreditation efforts.

The examples in this text of how CQI has spread and evolved are by no means exhaustive; improvements will continue to evolve at a pace that is difficult to capture in any snapshot in time. But the patterns of change that are described in this text provide a strong basis for future health improvement models and the challenges that come with these future models, as they address the questions of quality and cost and the issues of "value-added" care, leading to further learning and innovation to meet customer needs and improved health outcomes across the globe.

References

AHRQ. (2012). Questions to ask your doctor. Rockville, MD: Agency for Healthcare Research and Quality. Retrieved May 1, 2018 from https://www.ahrq.gov

AmStat News. (1993). W. Edwards Deming to address members in San Francisco. Washington, DC: American Statistical Association.

Avelling, E., McCulloch, P., & Dixon-Woods, M. (2013). A qualitative study comparing experiences of the surgical safety checklist in hospitals in high-income and low-income countries. British Medical Journal Open, 3, e003039. Retrieved December 15, 2017, from http://dx.doi.org/10.1136/bmjopoen-2013-003039

Baker, G. R., Norton P. G., Flintoft, V., Blais, R., Brown, A., Cox J., ... Tamblyn R. (2004). The Canadian adverse events study: The incidence of adverse events among hospital patients in Canada. Canadian Medical Association Journal, 170, 1678–1686.

Barratt, A. (2008). Evidence-based medicine and shared decision making: The challenge of getting both the evidence and preferences into health care. Patient Education and Counseling, 73, 407–412.

Batalden, P., & Stoltz, P. (1993). Performance improvement in health care organizations. A framework for the continual improvement of health care: Building and applying professional and improvement knowledge to test changes in daily work. *Joint Commission Journal of Quality Improvement, 19,* 424–452.

Batalden, P., & Davidoff, F. (2007). What is quality improvement and how can it transform health care? *Quality and Safety in Health Care, 16,* 2–3

Berwick, D. M. (1996). A primer on leading the improvement of systems. *British Medical Journal, 312,* 619–622.

Berwick, D. M. (2009). What "patient-centered" should mean: Confessions of an extremist. *Health Affairs, 28*(4), w555–w565.

Berwick, D. M., Nolan, T. W., & Whittington, J. (2008). The triple aim: Care, health, and cost. *Health Affairs, 27*(3), 759–769.

Blumenthal, D., Abrams, M., & Nuzum, R. (2015). The Affordable Care Act at 5 years. *The New England Journal of Medicine, 372,* 2451–2458. Retrieved December 11, 2017, at http://www.nejm.org/doi/full/10.1056/NEJMhpr1503614#t=article

Bosk, C. L., Dixon-Woods, M., Goeschel, C. A., & Pronovost, P. J. (2009). The art of medicine: Reality check for checklists. *The Lancet, 374,* 444–445.

Boynton, A. C., Victor, B., & Pine, B. J. (1993). New competitive strategies: Challenges to organizations and information technology. *IBM Systems Journal, 32*(1), 40–64.

Brennan, T. A., Leape, L. L., Laird, N. M., Hebert, L., Localio, A. R., Lawthers, A. G., ... Harvard Medical Practice Study I. (2004). Incidence of adverse events and negligence in hospitalized patients: Results of the Harvard medical practice study I. *Quality and Safety in Health Care, 13*(2), 145–151.

Brook, R. H. (2010). The end of the quality improvement movement: Long live improving value. *Journal of the American Medical Association, 304*(16), 1831–1832.

Brown, M. (1999). *Strategic thinking: considerations for public health—a personal perspective.* Paper presented at the Symposium on Public Health Leadership, School of Public Health, University of North Carolina at Chapel Hill.

Cohen, I. B. (1984). Florence Nightingale. *Scientific American, 250,* 128–137.

Crawley, J. (2010). Toyota's top U.S. exec warned about quality in 2006. Washington, DC: Reuters (March 2). Retrieved February 19, 2011, from http://www.reuters.com

Crosby, P. B. (1979). *Quality is free: The art of making quality certain.* New York, NY: Mentor.

Davis, P., Lay-Yee, R., Briant, R., Ali, W., Scott, A., & Schug, S. (2002). Adverse events in New Zealand public hospitals I: Occurrence and impact. *New Zealand Journal of Medicine, 115*(1167), U268.

Dawson, C., & Takahashi, Y. (2011). Toyota makes a new push to avoid recalls. *The Wall Street Journal* (Feb. 24). Retrieved December 15, 2017, from https://www.wsj.com

Day, L., & Smith, E. (2007). Integrating quality and safety content into clinical teaching in the acute care setting. *Nursing Outlook, 55,* 138–143.

Deming, W. E. (1986). *Out of the crisis.* Cambridge, MA: Massachusetts Institute of Technology Center for Advanced Engineering Study.

Deming, W. E. (1993). *The new economics for industry, government, education.* Cambridge, MA: Massachusetts Institute of Technology Center for Advanced Engineering Study.

de Vries, E. N., Prins, H. A., Crolla, R. M., den Outer A. J., van Andel G., van Helden S. H., ... SURPASS Collaborative Group. (2010). Effect of a comprehensive surgical safety system on patient outcomes. *The New England Journal of Medicine, 363,* 1928–1937.

Dixon-Woods, M., & Martin G. P. (2016). Does quality improvement improve quality? *Future Hospital Journal, 3*(3), 191–194.

Donabedian, A. (1993). *Models of quality assurance.* Leonard S. Rosenfeld Memorial Lecture, School of Public Health, University of North Carolina at Chapel Hill, February 26.

Gawande, A. (2009). *The checklist manifesto.* New York, NY: Metropolitan Books.

Hamburg, M. A., & Collins, F. S. (2010). The path to personalized medicine. *The New England Journal of Medicine, 363,* 301–304.

Hart, C. (1993). Handout, Northern Telecom. University Quality Forum, Research Triangle Park, North Carolina.

Haynes, A. B., Weiser, T. G., Berry, W. R., Lipsitz S. R., Breizat A. H., Dellinger E. P., ... Safe Surgery Saves Lives Study Group. (2009). A surgical safety checklist to reduce morbidity and mortality in a global population. *The New England Journal of Medicine, 360,* 491–499.

Hertz, H. S., Reimann, C. W., & Bostwick, M. C. (1994). The Malcolm Baldrige National Quality Award concept: Could it help stimulate or accelerate health care quality improvement? *Quality Management in Health Care, 2*(4), 63–72.

Houpt, J. L., Gilkey, R. W., & Ehringhaus, S. H. (2015). *Learning to lead in the academic medical center.* Cham, Switzerland: Springer.

Imai, M. (1986). *Kaizen: The key to Japan's competitive success.* New York, NY: Random House.

Institute of Medicine (IOM), National Academies of Sciences. (2000). *To err is human: Building a safer health system.* Washington, DC: National Academies Press.

Institute of Medicine (IOM), National Academies of Sciences. (2001). *Crossing the quality chasm: A new health paradigm for the 21st century.* Washington, DC: National Academies Press.

Kable, A. K., Gibbard, R., & Spigelman, A. (2002). Adverse events in surgical patients in Australia. *International Journal of Quality in Health Care, 14,* 269–276.

Kongstvedt, P. R. (1997). *Essentials of managed health care*, 2nd ed. Gaithersburg, MD: Aspen Publishers.

Kumar, A. (2007). From mass customization to mass personalization. *International Journal of Flexible Manufacturing Systems*, 19, 533–547.

Landrigan, C. P., Parry, G. J., Bones, C. B., Hackbarth A. D., Goldmann D. A., & Sharek P. J. (2010). Temporal trends in rates of patient harm resulting from medical care. *The New England Journal of Medicine*, 363(22), 2124–2134.

Langley, G. L., Moen, R. D., Nolan, K. M., Nolan, T. W., Norman, C. L., & Provost, L. P. (2009). *The improvement guide: A practical approach to enhancing organizational performance*, 2nd ed. San Francisco, CA: Jossey-Bass.

Leonhardt, D. (2009). Making health care better. *The New York Times*, November 8. Retrieved February 19, 2011, from http://www.nytimes.com

Linder, J. (1991). Outcomes measurement: Compliance tool or strategic initiative. *Health Care Management Reviews*, 16(4), 21–33.

McLaughlin, C. P. (1996). Why variation reduction is not everything: A new paradigm for service operations. *International Journal of Service Industry Management*, 7(3), 17–30.

McLaughlin, C. P., Johnson, J. K., & Sollecito, W. A. (Eds.). (2012). *Implementing continuous quality improvement in health care: A global casebook*. Sudbury, MA: Jones & Bartlett Learning.

McLaughlin, C. P., & A. D. Kaluzny. (2002). Missing the middleman: Disintermediation challenges to the doctor-patient relationship. *MGMA Connexion* 2(4), 48–52.

McLaughlin, C. P., & Kaluzny, A. D. (Eds.). (2006). *Continuous quality improvement in health care*, 3rd ed. Sudbury, MA: Jones and Bartlett Publishers.

Michaels, R. K., Makary, M. A., Dahab, Y., Frassica F. J., Heitmiller E., Rowen L. C., ... Pronovost, P. J. (2007). Achieving the National Quality Forum's "never events": Prevention of wrong site, wrong procedure, and wrong patient operations. *Annals of Surgery*, 245, 526–532.

Millenson, M. L. (2003). The silence on clinical quality failure. *Health Affairs*, 22(2), 103–112.

National Cancer Institute. (n.d.). NCI contact center— cancer information service. Bethesda, MD: U.S. Department of Health and Human Services. Retrieved May 1, 2018, from www.cancer.gov/contact /contact-center

Pfaff, H., Driller, E., Ernstmann, U., Karbach, U., Kowalski, C., Scheibler, F., & Ommen, O. (2010). Standardization and individualization in care for the elderly: Proactive behavior through individualized standardization. *Open Longevity Science*, 4, 51–57.

Pronovost, P. J., Needham, D., Berenholtz, S., Sinopoli, D., Chu, H., Cosgrove, S., ... Goeschel, C. (2006). An intervention to reduce catheter-related bloodstream infections in the ICU. *The New England Journal of Medicine*, 355, 2725–2732.

Rastegar, D. A. (2004). Health care becomes an industry. *Annals of Family Medicine*, 22, 79–83.

Rechtin, M. (2014). What Toyota learned from its recall crisis. *Automotive News* (May 25). Retrieved December 15, 2017, from http://www.autonews.com

Robinson, J. H., Callister, L. C., Berry, J. A., & Dearing, K. A. (2008). Patient-centered care and adherence: Definitions and applications to improve outcomes. *Journal of the American Academy of Nurse Practitioners*, 20, 600–607.

Ross, T. K. (2014). *Health care quality management—Tools and applications*. San Francisco, CA: Jossey-Bass.

Sackett, D. (1996). Evidence-based medicine: What it is and what it isn't. *British Medical Journal*, 312, 71–72.

Satterfield, J. M., Spring, B., Brownson, R. C., et.al. (2009). Toward a transdisciplinary model of evidence based practice. *The Millbank Quarterly*, 87(2).

Schlesinger, M. (2002). A loss of faith: The source of reduced political legitimacy for the American medical profession. *The Milbank Quarterly*, 80(2), 185–235.

Schenck, A. P., McArdle, J., & Weiser, R. (2013). Quality Improvement Organizations and continuous quality improvement in Medicare. In W. A. Sollecito & J. K. Johnson (Eds.), *Continuous quality improvement in health care*, 4th ed. Sudbury, MA: Jones and Bartlett Publishers.

Sherwood, G., & Jones, C. B. (2013). Quality Improvement in Nursing. In W. A. Sollecito & J. K. Johnson (Eds.), *Continuous quality improvement in health care*, 4th ed. Sudbury, MA: Jones and Bartlett Publishers.

Shewhart, W. A. (1931). *Economic control of quality of manufactured product*. Princeton, NJ: Van Nostrand Reinhold.

Somander, T. (2015). 4 Ways the Affordable Care Act is improving the quality of health care in America. Retrieved November 3, 2017, from https:// obamawhitehouse.archives.gov

Spath, P. L., & Kelly, D. L. (2017). *Applying quality management in healthcare: A systems approach*, 4th ed. Chicago, IL: Health Administration Press.

Spector, N., & Blackwell, K. (2009). Understanding the mechanisms behind trastuzumab therapy for human epidermal growth factor receptor 2–positive breast cancer. *Journal of Clinical Oncology*, 27(34), 5838–5847.

Speroff, T., James, B., Nelson, E., Headrick, L. A., & Brommels, M. (2004). Guidelines for the appraisal and publication of PDSA quality improvement. *Quality management in health care*, 13(1), 33–39.

Starr, P. (1982). *The social transformation of american medicine*. New York, NY: Basic Books.

Taylor, M.J., McNicholas, C., Nicolay, C., Darzi, A., Bell, D. & Reed, J. E. (2014). Systematic review of the application of the plan-do-study-act method to improve quality in healthcare. *BMJ Quality & Safety, 23,* 290–298.

Tseng, M. T., & Piller, F. T. (Eds.). (2003). *The customer centric enterprise: Advances in mass customization and personalization.* Berlin: Springer-Verlag.

Victor, B., & Boynton, A. C. (1998). *Invented here: Maximizing your organization's internal growth and profitability.* Boston, MA: Harvard Business School Press.

Wagner, E. (1996). Improving outcomes in chronic illness. *Managed Care Quarterly, 4*(2), 12–25.

Wandersman, A., Alia, K., Cook, B. S., Hsu, L. L., & Ramaswamy, R. (2016). Evidence based interventions are necessary but not sufficient for achieving outcomes in each setting in a complex world: Empowerment evaluation, getting to outcomes, and demonstrating accountability. *American Journal of Evaluation, 37*(4), 544–561.

World Health Organization. (2017). What is Quality of Care and why is it important. Retrieved December 8, 2017, from http://www.who.int

CHAPTER 2

Factors Influencing the Application and Diffusion of CQI in Health Care

William A. Sollecito and Julie K. Johnson

Change is not merely necessary to life — it is life.
—Alvin Toffler (Futurist)

ontinuous quality improvement (CQI) has gained acceptance within all sectors of health care and across geographic and economic boundaries. It has evolved as a global strategy for improving health care in a variety of settings, spanning a broad number of issues and improving services to a variety of customers ranging from individual patients to communities. The range of applications covers not only direct patient care in primary care or hospital settings, but also disease prevention and population initiatives—such as HIV, childhood obesity, and influenza vaccination programs—under the domain of public health agencies at the local, national, and international levels. These applications are characterized by continuous, ongoing learning and sharing among disciplines about ways to use CQI philosophies, processes, and tools in a variety of settings. New applications continue

to emerge, but at the same time, there are new challenges to the broad application of CQI. In this chapter, we examine the factors and processes that facilitate or impede the implementation of CQI as a dynamic programmatic innovation within a health care setting.

While many of the barriers to more rapid adoption of CQI in health care were reduced during the first decade of the 21st century, we continued to face many challenges to the widespread adoption of CQI. Some of these challenges were due to the scientific method—for example, the definition of evidence-based practice and how it varied across different areas of health care, with medicine perhaps being the most rigid due to an over-emphasis on randomized, controlled trials. Satterfield et al. (2009) reviewed this issue, noting that the interdisciplinary nature of health care research requires a new broader definition of evidence-based practice. This broader model represents a transformation in thinking that might increase the flexibility and the range of methodologies that are used to make scientific decisions, for example through the greater use of quasi-experimentation, and one effect of this model's adoption might be an increase in CQI initiatives. Other transformations that have occurred include the greater emphasis on translational research and the introduction of implementation research (see Chapter 3).

Since 2010, progress in CQI has been made at the system level in the United States, as a direct consequence of national initiatives including, but not limited to, the Affordable Care Act (ACA), which includes incentives that could serve as a catalyst for innovation such as those directed at lowering hospital acquired infections; and the implementation of new care models such as "primary medical care homes" (Somander, 2015). Also since 2011, the National Quality Strategy has been in place in the United States; this initiative, led by the Agency for Healthcare Research and Quality (AHRQ) is a transdisciplinary strategy to improve quality of care (AHRQ, 2017). Another major factor influencing system-wide CQI implementation, especially in public health, has been accreditation initiatives (see Chapters 11 and 12). Also noteworthy on a global scale has been progress made to expand CQI at a greater pace in resource-poor countries (see Chapter 13).

While progress has been made in understanding and implementing CQI, new challenges have arisen, and old challenges persist. For example, despite incentives for prevention, significant challenges remain in reducing medical errors; these are addressed further in Chapters 9 and 10. And some of the advances in technology, which are intended, at least in part, to facilitate greater adoption of CQI at the system level, have had a negative effect on individual health care providers' motivation to implement CQI. These include the more widespread use of electronic health records and electronic patient satisfaction surveys; these are discussed further later in this chapter as well as in Chapter 4. As a result, some important questions remain about the adaptation and diffusion of quality improvement methods,

especially in regard to the central role of individual health care providers. These include questions such as:

- Why aren't more health care providers using CQI tools and processes?
- Why is the gap between knowledge and practice so large?
- Why don't clinical systems incorporate the findings of clinical science or copy the "best known" practices reliably, quickly, and even gratefully into their daily work simply as a matter of course?

The answers to these questions, which have been raised by CQI leaders such as Dr. Brent James (Leonhardt, 2009) and Dr. Donald Berwick (2003), are multifaceted. Central to this issue is the question of how to influence practitioners to adopt new ideas and the broader topic of diffusion of innovation in health care.

The remainder of this chapter will address several questions:

- What is the current state of quality in health care, and what are the problems regarding implementation of CQI in health care?
- Given the widespread application of CQI in recent years, what are the factors that contribute to the implementation of CQI across industries and settings?
- Specifically for our application in health care, what are the factors that have influenced the rate of diffusion and spread of CQI in health care?
- What steps are needed to develop a culture in health care where CQI is the norm?

▶ The Current State of CQI in Health Care

There has been progress in improving quality and safety of patient care since the publication of the Institute of Medicine's landmark reports

To Err Is Human (IOM, 2000) and *Crossing the Quality Chasm* (IOM, 2001). Although there is evidence that there are global trends leading to ongoing improvements in health care, an earlier assessment of the state of health in the United States (Swensen et al., 2010, p. e12[1]) still persists today:

> U.S. health care is broken. Although other industries have transformed themselves using tools such as standardization of value-generating processes, performance measurement, and transparent reporting of quality, the application of these tools to health care is controversial, evoking fears of "cookbook medicine," loss of professional autonomy, a misinformed focus on the wrong care, or a loss of individual attention and the personal touch in care delivery. ... Our current health care system is essentially a cottage industry of nonintegrated, dedicated artisans who eschew standardization. ... Growing evidence highlights the dangers of continuing to operate in a cottage-industry mode. Fragmentation of care has led to suboptimal performance.

These statements were made at a time when the United States was launching the most major health reform in its history, the ACA, amid great opposition—opposition that still continues today. The challenge of the coming years continues to be how to build on the gains that we have made in the past and how to fix what many still consider a broken system.

Rather than assume that we have any easy answers—which we do not—some time will be devoted in this chapter to examples of successes, with a particular focus on CQI philosophies and processes, as models of how to generalize these successes more widely. Hopefully this will give us some direction toward a set of ideas to expand the implementation of CQI across a broader range of providers.

Dr. Brent James, former Executive Director of the Institute for Health Care Delivery Research and Vice President of Medical Research and Continuing Medical Education at Intermountain Health Care, in an interview with the *New York Times*, gave several examples of how Intermountain Health Care led the way to value-based care through the use of CQI processes. He identified the lack of widespread change as being directly related to the complexity of the health care system; a clear symptom of the depth of problems that persist is that the American health care system is vastly more expensive, but not vastly better, than the health systems of other countries (Leonhardt, 2009). Intermountain Health Care has also led the way to the future by implementing innovations that are rooted in past philosophies and processes of CQI, most notably Deming's process management theories. In a 2011 report, they demonstrated the basic CQI principle that the most effective way to reduce health care costs is to increase quality, using methodologies that are sustainable and generalizable to the entire nation, and which could facilitate the greater and more effective implementation of the ACA (James & Savitz, 2011). (Further details and ideas for academic discussion of the process for achieving success at Intermountain Health Care can be found in a case study describing the "Intermountain Way to Positively Impact Costs and Quality" [Savitz, 2012].)

Dr. Donald Berwick founded the Institute for Healthcare Improvement (IHI) more than 25 years ago and has also served as Administrator of the Centers for Medicare and Medicaid Services (CMS). In 2003, he noted "Americans spend almost 40% more per capita for health care than any other country, yet rank 27th in infant mortality, 27th in life expectancy, and are less satisfied with their care than the English, Canadians, or Germans" (Berwick 2003, p. 69). Two of the important issues at the heart of this problem, complexity and cost, were also key factors in the debate about health reform in the United States in 2009; they are also contributors to the explanation of why CQI has not been more widely adopted. He also addressed the issues of complexity and cost is his introduction of the Triple Aim of health care, to be discussed in greater detail later in this chapter (Berwick, Nolan, & Whittington, 2008).

The complexity of the health care system is both a challenge and a source of ideas for how to make improvements (Plsek & Greenhalgh, 2001). Health care can be described as a complex adaptive system, a concept that has implications for how to improve the system. For example, the importance of leadership is critical, as are incentives for improvement. As a complex adaptive system, health care can only be designed to a certain extent and cannot be designed around minimizing costs; rather, the focus must be on maximizing value (Rouse, 2008; Spath & Kelly, 2017).

▶ CQI and the Science of Innovation

While health care is unique in many ways, one commonality that it has with other complex endeavors is the difficulty surrounding diffusion of innovation, starting with simple resistance to change but including many other complex factors. Understanding these issues helps to provide pathways toward greater diffusion of CQI in health care. The research and principles that are specific to diffusion of innovation of health services are summarized in a systematic review of the literature presented by Greenhalgh et al. (2005). From this review, it is noted that there is a wide range of literature using a variety of concepts and approaches that describe how to move along the spectrum from the initiation of a concept for change to the spread, diffusion, and institutionalization of innovation.

Diffusion theory is useful in understanding the factors that thwart or support the adoption of CQI in health care. Because of the complexity of health care and the added complexity of CQI, as alluded to earlier in this chapter, there

are no simple answers about how to move CQI innovations into the mainstream of health care more quickly and efficiently. Complexity must be considered in understanding innovation. Although there are competing theories about how and why, innovation clearly does happen in "complex zones." There is some evidence that while innovation may not be susceptible to being managed, it is possible to design and control organizational conditions that "enhance the possibility of innovation occurring and spreading" (Greenhalgh, Robert, Bate, Macfarlane, & Kyriakidou, 2005, p. 80). Addressing this complexity requires, first and foremost, leadership, but also the creation of a receptive and even enthusiastic culture; one excellent example of how this has been accomplished in CQI in health care is the formation of quality improvement collaboratives, such as the SURPASS collaborative group, which among many accomplishments includes the successful application of surgical checklists to improve patient safety (de Vries et al., 2010).

The speed and overall adoption of any change, including CQI, can be influenced by the characteristics of the change and how it is perceived by those responsible for implementation. These characteristics include relative advantage, compatibility, simplicity, trialability, and observability (Rogers, 1995). All of these characteristics relate to changes and improvements in health care, and two are particularly relevant to health care: *compatibility*, which relates to how closely the change ideas align with the existing culture and environment, and *trialability*, which addresses how the changes can be adapted and tested in the new environments in which they are being spread.

A further extension of these change concepts yields the following seven rules for dissemination of innovation in health care (Berwick, 2003):

1. Find sound innovations.
2. Find and support innovators.
3. Invest in early adopters.

4. Make early-adopter activity observable.
5. Trust and enable reinvention.
6. Create slack for change.
7. Lead by example.

All of these rules are applicable to innovations around CQI; leadership, trust, and reinvention are fundamental. Reinvention has to do with the cross-disciplinary learning concept that has permeated CQI and is responsible for its evolution across industries and across the globe. CQI cannot be a top-down mandate. It must be part of the vision of an organization and accepted by all who must implement CQI, thus requiring trust at all levels, which comes from leadership, teamwork, and Deming's concept of "constancy of purpose." Top leadership must be involved, supporting and communicating the vision for innovation and change; however, participation, buy-in, and support from opinion leaders at all levels within an organization are critical for successful implementation and the process of reinvention.

One size will not fit all. As described by Berwick, "To work, changes must be not only adopted locally, but also locally adapted" (2003, p. 1974). Berwick asserts that for this to happen, there must be reinvention. In his words, "Reinvention is a form of learning, and, in its own way, it is an act of both creativity and courage. Leaders who want to foster innovation … should showcase and celebrate individuals who take ideas from elsewhere and adapt them to make them their own" (Berwick, 2003, p. 1974).

The checklist tool cited in Chapters 1 and 8 of this book is a clear illustration of this process of reinvention and leadership. It was adapted from the airline and other industries, first to intensive care and later to surgery, with trusted leaders in their fields and disseminating their ideas and successes via scientific venues. The fact that these evidence-based tools are not fully accepted and used returns us to the point that health care is complex and requires diligence to

spread the improvement process. The systematic review of diffusion of innovation in health services identifies complexity as one of the key elements that is inversely associated with successful diffusion. Quite often, due to the complex nature of health care systems, equally complex quality improvement strategies are required, thus lessening their quick and easy adoption. This helps to explain why simpler quality improvement processes, such as the use of PDSA cycles, have enjoyed broad success. But other factors may need to be considered to overcome resistance to changes in health care procedures and understand how these changes truly lead to improvements (Langley et al., 2009). For example, a prospective study of the attributes of 42 clinical practice recommendations in gynecology (Foy et al., 2002) helps to explain what these factors may be. After review of almost 5,000 patient records, findings indicate two relevant outcomes that explain why there may be unexpected resistance to change. First, recommendations that were compatible with clinician values and did not require changes to fixed routines were associated with greater compliance. Second, initial noncompliance could be reversed after audit and feedback stages were carried out, indicating that perhaps more time will yield greater compliance. This is especially to be considered when evaluating improvements in outcomes (vs. processes), which may require more time and repeated cycles of process changes to take hold and be sustained.

The techniques and philosophies described throughout this book provide some other examples of progress that has been made in specific segments of health care and also describe models that can be considered to increase diffusion of CQI ideas. For example, social marketing has been documented as being an effective tool for understanding ways to improve the impact of innovations in health care in general (Greenhalgh et al., 2005). In Chapter 8 of this text and in an illustrative case study (Breland, 2012), a novel social marketing approach is proposed as a technique for increasing compliance with use of surgical checklists and other CQI innovations.

▶ The Business Case for CQI

Health care delivery systems are large, decentralized, and complex, yet at their core they involve a fundamental personal relationship between providers and patients. Moreover, if this were not a sufficient challenge, rapid and uncertain changes in the structure and processes of providing and paying for care make measuring the effect of any single management intervention over time very difficult, if not impossible. Although evidence has been accumulated from both controlled trials (Goldberg, Wagner, & Finh, 1998; Mehta et al., 2000; Solberg, 1993) and survey data (Shortell, Bennett, & Byck, 1998) on the implementation process and perceived impact, much of the evidence remains anecdotal (Arndt & Bigelow, 1995; Bigelow & Arndt, 1995). Leatherman et al. (2003), for example, argue that the "business case" for quality improvement is yet to be proven, even while evidence mounts for the overall societal and economic benefits:

> A *business case* for a health care improvement intervention exists if the entity that invests in the intervention realizes a financial return on its investment in a reasonable time frame, using a reasonable rate of discounting. This may be realized as "bankable dollars" (profit), a reduction in losses for a given program or population, or avoided costs. In addition, a *business case* may exist if the investing entity believes that a positive indirect impact on organization function and sustainability will accrue within a reasonable time frame. (p. 18)

These arguments continue; the economic case includes the returns to all the actors, not just the individual investing business unit. The social case, as they define it, is one of measuring benefits, but not requiring positive returns on the investment. That has been overriding the consideration in the battle to control medical variation and medical errors (McGlynn, Asch, & Adams, 2003). The business case for quality improvement suffers from the same negative factors as the business case for other preventive health care measures—namely, all or part of the benefits accruing to other business units or patients, and delayed impacts that get discounted heavily in the reckoning (Leatherman et al., 2003). The regulatory arguments for quality improvement efforts have generally been justified on the basis of social and economic benefits such as lives saved and overall cost reductions, but these arguments are not necessarily profitable to the investor. These authors also present a whole array of public policy measures that would overcome the barriers to a positive business case and encourage wider and more assertive implementation of quality improvement methods. Clearly, economics alone does not provide an argument strongly for or against the use of CQI, but it does add to the complexity that pervades the wider and more rapid implementation of CQI in health care.

In summary, this brief overview indicates that a strong business case for CQI in health care cannot be made. Looking back over the past 40 years, Robert Brook, UCLA Professor of Medicine and Health Services and Distinguished Chair in Health Care Services for the RAND Corporation, observes, "Although there are some examples in the literature to support the concept that better quality of care is less expensive, few studies have produced information that could be generalized across time and institutional settings" (Brook, 2010, p. 1831). Building on the traditional business concepts that have been discussed and in consideration of the limited evidence to support the business case for CQI, a transformation that may support greater diffusion of CQI and the continuing need to bridge the quality chasm is to consider a more value-based approach to CQI in health care. This approach argues for simultaneous goals of higher quality and lower cost, which will only be achieved when there is a reorientation among CQI proponents that includes a thorough understanding of how to achieve a positive return on investment (Brook, 2010). This view is consistent with the Triple Aim of Health Care described by Berwick, Nolan, and Whittington (2008) and its most recent recommended enhancement, the Quadruple Aim (Bodenheimer & Sinsky, 2014); it will be discussed in greater detail in the final chapter of this text (Chapter 14), which will address future quality trends in health care.

▶ Factors Associated with Successful CQI Applications

Despite the need for greater diffusion of CQI in health care, much progress has been made, suggesting a broad array of factors that can be associated with successful CQI implementation. The key to greater diffusion is understanding and emphasizing those factors that work while exploring new concepts, such as the value focus described previously. This analysis starts with regulatory (e.g., accreditation) factors and organizational factors such as leadership, organizational culture, and teamwork; and finishes with individual providers' internal/intrinsic motivation, perhaps the most important factor for adoption of innovations and CQI.

Capturing the Intellectual Capital of the Workforce

Industrial managers are increasingly recognizing that frontline workers know their work processes better than the management does. Therefore, management encourages workers to apply that knowledge and insight to the firm's processes. This is especially true in health care, where the professionals employed by or practicing in the institution control the technological core of the organization. Management that does not capitalize on this available pool of professional and specialized knowledge within the organization is naive at best.

Reducing Managerial Overhead

Some companies have been able to remove layers of management as work groups have taken responsibility for their own processes. Health care organizations are actually already limited in the number of staff positions, mostly because the professionals, rather than the corporate staff, have clinical process knowledge. Indeed, one might view the new investments in CQI as a catching-up process for the lack of process-oriented staff that are involved in process enhancement in most other industries. This is but another example of how the incentives in health care are misaligned. Since physicians are not employees in most community hospitals, they are not at risk when processes are suboptimal, unless the situation is so bad that it prompts a lawsuit.

Lateral Linkages

Health care organizations are characterized by their many medical specialties, each organized into its own professional fiefdom. Specialization is just one response to an information overload in the organization (Galbraith, 1973). By specializing, each unit tends to learn more and more about less and less. One way to offset the effects of this specialization is to provide lateral linkages—coordinators, integrating mechanisms—to get the information moving across the organization as well as up and down the chain of command (Galbraith, 1973; Lawrence & Lorsch, 1967). So far, that has proved very difficult in health care institutions. CQI, through its use of interdisciplinary teams and its focus on a broader definition of process and system as it affects customers rather than professional groups, presents one way to establish linkages. The technology of CQI focuses as much on coordination of the change process as on its motivation. In modern medicine, as practiced in the 21st century, this coordination and motivation of CQI is bolstered by the need for greater coordination in medical care in general and is therefore quite natural. There is a greater emphasis on interdisciplinary care, which leads to fostering interdependence and, in turn, better teamwork, including greater employee engagement and improvements in the patient experience and the financial performance of practices (Swensen et al., 2010).

Regulatory Agencies and Accreditation

Regulatory mechanisms such as accreditation are key factors that have led to greater diffusion of CQI and will continue to do so in the future as a direct result of mandated measurement and improvement of the quality of care. Chapter 12 will provide a broad overview of accreditation and its impact across the globe, but for the purposes of this discussion, a focus on the United States is illustrative.

In the United States, the efforts of The Joint Commission (TJC) and CMS have led to the implementation of a series of initiatives that require hospitals to report on quality measures; after a period of strong resistance, routine reporting of key metrics is now commonplace and required for accreditation by TJC; and has been reinforced by provisions in the ACA (Somander, 2015). Also, as described in Chapters 11 and 12 of this text, accreditation initiatives at the national and state levels have served as an impetus for CQI in public health agencies in the United States. The local health department accreditation system in North Carolina also serves as an example of CQI innovation at a state-wide level, as it was one of the first states to implement mandatory public health accreditation, which

has led to sustainable CQI efforts (Stone & Davis, 2012).

Likewise, CMS generates extensive CQI activities and associated reporting of findings via the efforts of Quality Improvement Organizations (QIOs). QIOs represent a clear example of diffusion of CQI in health care and continue to play an important role in ensuring the highest quality of care to the millions of beneficiaries covered by Medicare in the United States. QIOs are a clear example of diffusion, as they grew from what they were in 1972 when they were termed Professional Standards Review Organizations (PSROs) (Schenck, McArdle, & Weiser, 2013). (For an in-depth discussion and to provide a series of academic questions to be considered for understanding how QIOs work, readers are referred to an illustrative case study provided by Rokoske, McCardle, and Schenck, 2012.)

The processes for each of these regulatory mechanisms provide evidence for factors to be considered, as well as lessons learned, in regard to further diffusion of CQI in health care. For example, the impact of the measurement requirements has been notable. In a review published by members of TJC, this impact was described as being due to the use of robust, evidence-based measures, which link process performance and patient outcomes (Chassin, Loeb, Schmaltz, & Wachter, 2010). Despite extensive documentation of successes in the article, these authors also note the need and define a direction for further improvement, centered on process measurement. They point out that the focus of this measurement process is entirely on hospital care, leaving much to be done in regard to ambulatory care. They also note that the measures in place are process measures, not outcome measures. In the spirit of continuous improvement, they offer guidance in improving the measures that are currently in place.

Once again, this program, while not without problems, is a good model for further diffusion of CQI; early resistance to measurement no longer exists, and now the issue is more about finding the most effective measures, with little resistance expected from hospitals and physicians. In the language of diffusion of innovation, TJC has passed the early adoption stage and is now well into the institutionalization stage, at least in the hospital sector, and relative to a subset of process measures. However, despite their optimism about the progress that has been made and the value of their proposed measurement framework, Chassin et al. (2010) close their discussion of these new accountability measures by realistically pointing out that perpetual vigilance is required to review and improve the measurement process via feedback from internal and external customers. So a partial answer to our question of how to "fix the broken system" is provided by accreditation, and much has been accomplished, with some guidance from TJC on what to do next. However, these comments are specific to measurement of processes in hospitals, and a more general answer is still needed to truly address the broader health care system and its subcomponents.

Motivational Factors

A number of motivational factors contribute to the sustained interest and enthusiasm for health care improvement. These factors have an impact on the motivation of the management of the organization and its employees. The first argument for CQI is its direct impact on quality, usually a net gain to the customer/patient and to the employees of the organization, the external and internal customers. The second argument relates to the set of benefits associated with a plan that empowers employees in health care through participation in decision making. These factors represent benefits for employees and management that can be classified as follows.

Internal/Intrinsic Motivation

With the proper internal or intrinsic motivation, the vast majority of health care workers

support the concept of quality care and would like to see improvements and participate in a meaningful quality improvement process. Allowing personnel to work on their own processes, permitting them to "do the right thing," and then rewarding them for that behavior is almost sure to increase intrinsic motivation in employees, if done properly. It is a classic case of empowerment and job enrichment for health care workers and follows the principle clearly delineated by Deming about the important role of internal (vs. external) motivation and employee engagement in CQI efforts. It should be noted that internal and intrinsic motivation will be used interchangeably throughout this text, representing the form of motivation that Deming describes as being linked to self-esteem and dignity (1993).

System of Profound Knowledge

It is well known that the system of profound knowledge and the original 14 points of Deming (see Chapter 1) emphasize high levels of trust, empowerment, and especially internal motivation and engagement as important factors associated with implementation of CQI initiatives (Deming, 1986,; 1993). This is clearly and succinctly emphasized in Deming's point number 12: "remove barriers that rob people of pride of workmanship" (Deming, 1986, p. 77). In health care, and especially in nursing and medicine, one indication of demotivation and lack of engagement is the increasing rate of burnout and work dissatisfaction in recent years (Shanafelt et al., 2015). A systematic review and meta-analysis reported in *The Lancet* in 2016 described physician burnout as reaching epidemic proportions (West, Dyrbye, Erwin, and Shanafelt, 2016). Burnout, which can be defined as the opposite of engagement, is indicated by emotional exhaustion, depersonalization and perceived lack of personal accomplishment; and in health care, burnout is manifested by diminished personal well-being and longevity and leads to decreased quality of patient care

(Chew et al., 2017). Provider burnout has also been linked to greater patient dissatisfaction and higher costs. Examples that have been cited of lower quality/safety of care resulting from burnout include prescribing inappropriate medications (Bodenheimer & Sinsky, 2014). Reports of physician burnout have been persistent during the second decade of the 21st century, as indicated by findings from two large studies, which reported prevalence of at least one symptom of burnout as high as 54.4% in 2014 (Shanafelt et al., 2015) compared to 45.5% in 2011 (Shanafelt et al., 2012). In both studies, the sample sizes consisted of over 3,000 responding physicians; although response rates were in the 20% range, which may compromise the ability these data have to serve as predictors of population parameters, the consistency and large sample size that these findings are based on are indicative of a long-term trend that burnout is consistent and may be worsening over the time period between these two studies. Other studies in the United States and Europe of a range of types of health care providers, including nurses and staff as well as physicians, yield similar findings. For example, one provider survey, in 2013, in the United States found that 60% of respondents reported burnout and 34% indicated that they planned to look for another job (Bodenheimer & Sinsky 2014). A 2015 survey of British physicians reported that 44% of respondents reported very low or low morale, with similar findings for nurses and health care staff (Sikka, Morath, & Leape, 2015).

Among the various factors that thwart innovation and CQI implementation, burnout and low morale are often mentioned not only for the sake of encouraging innovation, but more importantly, to improve the health and well-being of health care providers. A key question for all in health care and specifically to address the topic of this chapter is how to reverse these trends; how to eliminate factors that may be causally related to burnout and how to identify factors that will increase the rate of innovation and CQI implementation.

From Triple Aim to Quadruple Aim

An important innovative concept that was first introduced in 2008 is the Triple Aim of Health Care (Berwick, Nolan, & Whittington, 2008). This innovation broadens the goals and definition of quality health care through the simultaneous pursuit of three aims: "improving the experience of care, improving the health of populations, and reducing the per capita costs of health care" (Berwick, Nolan, & Whittington, 2008, p. 759). Since its introduction, the adoption of the Triple Aim has become a goal of many health care providers both nationally and globally and can be viewed as a new stage in the ongoing evolution of CQI in health care; it has done so by using a systems optimization perspective and has taken advantage of associated innovations that have facilitated the implementation of systems to pursue the Triple Aim. For example, adoption of the Triple Aim has benefited from improvements in technology, such as the broader overall use and the institutionalization, at least in large hospital systems, of electronic health records. It has also benefited from CQI tools and techniques that have become more widely adopted in recent years such as elimination of waste in health care processes via LEAN/Six Sigma, described in Chapter 5.

The introduction of the Triple Aim is an example of innovation in health care systems, and the application of a systems approach utilizing synergy derived from the interdependence of the three aims. However, this interdependence requires careful attention to system optimization since changing any one has a direct impact on the other two aims. This important characteristic has direct implications on the further adoption of CQI in health care, which requires that intrinsic motivation for change and improvement is maintained by providers. For example, if cost reductions lead to overburdening busy providers with lower leverage tasks, then they may not be motivated to identify and implement new CQI ideas. The cost-reduction mentality that is described in some business models as "doing more with less" can also lead, in health care, to poorer quality and lower patient satisfaction if tradeoffs are not carefully understood and managed.

Quadruple Aim

Although many health care providers have adopted the Triple Aim, others have not been able to do so successfully. One explanation for less than full implementation may be that "practices working toward the Triple Aim may increase physician burnout and thereby reduce their chances of success" (Bodenheimer & Sinsky, 2014, p. 575). A partial explanation for this trend is that some of the very same factors that lead to successful adoption of the Triple Aim may have inadvertently led to burnout and demotivation among some health care providers. For example, the widespread increase in utilization of electronic health records, a plus factor for implementing the Triple Aim, has been shown to lead to increases in burnout (Babbott et al., 2014).

Provider burnout and dissatisfaction, the opposite of internal motivation and engagement, may also lead to a reluctance to adopt or lead the development of innovations/CQI initiatives. Because of its possible causative links to burnout, the Triple Aim, while by definition designed to lead to greater CQI implementation and innovation in health care, may inadvertently have the opposite effect, at least in some cases.

To address this conflict in positive and negative effects of pursuing the Triple Aim, one solution that has been proposed is to expand the Triple Aim by adding a fourth aim—improving the work life of clinicians and health care staff and increasing the experience of joy and meaning in health care work (Bodenheimer & Sinsky, 2014; Sikka, Morath, & Leape, 2015). The key question is, how?

As with many CQI initiatives the solution of expanding from a Triple Aim to a Quadruple Aim must start with a system-level focus. For example, one form of system optimization that is proposed to implement the Quadruple Aim for primary care is to shift relevant responsibilities from physicians to practice staff but at the same time ensuring that "staff who assume new responsibilities are well trained and understand that they are contributing to the health of their patients and that unnecessary work is reengineered out of the practice" (Bodenheimer & Sinsky, 2014, p. 575). This approach represents just one of many possible system changes that can be included under the umbrella of empowerment, a well-established, cost-effective approach to improve internal motivation and engagement (Daft, 2015). It also requires attention to the concept of task-relevant maturity for ensuring that those who are empowered are prepared to accept greater responsibility, including receiving adequate training (Grove, 1995). The successful application of these concepts may require an initial investment in dollars and time that will offer a future return on investment. And most important, it requires a culture that is open to transformational leadership concepts (Daft, 2015) such as empowerment and a vision that embraces innovation and improvement; such a culture is described in the next section of this chapter.

In summary, the concept and effectiveness of the Triple Aim will be further improved by the addition of a fourth aim that focuses on the welfare of providers because "maintaining a balance between workforce satisfaction and patient satisfaction will be critical in achieving the fourth aim. Reductions in physician and staff burnout will support the primary goal of the Triple Aim, improving population health" (AHRQ, 2015). Stated more succinctly, "health care is a relationship between those who provide care and those who seek care, a relationship that can only thrive if it is symbiotic" (Bodenheimer & Sinsky, 2014, p. 575). And this symbiotic relationship is at the core of successful CQI implementation.

▶ Culture of Excellence

Throughout the history of the application of CQI, one of the most important factors associated with successful applications of CQI has been the interaction of leadership, organizational culture, teamwork and internal motivation. Transformational leadership, distinguished by its emphasis on vision, is a starting point and a consistent force in motivating change and improvement. "Transformational leadership is characterized by the ability to bring about significant change in both followers and the organization. Transformational leaders have the ability to lead changes in the organization's vison, strategy and culture as well as promote innovation in products and technologies" (Daft, 2015, p. 360). To ensure CQI, the most important role of a leader is transformation (Deming, 1993), which starts with a motivating vision that must be developed, communicated, and embraced by all in the organization, and which in turn leads to high levels of commitment to the vision of change and improvement (Melum & Sinioris, 1993; Tichy & Devanna, 1986). Leaders ensure commitment to the vision by shaping a culture that not only accepts but embraces change (Balestracci, 2009; Schein, 1991). **FIGURE 2.1** describes the way in which this is accomplished in an organization that is dedicated to CQI and

thereby defines a set of factors that are critical to the greater diffusion of CQI in health care.

The development of and commitment to a vision leads to what Deming called constancy of purpose for all in the organization, referring to a clear sense of where the organization is going or what a system is intended to accomplish (Deming, 1986). The type of culture that is needed to succeed in an organization whose goal is to continuously improve can be called a "culture of excellence." This concept is similar to a "safety culture," defined as a culture in which "a commitment to safety permeates all levels of the organization from frontline personnel to executive management" (AHRQ, 2011). Also similar is a clearly defined, shared vision that translates into detailed procedures, decision-making processes based on teamwork, and strategic actions that lead to achievement of the vision of quality and safety. A culture of excellence is one that ensures high quality at every customer interface and in which a commitment to the highest quality—and CQI, in particular—is shared by all in the organization.

Underlying the creation of a culture of excellence is a need for a systems view. A systems view of health care emphasizes the importance of adding value and the importance of leadership rather than management, influence rather than power, and the alignment of incentives focused on quality rather than quantity of services (Rouse, 2008). A culture of excellence

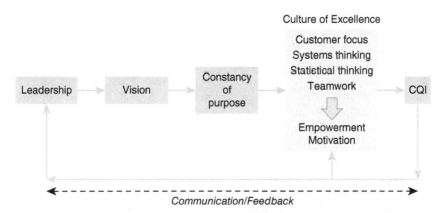

FIGURE 2.1 A Cultural Model to Ensure Successful CQI Implementation

embraces this view, is performance oriented, and at a minimum adopts a CQI philosophy (as defined in Chapter 1). It exemplifies the following elements outlined in Figure 2.1:

- *Customer focus:* Emphasizing the importance of both internal and external customers (see Chapter 1). It should be noted here that in defining the population who will ultimately benefit from health care innovations and CQI (i.e., the external customer), there may be some discomfort with the generic term "customer," especially among physicians and nurses (Houpt, Gilkey, & Ehringhaus, 2015). There should be awareness of this issue, especially when developing a culture to embrace the ideas presented here, but for simplicity and consistency with terminology presented here and in the CQI literature in general, the term *customer* will continue to be used—as a term that denotes the highest respect for the patients, their families and communities served in health care.
- *Systems thinking:* Maintaining a goal of optimizing the system as a whole and thereby creating synergy (Deming, 1986; Spath & Kelly, 2017).
- *Statistical thinking:* Understanding causes of variation and the importance of learning from measurement; having the ability to use data to make decisions (see Chapter 4 and Balestracci, 2009).
- *Teamwork:* Teams of peers working together to ensure empowerment, thereby creating the highest levels of motivation to ensure alignment of the organization, the team, and the individual around the CQI vision (see Chapter 6 and Grove, 1995).
- *Motivation and empowerment:* A key component of the culture of excellence is its ability to increase empowerment and internal motivation necessary for any successful CQI initiative (Deming, 1986, 1993). Ultimately, this will lead to higher

levels of engagement. "The most recent thinking about motivation considers what factors contribute to people's willingness to be fully engaged at work and "go the extra mile" to contribute their creativity, energy and passion on the job. One approach is to foster an organizational environment that helps people find true value and meaning in their work. One path to meaning is through employee engagement" (Daft, 2015, pp. 245–246). A culture of excellence creates an environment where empowerment, motivation and engagement are the norm. It should ultimately address the need for "joy in work" by providing a platform for the Quadruple Aim to be achieved; and in a cyclical manner this will in turn further increase the motivation of health care providers to be innovative and embrace CQI initiatives.

- *Communication and feedback:* Maintaining open channels of communication and feedback to make adjustments as needed, including modifying the vision to achieve higher levels of quality in a manner consistent with a learning organization (Senge, 1990), including feedback that is fact-based and given with true concern for individuals' organizational success (Balestracci, 2009). Open communication and feedback are key characteristics of the team approach necessary to achieve the goals of CQI (see Chapter 6).

Leadership and Diffusion

In discussing factors that support the implementation of CQI, the theory of diffusion of innovation clearly supports the important role of leadership in CQI. A capacity for innovation, as described in the literature of organizational psychology, is seen as critically dependent on good leadership; one of the key factors to the implementation and routinization of innovation once adopted is the consultation and active involvement of leaders—and especially leadership by example. Furthermore, organizational leadership is critical to the development of a culture that fosters innovation (Greenhalgh et al., 2005). CQI is a form of change and innovation that also requires cultural change driven by leadership. As Greenhalgh et al. explain, "Leaders within organizations are critical firstly in creating a cultural context that fosters innovation and secondly, establishing organizational strategy, structure, and systems that facilitate innovation" (2005, p. 69). This perspective ties directly back to Deming's point about leadership: leaders must know and understand the processes they are responsible for and lead by example, acting as part of the improvement effort and on the "corrections" required (Deming, 1986). This point was emphasized by Gawande (2009, p. 146) in describing how the initial adoption of surgical checklists was accomplished:

> Using the checklist involved a major cultural change, as well—a shift in authority, responsibility, and expectations about care—and the hospitals needed to recognize that. We gambled that their staff would be far more likely to adopt the checklist if they saw their leadership accepting it from the outset.

Leaders at All Levels

Various types of leaders can contribute to (or detract from) the innovation process. Traditional organizational and team leaders are most often associated with CQI initiatives; however, in regard to innovations, the terminology of "leader" can be expanded to include opinion leaders, champions, and boundary spanners.

Opinion leaders represent a broad range of leaders "within the ranks" as well as those at the top level. In clinical settings, opinion leaders have influence on the beliefs and actions of their colleagues, either positive or negative in regard to embracing innovation. Opinion leaders may be experts who are respected for their formal academic authority in regard to a particular innovation; their support represents a form of evidence-based knowledge. Opinion leaders may also be peers who are respected for their know-how and understanding of the realities of clinical practice (Greenhalgh et al., 2005).

Unlike opinion leaders, who may support or oppose an innovation, *champions* persistently support new ideas. They may come from the top management of an organization, including technical or business experts. Champions include team and project leaders and others who have perseverance to fight both resistance and/or indifference to promote the acceptance of a new idea or to achieve project goals (Greenhalgh et al., 2005).

Boundary spanners represent a combination of these various types of leaders and are distinguished by the fact that they have influence across organizational and other boundaries (Greenhalgh et al., 2005; Kaluzny, Veney, & Gentry, 1974). Boundary spanners play an important role in multi-organizational innovations and quality improvement initiatives, such as quality improvement collaboratives. Each of these types of leaders is found in the adoption of quality improvement initiatives in health care, and often these various types of leaders are found in combination.

Teamwork

CQI in health care is a team game. These teams are composed of peers who are highly trained technical experts supporting each other and empowered to take a leadership role as required to meet the needs of customers. Teamwork is one of the most important components of all successful CQI initiatives; team building centers on the ability to create teams of empowered and motivated people who are leaders themselves and who will take the lead as needed to foster change, innovation, and improvement (Byham & Cox, 1998; Grove 1995; Kotter, 1996). The glue that holds a culture of excellence together and that ensures there will be quality at every interface is the link between leadership and teamwork—with leadership exhibited as called for at all levels within a team. As Deming states, "There is no substitute for teamwork and good leaders of teams to bring consistency of effort along with knowledge" (1986, p. 19).

Motivation and Empowerment

Inherent in teamwork is a high level of empowerment of team members, which in turn leads to high levels of motivation. Empowerment implies that levels of authority match levels of responsibility and training. For example, suggestions and interventions can be made to allow improvements and prevent problems or errors. This initiative goes beyond simply allowing team members to speak up; it means ensuring they are comfortable speaking up when something seems wrong (Byham & Cox, 1998; Deming, 1986; Grove, 1995).

Improved motivation is the direct result of transformational leadership and especially its emphasis on empowerment. Motivation and empowerment both will interact to lead to higher quality; but to work, these elements require another aspect of cultural change and associated leadership responsibility—building a culture of trust. This is emphasized in Deming's 14 points, namely point number 8: Drive out fear. Create trust. Create a climate for innovation (see Chapter 1). Deming explains, "No one can put in his best performance unless he feels secure. ... Secure means without fear, not afraid to express ideas, not afraid to ask questions" (1986, p. 59). This ties directly back to the surgical checklist example as well as the airline safety tradition, where use of a checklist implies responsibility to communicate and question each other as part of the checklist process, regardless of the team member's rank. A leader's goal must be to create a culture where people are empowered to do their jobs

to the best of their abilities, with trust and a clear understanding of the vision that creates the constancy of purpose needed to achieve the highest quality.

Training is critical to the success of leaders and the ability to achieve constancy of purpose, not only training of employees in the skills required to do their jobs, which removes barriers to motivation, but also training the future leaders of the organization, which creates further motivation. Training of future leaders is one of the most important responsibilities of a leader (Tichy, 1997). And it is a key characteristic of transformational leadership; "transformational leadership inspires followers ... motivates people to do more than originally expected ... develops followers into leaders" (Daft, 2015, p. 361). Gawande (2009) addresses this issue in describing the process for testing and implementing the surgical safety checklist. Despite the obvious key role of the surgeon, it was decided that the "circulating nurse" on the surgery team would be the one to start the checklist process at the beginning of a surgery. This was done for several reasons, but one of the most important was "to spread responsibility and the power to question" (p. 137).

Examples of Leadership and Teamwork in CQI

The linkage between leadership and teamwork to ensure success in quality improvement in health care has been demonstrated in many instances, including the very successful implementation of quality improvement collaboratives (QICs). QICs represent a form of virtual organizations (Byrne, 1993) the effectiveness of which have been demonstrated in industry for many years. Part of the success of QICs can be tied to this effective team structure. For example, in describing the successful application of a QIC using the IHI Breakthrough series (Kilo, 1998) in 40 U.S. hospitals to reduce adverse drug events, Leape et al. (2000) identify strong leadership and teamwork among their most important success factors: "Success in making significant changes was associated with strong leadership, effective processes, and appropriate choice of intervention. Successful teams were able to define, clearly state, and relentlessly pursue their aims, and then chose practical interventions and moved early into changing a process" (Greenhalgh et al., 2005, p. 165). Further examples of QICs and their importanace in the future of CQI in health care are presented in Chapter 14.

In summary, leadership, effective team-work, and the empowerment of teams, which lead to higher levels of internal motivation, have been critical factors in the evolution of CQI in health care and are directly related to the pace and broad adoption of CQI in health care in recent years. Chapter 6 provides a detailed description of how to build teams and ensure that they operate most effectively to improve quality in health care. Grove (1995) provides examples of how to create an organizational structure that supports multiple teams working in parallel and how to ensure efficiency in doing so.

▶ Kotter's Change Model

A traditional model that is used to define a culture of change and in particular the role of vision and leadership is the eight-stage change model developed by John Kotter (1996), which is outlined in BOX 2.1. The discussion of leadership, organizational culture, and teamwork presented previously described "what is" the type of culture that is needed to implement successful CQI initiatives; Kotter's model describes "how to" implement major change and also provides guidance on traditional errors to avoid. These two approaches are closely related. There is clear overlap between Kotter's model and the factors defined in Figure 2.1, which describe the culture of excellence. These common elements include empowerment, communication, feedback loops to produce more change, and, most important, the central role of vision and anchoring change in the

culture. The presentation of Kotter's model, which is well known with widespread application beyond health care, also serves as validation for the basic concepts of the Culture of Excellence Model.

One key point of Kotter's model that is worthy of a bit more discussion here is his first point: "Establishing a sense of urgency." This point relates to an earlier discussion about how long it takes, or should take, to implement CQI concepts. The emphasis is not that decisions should be rushed, but that complacency is to be avoided. Complacency may be due to many reasons that can be associated with the need for CQI in health care. These include, according to Kotter, "too much past success, lack of visible crises, low performance standards, [and] insufficient feedback from external constituencies. ... Without a sense of urgency, people won't give that extra effort that is essential. They won't make needed sacrifices. Instead they cling to the status quo and resist initiatives from above" (1996, p. 5). This point directly relates to CQI in health care; the importance of ensuring safety and quality in health care requires a sense of urgency.

See Kotter's text for a comprehensive description of the elements in Box 2.1 and the broader subject of how to implement organizational change.

▶ Conclusions

Despite the increased use of CQI and a good understanding of the philosophy and processes of CQI, its effectiveness and further adoption in health care remain subjects of ongoing concern. The literature on diffusion of innovation suggests some guidelines to understand factors that influence the adoption of CQI. Understanding the factors that enable or influence adoption of CQI, as well as the factors that present barriers, is particularly important as more countries around the world are utilizing CQI to solve health challenges, including resource-poor countries and as national health initiatives are being modified or introduced around the world, including in the United States.

Among the factors that are gaining greater attention is the emphasis on cost, efficiency and value. The emphasis on value is directly correlated with concerns about the costs of quality health care and has led to novel concepts such as the Triple Aim of health care—simultaneously focusing on care, health, and cost. At the same time, the critical role of internal motivation, that was emphasized by CQI pioneers, such as W. Edwards Deming, as central to ongoing implementation of CQI, leads to consideration of a fourth aim, improving the motivation and work life of health care providers. This consideration has been driven in part by demotivation resulting from increasing rates of burnout that have been reported among health care providers. Central to promoting the diffusion of innovation, and in particular CQI, is leadership, vision, and teamwork, resulting in empowerment and motivation of the health care workforce. A model that combines these factors to ensure the continuing adoption of CQI in health care, and including the goals of the Quadruple Aim, is the implementation of a culture of excellence as described and defined in this chapter.

References

AHRQ Patient Safety Network. (2011). Glossary: Safety culture. Rockville, MD: Agency for Healthcare Research and Quality. Retrieved January 1, 2011, from http://psnet.ahrq.gov

AHRQ. (2015). Quadruple aim proposed to address workforce burnout. Rockville, MD: Agency for Healthcare Research and Quality. Retrieved October 27, 2017, from https://integrationacademy.ahrq.gov

AHRQ. (2017). About the National Quality Strategy. Rockville, MD: Agency for Healthcare Research and Quality. Retrieved November 3, 2017, from http://www.ahrq.gov

Arndt, M., & Bigelow, B. (1995). The implementation of total quality management in hospitals. *Health Care Management Reviews, 20,* 3–14.

Babbott, S., Manwell, L. B., Brown R., Montague, E., Williams, E., Schwartz, M., ... Linzer, M. (2014). Electronic medical records and physician stress in primary care: results of the MFMO Study. *Journal of the American Medical Informatics Association, 21*(e1), e100–e106.

Balestracci, D. (2009). *Data sanity: A quantum leap to unprecedented results.* Englewood, CO: Medical Group Management Association.

Berwick, D. M. (2003). Disseminating innovations in health care. *Journal of the American Medical Association, 289,* 1969–1975.

Berwick, D. M., Nolan, T. W., & Whittington, J. (2008). The Triple Aim: Care, health and cost. *Health Affairs, 27*(3), 759–769.

Bigelow, B., & Arndt, M. (1995). Total quality management: Field of dreams? *Health Care Management Reviews, 20,* 15–25.

Bodenheimer, T., & Sinsky, C. (2014). From triple to Quadruple Aim: Care of the patient requires care of the provider. *Annals of Family Medicine, 12*(6), 573–576.

Breland, C. (2012). Forthright Medical Center: Social marketing and the surgical checklist: In C. P. McLaughlin, J. K. Johnson, & W. A. Sollecito (Eds.), *Implementing continuous quality improvement in health care: A global casebook.* Sudbury, MA: Jones & Bartlett Learning.

Brook, R. H. (2010). The end of the quality improvement movement: Long live improving value. *Journal of the American Medical Association, 304*(16), 1831–1832.

Byham, J. C., & Cox, J. (1998). *Zapp! The lightning of empowerment—How to improve quality, productivity and employee satisfaction.* New York, NY: Fawcett Ballantine, The Ballantine Publishing Group.

Byrne, J. (1993). The virtual corporation. *Business Week, 3304,* 98–102.

Chassin, M. R., Loeb, J. M., Schmaltz, S. P., & Wachter, R. M. (2010). Accountability measures: Using measurement to promote quality improvement. *The New England Journal of Medicine, 363,* 683–688.

Chew, F. S., Mulcahy, M. J., Porrino J. A., Mulcahy, H., & Relyea-Chew, A. (2017). Prevalence of burnout among musculoskeletal radiologists. *Skeletal Radiology, 46,* 497–506.

Daft, R. L. (2015). *The leadership experience,* 6th ed. Mason, OH: Cengage Learning.

Deming, W. E. (1986). *Out of the crisis.* Cambridge, MA: Massachusetts Institute of Technology Center for Advanced Engineering Study.

Deming, W. E. (1993). *The new economics for industry, government, education.* Cambridge, MA: Massachusetts Institute of Technology Center for Advanced Engineering Study.

de Vries, E. N., Prins, H. A., Crolla, R. M., den Outer A. J., van Andel G., van Helden S. H., ... SURPASS Collaborative Group. (2010). Effect of a comprehensive surgical safety system on patient outcomes. *The New England Journal of Medicine, 363,* 1928–1937.

Foy, R., MacLennan, G., Grimshaw, J., Penney, G., Campbell, M., & Grol, R. (2002). Attributes of clinical recommendations that influence change in practice following audit and feedback. *Journal of Clinical Epidemiology, 55,* 717–722.

Galbraith, J. (1973). *Designing complex organizations.* Reading, MA: Addison-Wesley.

Gawande, A. (2009). *The checklist manifesto.* New York, NY: Metropolitan Books.

Goldberg, H. I., Wagner, E. H., & Finh, S. D. (1998). A randomized controlled trial of CQI teams and academic detailing: Can they alter compliance with guidelines? *Joint Commission Journal of Quality Improvement, 24,* 130–142.

Greenhalgh, T. E., Robert, G., Bate, P., Macfarlane, F., & Kyriakidou, O. (2005). Diffusion of innovations in health service organizations: A systematic literature review. Oxford, UK: Blackwell Publishing.

Grove, A. S. (1995). *High output management.* New York, NY: Vintage Books.

Houpt, J. L., Gilkey, R. W., & Ehringhaus, S. H. (2015). *Learning to lead in the academic medical center—A practical guide.* Switzerland: Springer International Publishing.

Institute of Medicine (IOM). (2000). *To err is human: Building a safer health system.* Washington, DC: National Academies Press.

Institute of Medicine (IOM). (2001). *Crossing the quality chasm: A new health paradigm for the 21st century.* Washington, DC: National Academies Press.

James, B. C., & Savitz, L. A. (2011). How Intermountain trimmed health care costs through robust quality improvement efforts. *Health Affairs, 30*(6), 1185–1191.

Kaluzny, A., Veney, J. A., & Gentry, J. T. (1974). Innovation of health services: A comparative study of hospitals and health departments. *Milbank Memorial Fund Quarterly: Health & Society, 52,* 51–82.

Kilo, C. M. (1998). A framework for collaborative improvement: Lessons from the Institute for Healthcare Improvement's breakthrough series. *Quality Management in Health Care, 6,* 1–13.

Kotter, J. P. (1996). *Leading change.* Boston, MA: Harvard Business School Press.

Langley, G. J., Moen, R. D., Nolan, K. M., Nolan, T. W., Norman, C. L., & Provost, L. P. (2009). *The improvement guide: A practical approach to enhancing organizational performance,* 2nd ed. San Francisco, CA: Jossey-Bass.

Lawrence, P. R., & Lorsch, J. W. (1967). *Organization and environment.* Boston, MA: Harvard University Press.

Leape, L. L., Kabcenell, A. I., Gandhi, T. K., Carver, P., Nolan, T. W., & Berwick, D. M. (2000). Reducing adverse drug events: Lessons from a breakthrough series collaborative. *Joint Commission Journal of Quality Improvement, 26,* 321–331.

Leatherman, S., Berwick, D., Iles, D., Lewin, L. S., Davidoff, F., Nolan, T., & Bisognano, M. (2003). The business case for quality: Case studies and an analysis. *Health Affairs, 22*(2), 17–30.

Leonhardt, D. (2009). Making health care better. *The New York Times,* November 24, 1–14. Retrieved April 25, 2018, from https://www.nytimes.com/

McGlynn, E. A., Asch, S. M., & Adams, J. (2003). The quality of health care delivered to adults in the United States. *The New England Journal of Medicine, 348,* 2635–2645.

Mehta, R. H., Das, S., Tsai, T. T., Nolan, E., Kearly, G., & Eagle, K. A. (2000). Quality improvement initiative and its impact on the management of patients with acute myocardial infarction. *Archives of Internal Medicine, 160,* 3057–3062.

Melum, M. M., & Sinioris, M. K. (1993). *Total quality management—The health care pioneers.* Chicago, IL: American Hospital Publishing.

Plsek, P., & Greenhalgh, T. (2001). The challenge of complexity in health care. *British Medical Journal, 323*(7313), 625–628.

Rogers, E. (1995). *Diffusion of innovations.* New York, NY: Free Press.

Rokoske, F., McArdle, J. A., & Schenck, A. P. (2012). Clemson's nursing home: Working with the state quality improvement organization's restraint reduction initiative. In C. P. McLaughlin, J. K. Johnson, & W. A. Sollecito (Eds.), *Implementing continuous quality improvement in health care: A global casebook.* Sudbury, MA: Jones & Bartlett Learning.

Rouse, W. B. (2008). Health care as a complex adaptive system. *Bridge, 38,* 17–25.

Satterfield, J. M., Spring, B., Brownson, R. C., Mullen, E. J., Newhouse, R. P., Walker, B. B., & Whitlock, E. P. (2009). Toward a transdisciplinary model of evidence-based practice. *The Milbank Quarterly, 87*(2), 368–390.

Savitz, L. (2012). The Intermountain way to positively impact costs and quality. In C. P. McLaughlin, J. K. Johnson, and W. A. Sollecito (Eds.), *Implementing continuous quality improvement in health care: A global casebook.* Sudbury, MA: Jones & Bartlett Learning.

Schein, E. H. (1991). *Organizational culture and leadership.* San Francisco, CA: Jossey-Bass.

Schenck, A. P., McArdle, J., & Weiser, R. (2013). Quality improvement organizations and continuous quality improvement in Medicare. In W. A. Sollecito & J. K. Johnson (Eds.), *Continuous quality improvement in health care,* 4th ed. Sudbury, MA: Jones & Bartlett Learning.

Senge, P. (1990). *The fifth discipline: The art and practice of a learning organization.* New York, NY: Doubleday.

Shanafelt, T. D., Boone, S., Tan, L., Dyrbye, L. N., Sotile, W., Satele, D., ... Oreskovich, M. R. (2012). Burnout and satisfaction with work-life balance among US physicians relative to the general US population. *Archives of Internal Medicine, 172*(18), 1377–1385.

Shanafelt, T. D., Hasan, O., Dyrbye, L. N., Sinsky, C., Satele, D., Sloan, J., & West, C. P. (2015). Changes in burnout and satisfaction with work-life balance in physicians and the general US working population between 2011–2014. *Mayo Clinic Proceedings, 90*(12), 1600–1613.

Shortell, S. M., Bennett, C. L., & Byck, G. R. (1998). Assessing the impact of continuous quality improvement on clinical practice: What will it take to accelerate programs. *The Milbank Quarterly, 76,* 593–624.

Sikka, R., Morath, J. M., & Leape, L. (2015). The Quadruple Aim: Care, health, cost and meaning in work. *BMJ Quality & Safety, 24,* 608–610. Retrieved October 4, 2017, from http://qualitysafety.bmj.com

Solberg, L. (1993). *Improving disease prevention in primary care.* Washington, DC: AHCPR Working Paper.

Somander, T. (2015). 4 Ways the Affordable Care Act is Improving the Quality of Health Care in America. Retrieved November 3, 2017, from https://obamawhitehouse.archives.gov

Spath, P. L., & Kelly, D. L. (2017). *Applying quality management in healthcare: A systems approach,* 4th ed. Chicago, IL: Health Administration Press.

Stone, D., & Davis, M. V. (2012). North Carolina local health accreditation program. In C. P. McLaughlin, J. K. Johnson, & W. A. Sollecito (Eds.), *Implementing continuous quality improvement in health care: A global casebook.* Sudbury, MA: Jones & Bartlett Learning.

Swensen, S. J., Meyer, G. S., Nelson, E. C., Hunt, G. C. Jr., Pryor, D. B., Weissberg, J. I., ... Berwick, D. M. (2010). Cottage industry to postindustrial care: The revolution in health care delivery. *The New England Journal of Medicine, 362,* e12(1)–e12(4).

Tichy, N. M. (1997). *The leadership engine.* New York, NY: Harper Business.

Tichy, N. M., & Devanna, M. A. (1986). *The transformational leader.* New York, NY: John Wiley and Sons.

West, C. P., Dyrbye, L. N., Erwin, P. J., & Shanafelt, T. D. (2016). Interventions to prevent and reduce physician burnout: A systematic review and meta-analysis. *The Lancet, 388,* 2272–2281.

CHAPTER 3

Integrating Implementation Science Approaches into Continuous Quality Improvement

Rohit Ramaswamy, Julie K. Johnson, and Lisa R. Hirschhorn

It is often difficult, and indeed not always helpful, to separate intervention from context to the extent that transplanting a programme in its entirety from one setting to another is rarely straightforward.

— **Mary Dixon-Woods**

The most consistent challenges to continuous quality improvement (CQI) throughout its evolution in health care have been ensuring the broadest adoption of evidence-based improvements in practice and motivating research into further improvements of processes and outcomes. The challenge of how to maximize adoption of CQI-proven practices is addressed in this chapter through an introduction to implementation science as a methodology to increase the adoption and implementation of innovations and improvements in health care-practice settings. Drawing on its multidisciplinary roots and applications, implementation science represents a next step in the evolution of CQI in health care.

▶ Implementation Science Defined

Implementation is "*a specified set of activities designed to put into practice, an activity, or program*" (NIRN, 2018). Even if we know the interventions needed to implement or improve a program, we still need a scientific approach to make sure that these activities are executed in a way that results in their effective use. We also need to learn from this experience to accelerate change more broadly.

The emerging field of implementation science involves the systematic study of how to improve the quality of implementation of interventions and programs that are known

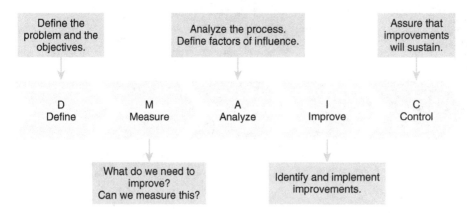

to work, typically in health care, public health, behavioral health, education, and other settings where sustainable solutions at scale are difficult to achieve. Implementation science has a number of definitions, but it can be understood as the "scientific study of methods to promote the systematic uptake of research findings and other evidence-based practices into routine practice, and, hence, to improve the quality and effectiveness of health services and care ... (this) field includes the study of influences on health care professional and organizational behavior." Recognizing the importance of how and where these interventions are implemented, the National Implementation Research Network (NIRN) also defines the field as "the study of factors that influence the full and effective use of innovations in practice" (NIRN, 2018). In this chapter, we describe the key principles of implementation science and how integrating these principles into improvement strategies can be a valuable step to helping quality improvement (QI) programs achieve their desired results.

While the use of QI methods such as Lean, Six Sigma (see Chapter 5), or the Model for Improvement (introduced in Chapter 1) to improve systems and processes in health care is now well established, there is still much debate about the effectiveness of these methods. For example, a recent systematic review of Lean methods concluded that there is little

evidence to support the claim that Lean leads to improved health care (Moraros, Lemstra, & Nwankwo, 2016). The lack of a systematic approach to implementation is one reason for this conclusion. The most common QI methodologies do not incorporate a systematic approach to the implementation of the improvement solution—a failing that can lead to an incorrect conclusion that the solution isn't effective. For example, Six Sigma's Define, Measure, Analyze, Improve, Control (DMAIC) process (**FIGURE 3.1**) moves directly from the *Improve* step (where improvement solutions are generated and prioritized) to the *Control* step (where the post-improvement process is monitored for stability) without any mention of the context-specific details needed to guide the implementation of the selected solutions. *The Wall Street Journal* reports that 60% of Six Sigma projects fail to achieve the desired results, because "in the middle stage of an improvement project—when the Six Sigma expert moves on to another project and top management turns it focus to another group of workers—implementation starts to wobble, and teams may find themselves struggling to maintain the gains they achieved early on" (Chakravorty, 2010). The three questions framing the Model for Improvement (**FIGURE 3.2**) are structured to help teams develop improvement solutions but do not address their implementation and often neglect the broader organizational changes needed for immediate success as well as sustainability of change.

In other words, it is not enough to use QI methods rigorously to come up with a solution that works. It is equally important to be rigorous about applying the approaches and tools from implementation science to put these solutions into effective practice and sustain the changes.

The key ingredients needed for interventions to achieve successful outcomes are summarized in **FIGURE 3.3** (Bertram, Blase, & Fixsen,

2015). Positive outcomes require an intervention that is appropriate to the context, which QI methods can help to develop. But the intervention is just one ingredient. An implementation approach appropriate to the setting and resources and a supportive organizational, policy, or funding environment are needed as well. The multiplicative nature of these "ingredients" means that failure in any of these steps will decrease the chance that desired outcomes are achieved.

FIGURE 3.4 shows how quality improvement methods and implementation science approaches can work together to achieve effective outcomes in health care and in public health. Systematic improvement methods help to create effective interventions (sometimes referred to as change packages) that fit the local context. Implementation science methods can be used to identify appropriate implementation strategies to ensure effective implementation of the change package.

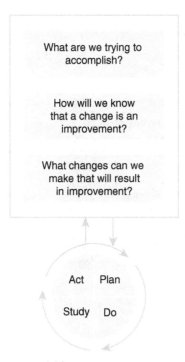

FIGURE 3.2 Model for Improvement

Reproduced from Langley, G.L., Nolan, K.M., Nolan, T.W., Norman, C.L. and Provost, L.P. (2009), The Improvement Guide: A Practical Approach to Enhancing Organizational Performance, 2nd ed., Jossey Bass, San Francisco.

▶ Integrating Implementation into QI: The Model for Improvement and Implementation

Incorporating the tools and methods of implementation science in a systematic way requires enhancing the Model for Improvement with implementation steps. We refer to this model,

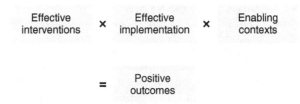

FIGURE 3.3 Key Ingredients for Achieving Outcomes

Modified from National Implementation Research Network

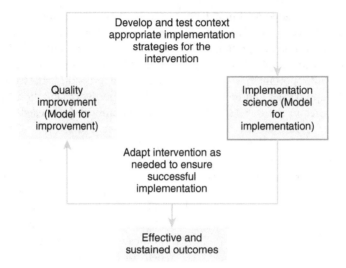

FIGURE 3.4 Integrating Improvement and Implementation

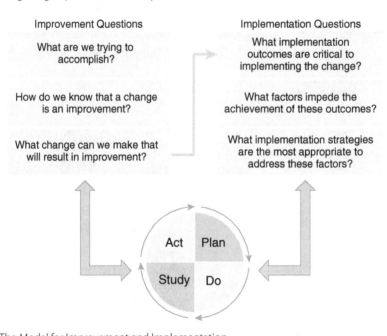

FIGURE 3.5 The Model for Improvement and Implementation

Modified from Langley, G.L., Nolan, K.M., Nolan, T.W., Norman, C.L. and Provost, L.P. (2009), The Improvement Guide: A Practical Approach to Enhancing Organizational Performance, 2nd ed., Jossey Bass, San Francisco.

shown in FIGURE 3.5, as the Model for Improvement and Implementation (MFII). This model incorporates three implementation questions into the traditional model for improvement.

The implementation questions begin with *implementation outcomes*, which are the desired results of the implementation of the change package. Analogous to improvement aims, these outcomes specify the *implementation aims* to ensure quality implementation in a particular setting or context, such as feasibility, fidelity, acceptability, or cost. The second question addresses *implementation determinants*, or factors that may affect the implementation outcomes in that context. And finally, the third question identifies *implementation strategies*, which are implementation interventions to address the determinants that may impede the achievement of the implementation and ultimately the QI outcomes. The Plan, Do, Study, Act (PDSA) cycles test and refine these strategies so that they fit the implementation context. As a result of this testing, it may become apparent that the change package is inappropriate for the context and may need to be modified or adapted. This will initiate the redesign of the change package and the creation of a new improvement solution. Improvement and implementation are thus intrinsically connected in the joint model.

Implementation Outcomes

The first implementation question of the MFII is intimately connected to the first improvement question, *What are we trying to accomplish?*, because we cannot achieve health improvement goals if improvement interventions are not implemented well. Implementation outcomes are defined as "the effects of deliberate and purposive actions to implement new treatments, practices, and services" (Proctor et al., 2011). In other words, implementation outcomes measure how well the implementation process worked, since the quality of the implementation process affects how well the QI intervention achieves the

desired health outcomes. There are more than 500 studies offering evidence that the quality of implementation affects health outcomes (Durlak & DuPre, 2008).

The link between implementation outcomes and quality of care outcomes (defined here as service outcome and patient/client outcomes) is shown in FIGURE 3.6 (from Proctor et al., 2011). There are eight implementation outcomes shown in the figure, and their definitions are provided in TABLE 3.1.

Quality improvement project teams can use Figure 3.6 to select the implementation outcomes most likely to affect the achievement of their improvement aims. For example, an improvement intervention that relies on fast ambulance services to improve referral processes affecting the timeliness of care may not be feasible or may be too expensive in low-resource settings where ambulance services are not easily available. In this context, *feasibility* and *cost* may be the most important implementation outcomes that affect the ability to improve timeliness of care. In the case of an intervention focusing on improving patient satisfaction by enhanced provider/patient communication, *acceptability* of new communication protocols by providers may be the primary implementation outcome of interest. For a hand-hygiene intervention, *adoption* by clinicians may affect the reduction in health care-associated infection (HCAI) prevalence. In this case, adoption may vary by facility and

Implementation outcomes	Service outcomes*	Client outcomes
Acceptability	Efficiency	Satisfaction
Adoption	Safety	Function
Appropriateness	Effectiveness	Symptomatology
Costs	Equity	
Feasibility	Patient-centeredness	
Fidelity	Timeliness	
Penetration		
Sustainability		

*IOM Standards of care

FIGURE 3.6 Implementation Outcomes

Reproduced from E. Proctor, 2011. *Adm Policy Ment Health*. 2011 Mar;38(2):65–76. doi: 10.1007/s10488-010-0319-7. Outcomes for implementation research: Conceptual distinctions, measurement challenges, and research agenda.

TABLE 3.1 Implementation Outcomes and Definitions	
Implementation Outcome	**Definition**
Acceptability	Perception that an intervention is agreeable or satisfactory.
Adoption	Uptake of an intervention by practitioners or providers.
Appropriateness	Fit of an intervention to a particular context or setting.
Cost	Money, resources, time, or effort needed to implement an intervention.
Feasibility	The extent to which organizational resources, motivation, and capabilities can support the implementation of an intervention.
Fidelity	The match between how an intervention is intended to be delivered and how it is actually delivered.
Penetration	The extent to which an intervention reaches the population for whom it is intended.
Sustainability	The extent to which an intervention becomes part of an organization's everyday practice.

the adoption rates may be affected by differences in *acceptability* of the intervention, and it therefore may be necessary to pay attention to both outcomes.

How should these implementation outcomes be integrated into the work of QI teams? After teams have defined the change package to be implemented as part of the QI initiative, they will consider the implementation questions in MFII and determine the implementation outcomes that are most relevant to the successful implementation of their change package. They will collect baseline measures for their selected outcomes and set targets for the implementation outcomes that will result in sustained achievement of the improvement outcome.

Implementation outcomes can be measured in a variety of ways. Perceptual measures such as feasibility, acceptability, appropriateness, or adoption can be measured through surveys or through semi-structured interviews or routine

measurement depending on the indicators chosen. Some of these measures may be integrated into the data collection plan of the QI project without the need for additional work. For most QI projects, a simple survey with a few questions might suffice. But if more rigor is needed, validated survey instruments exist for these outcomes (Weiner et al., 2017; Roberts, Becker, & Seay, 1997). Fidelity can be measured through observations of adherence (Carroll et al., 2007) to a practice or protocol using checklists (Breitenstein et al., 2010). Cost and reach can be measured through reviews of operational documents (e.g., admissions registers or accounting records). Lewis and colleagues (Lewis et al., 2015) identified 104 instruments for measuring one or more implementation outcomes.

BOX 3.1 illustrates the use of implementation outcomes in improvement work at a hypothetical hospital. "Mercy Hospital" is a tertiary hospital with a mature QI program. They have been very successful at initiating QI projects, but have had trouble making them stick in their organization. Guided by implementation scientists, Mercy Hospital QI teams are beginning to use the MFII to improve their quality of implementation. The evidence-based communication protocol is their first project to use the enhanced model.

Implementation Determinants

The second implementation question in the MFII asks, *What are the factors that facilitate and impede the achievement of the implementation aim?* These are referred to as *implementation determinants* in the implementation science literature. In a comprehensive review of the literature, Durlak and Dupre (2008) identified 23 contextual factors that affect implementation. A partial listing, from Durlak (Durlak & DuPre, 2008), is shown in TABLE 3.2.

As shown in Table 3.2, the factors affecting implementation can depend on a variety of characteristics such as the practitioner, the process, the organization, the program and the environment. Sorting through these and identifying the factors that are most relevant for a specific QI program in a specific context could be a formidable task. Implementation researchers have developed a variety of frameworks that facilitate a systematic approach. Nilsen (2015) identified 13

"determinant" frameworks in which the "aim is to understand and/or explain influences on implementation outcomes, e.g., predicting outcomes or interpreting outcomes retrospectively." One of the most widely accepted of these is the Consolidated Framework for Implementation Research (Damschroder et al., 2009), commonly referred to as CFIR. The framework has been tested widely in many different contexts. A systematic review identified 26 studies that have used the framework (Kirk et al., 2016).

FIGURE 3.7 shows the graphic of the framework, which consists of 39 factors affecting implementation organized by five domains that are similar to those described in Table 3.2. Definitions of each of the factors are provided in APPENDIX 3.1. Extensive documentation to support the use of the framework by practitioners and researchers is available at the CFIR website. To explore how CFIR can be used to identify factors that affect implementation outcomes, BOX 3.2 returns to the hypothetical example of implementing provider/patient communication protocols described earlier.

CFIR was developed to assist implementation researchers, though it is also a useful framework for practitioners. Another set of frameworks oriented primarily toward practitioners is the five Active Implementation Frameworks (AIF) (Metz & Bartley, 2012; Blanchard et al., 2017) created by the

TABLE 3.2 Selected List of Factors Affecting Implementation

Community-wide or Societal Factors	Practitioner Characteristics	Characteristics of the Program	Factors Related to the Organization Hosting the Program	Factors Specific to the Implementation Process
Scientific theory and research	Perceived need for the program	Its compatibility or fit with the local setting	The organization's openness to change and innovation	Successful training
Availability of funding	Perceived benefits of the program	Its adaptability (can parts of the program be modified if needed?)	Shared vision and consensus about the program	On-going technical assistance
Policy			Effective leadership	

Data from: Durlak, J. A., & DuPre, E. P. (2008). Implementation matters: A review of research on the influence of implementation on program outcomes and the factors affecting implementation. *American Journal of Community Psychology, 41*(3-4), 327–350. doi:10.1007/s10464-008-9165-0

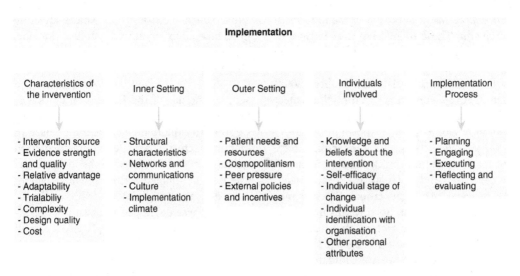

Implementation

Characteristics of the invervention	Inner Setting	Outer Setting	Individuals involved	Implementation Process
- Intervention source - Evidence strength and quality - Relative advantage - Adaptability - Trialabiliy - Complexity - Design quality - Cost	- Structural characteristics - Networks and communications - Culture - Implementation climate	- Patient needs and resources - Cosmopolitanism - Peer pressure - External policies and incentives	- Knowledge and beliefs about the intervention - Self-efficacy - Individual stage of change - Individual identification with organisation - Other personal attributes	- Planning - Engaging - Executing - Reflecting and evaluating

FIGURE 3.7 Consolidated Framework for Implementation

Based on Laura J Damschroder, David C Aron, Rosalind E Keith, Susan R Kirsh, Jeffery A Alexander and Julie C Lowery, "Fostering implementation of health services research findings into practice: a consolidated framework for advancing implementation science", © Damschroder et al., licensee BioMed Central Ltd. 2009.

BOX 3.2 Implementing an Evidence-Based Communication Protocol, Part 2

Recall that the implementation outcome of interest at Mercy Hospital was the acceptability of the communication protocol to providers. The CFIR domains provide a systematic way of identifying the most important barriers to acceptability. Reviewing the results from the staff survey, the team determines that the *individuals involved* and the *inner setting* (i.e., organizational characteristics) are the most important determinants affecting the acceptability of the protocol. These include service provider knowledge regarding the communication protocol, their beliefs about their ability to implement it, and organizational attitudes towards change. To get a deeper understanding or these determinants, the team may conduct additional interviews with the staff and leadership of the facilities or use questionnaires to measure organizational readiness for change. Simple, locally developed questionnaires might suffice, but for those requiring rigor, several validated instruments such as the *Acceptance of Change Scale* (ACS) to measure individual attitudes (Di Fabio & Gori, 2016), or the *Organizational Readiness to Implement Change* (ORIC) instrument (Shea, Jacobs, Esserman, Bruce, & Weiner, 2014) to assess organizational motivation and capacity for implementation are available in the literature.

National Implementation Research Network (NIRN). Together, these frameworks address all the components needed to realize outcomes through the successful implementation of interventions. The five frameworks are: (1) Usable interventions, defining the characteristics of interventions that are most suitable for implementation; (2) implementation stages, reflecting the process needed to plan and execute implementation of an intervention; (3) implementation drivers, which are defined as "key components of capacity and infrastructure that influence a program's success" (Metz & Bartley, 2012); (4) implementation teams to support the implementation; and (5) improvement cycles to ensure that the implementation is adapted to local contexts. The frameworks and their definitions are shown in **FIGURE 3.8**. As with the CFIR, extensive resources, training modules, and tools describing the use of these frameworks are available on the NIRN website.

Among the five AIFs, the implementation drivers (Bertram et al., 2015) are most directly related to the factors affecting implementation. The drivers are shown in **FIGURE 3.9** and are categorized into competencies (hiring, training, and support needed to ensure that staff are well equipped

to implement), leadership (ensuring that leaders have both the management skills and the ability to adapt to changing implementation environments) and organization (use of data to drive decisions, organizational support for change, and integration of the implementation with other external policy and resource priorities). These drivers can be mapped on to the CFIR components of inner setting, outer setting, individuals involved and the implementation process.

Implementation Strategies

The third implementation question of the MFII—*What implementation strategies can we use to improve implementation of the chosen intervention?*—addresses the actions that a QI team needs to take to enhance the implementation quality of the QI intervention. Implementation strategies are defined as "methods or techniques used to enhance the adoption, implementation, and sustainability" (Powell et al., 2015). Powell and his colleagues used an expert consensus building process to identify 73 discrete implementation strategies that are typically used for implementing program and practices (shown in **APPENDIX 3.2**). In a further study, these strategies were aggregated

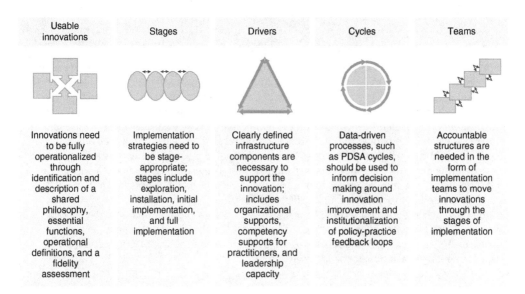

Usable innovations	Stages	Drivers	Cycles	Teams
Innovations need to be fully operationalized through identification and description of a shared philosophy, essential functions, operational definitions, and a fidelity assessment	Implementation strategies need to be stage-appropriate; stages include exploration, installation, initial implementation, and full implementation	Clearly defined infrastructure components are necessary to support the innovation; includes organizational supports, competency supports for practitioners, and leadership capacity	Data-driven processes, such as PDSA cycles, should be used to inform decision making around innovation improvement and institutionalization of policy-practice feedback loops	Accountable structures are needed in the form of implementation teams to move innovations through the stages of implementation

FIGURE 3.8 Active Implementation Frameworks

Reproduced from: Blanchard et al, 2017. *Res Social Adm Pharm*. 2017 Sep – Oct;13(5):922–929. doi: 10.1016/j.sapharm.2017.05.006. Epub 2017 May 22. The Active Implementation Frameworks: A roadmap for advancing implementation of Comprehensive Medication Management in Primary care.

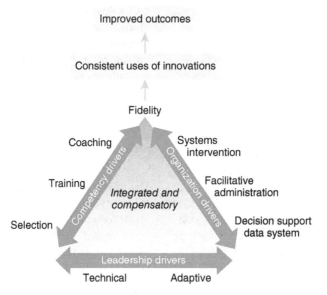

FIGURE 3.9 Implementation Drivers

Reproduced from: Bertram, R. M., Blase, K. A., & Fixsen, D. L. (2015). Improving programs and outcomes. Research on Social Work Practice, 25(4), 477–487. doi:10.1177/1049731514537687

into nine categories (Waltz et al., 2015) shown in **TABLE 3.3**. The categories and the discrete strategies are shown in **APPENDIX 3.3**. This list is a useful guide for teams seeking to determine approaches to improve the quality of implementation of their QI interventions. Different strategies may need to be combined depending on the context in which

TABLE 3.3 Implementation Strategies and Key Activities

Strategy Category	Key Activities
Engage consumers	Involve patients and family members to be active participants in the intervention to increase uptake and sustainability.
Use evaluative and iterative strategies	Monitor the quality of implementation and use iterative methods (such as PDSA cycles) to improve implementation quality.
Provide technical assistance	Provide local and/or facilitation and technical assistance to support the implementation.
Adapt and tailor to the context	Use data to adapt and modify strategies to the context.
Develop stakeholder relationships	Build coalitions, identify local champions, advisory boards and academic partners, train leadership, use early adopters and opinion leaders, capture and share local knowledge, etc.
Train and educate stakeholders	Conduct educational outreach, prepare training materials, train trainers, etc.
Support clinicians (and service providers)	Redesign clinical teams, provide timely data to service providers, develop resource-sharing agreements, develop clinician reminders, etc.
Utilize financial strategies	Provide financial incentives and disincentives (new funding, altered payment schemes, support for innovation, etc.)
Change infrastructure	Change accreditation requirements, liability laws, physical structure and equipment, licensing standards, service sites, etc.

the QI initiative is implemented. **TABLE 3.4** shows how strategies map to implementation outcomes. A similar map between the CFIR domains and strategies is shown in **TABLE 3.5**. Another set of strategies was developed by Michie and is drawn from a distillation of theories related to behavior change (Michie et al., 2013). The result of this distillation is a list of behavior change strategies shown in **APPENDIX 3.4**.

To illustrate how Tables 3.3, 3.4, and 3.5 might be used in practice, let us return to the patient-centered communication protocol example at Mercy Hospital, shown in **BOX 3.3**.

TABLE 3.4 Mapping Implementation Outcomes to Strategies

Implementation Outcome	Typical Strategy Categories
Acceptability	Engaging customers, developing stakeholder interrelationships
Appropriateness	Adapting and tailoring, using evaluative and iterative strategies
Adoption	Training and educating stakeholders, providing technical assistance
Feasibility	Supporting clinicians
Fidelity	Providing technical assistance, supporting clinicians
Cost	Changing infrastructure
Penetration	Engaging customers, developing stakeholder relationships
Sustainability	Changing infrastructure, using evaluative and iterative strategies, utilizing financial strategies

TABLE 3.5 Mapping CFIR Domains to Strategies

CFIR Domain	Typical Strategy Categories
Characteristics of the Innovation	Adapting and tailoring
Inner Setting	Training and educating stakeholders, providing technical assistance, supporting clinicians
Outer setting	Engaging customers, changing infrastructure, developing stakeholder interrelationships
Individuals Involved	Using financial strategies
Implementation process	Using evaluative and iterative strategies

Recall that the most relevant implementation outcome was *acceptability* of the protocol and that surveys and interviews conducted by the QI team identified the individuals involved and the inner settings as the CFIR domains of interest. Based on Table 3.4 and 3.5, the QI team may select *developing stakeholder interrelationships, training and educating stakeholders,* and some *financial incentives or disincentives* as categories from which to create a collection of implementation strategies. From Appendix 3.3, the team may select applicable detailed strategies.

TABLE 3.6 shows the strategy categories and the detailed strategies that may be used as defined in Powell (2015).

As shown in Figure 3.4, the selected implementation strategies are tested, refined, and tailored for to the implementation context using PDSA cycles. The third column of Table 3.6 describes how this leads to particular adaptation of the strategy to implement the communication protocol in the context of Mercy Hospital.

TABLE 3.6 Collection of Strategies to Implement Communication Protocol

Strategy Category	Discrete Strategy	Adapted Strategy
Developing stakeholder relationships	▪ Identifying and preparing championsOrganizing clinical implementation team meetings	▪ Select leaders from the physician and nursing staff who are enthusiastic about the protocol to champion the intervention.Use these champions to present the details about the implementation of the protocol at staff meetings.
Training and educating stakeholders	▪ Creating a learning collaborative	▪ Organize learning sessions where staff from different departments share their experiences with the implementation of the protocol.
Utilizing financial strategies	▪ Developing disincentives	▪ Link the implementation and use of the protocol to annual staff performance review.

▶ Implementing Well: Using Frameworks for Implementation

Even the best implementation strategies will not be of use unless they are implemented well. Several frameworks for guiding the implementation process exist in the implementation science literature. We will describe two that are useful to practitioners: *Stages of Implementation*, which is one of the AIFs described earlier, and the *Interactive Systems Framework for Dissemination and Implementation.*

The NIRN stages of implementation framework describes four stages through

Implementation stages

2–4 Years

Exploration	Installation	Initial implementation	Full implementation
• Assess needs • Examine intervention components • Consider implementation drivers • Assess fit	• Acquire resources • Prepare organization • Prepare implementation drivers • Prepare staff	• Adjust implementation drivers • Manage change • Deploy data systems • Initiate improvement cycles	• Monitor, manage implementation drivers • Achieve fidelity and outcome benchmarks • Further improve fidelity and outcomes

FIGURE 3.10 Stages of Implementation

Reproduced from Bertram, R. M., Blase, K. A., & Fixsen, D. L. (2015). Improving programs and outcomes. Research on Social Work Practice, 25(4), 477–487. doi:10.1177/1049731514537687

which the implementation of an intervention takes place (Bertram et al., 2015). The stages are shown in **FIGURE 3.10**. The Exploration Stage overlaps with some of the planning activities mentioned previously to assess organizational readiness for implementation, identify key factors affecting implementation, and develop implementation strategies. During the Installation Stage, resources for carrying out the implementation strategies are acquired, both for the actual implementation itself and for any technical support that may be required. Training of staff may also take place at this stage. The Initial Implementation is where the intervention is implemented for the first time, using the implementation strategies. The strategies themselves may be tested and adapted during this stage, and any changes to the intervention may be considered. During Full Implementation, ongoing testing and refinement may take place, but the intervention begins to get embedded in the organization and becomes part of everyday work.

It is important to understand that while the stages are represented as a linear progression, in reality this is a nonlinear process. The stages overlap with each other, and there may be situations where there may be the need to cycle back to earlier stages based on the results of tests of strategies (e.g., if it is apparent during initial implementation that staff have not been trained adequately or are not motivated, it may be necessary to go back to some of the installation and exploration activities of staff preparation and readiness building).

The Interactive Systems Framework (Wandersman et al., 2008; Scaccia et al., 2015) shown in **FIGURE 3.11** conceptualizes implementation occurring through interactions between three systems: the *synthesis and translation system*, the *support system*, and the *delivery system*. The synthesis and translation system adapts an intervention (or an implementation strategy) and tailors (translates) it to fit the local context. The support system provides training, coaching, tools, and technical assistance needed for implementation. The delivery system is where the work gets done. According to the framework, successful implementation requires an appropriate implementation strategy, and motivation and capacities to both support the implementation and to deliver it in practice. The framework distinguishes between general

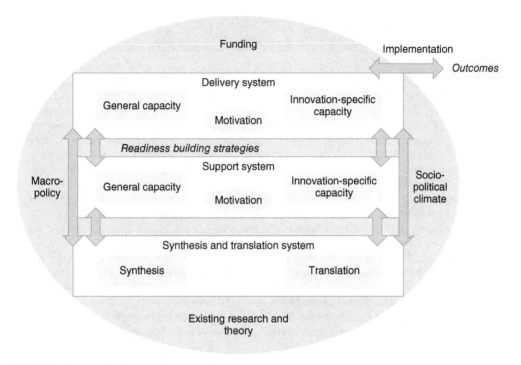

FIGURE 3.11 Interactive Systems Framework

Reproduced from: Scaccia, 2015. *J Community Psychol*. Apr;43(4):484–501. Epub 2015 Apr 13. A practical implementation science heuristic for organizational readiness: R = MC².

capacities and innovation-specific capacities. The former relate to overall organizational capabilities and include factors such as leadership, adequate resources, organizational readiness to change and innovate, and effective processes for support and delivery that are needed for the successful implementation of any intervention. The latter refer to knowledge, skills and abilities and organizational support that are unique to the intervention itself. For example, in the case of a hand-hygiene intervention, this could be knowledge about hand-washing techniques and organizational support for a hand-hygiene program.

How can these frameworks be used in practice to improve the quality of implementation of a QI intervention? As described by Leeman et al. (2017), a collection of selected implementation strategies such as the one shown in Table 3.6 is nothing more than a list until the strategies can be embedded in the implementation process. For implementation to be successful, different strategies need to be used at different implementation stages and in different systems, and the frameworks provide guidance on how to do this. Let's return to the example of the communication protocol (BOX 3.4). We show how the two frameworks described above can be used to develop an implementation plan based on the strategies in Table 3.6. TABLE 3.7 shows the strategies from Table 3.6 organized by implementation stage. TABLE 3.8 shows how the Interactive Systems Framework (ISF) may be used for implementation planning.

▶ Conclusions

The purpose of this chapter is to introduce quality improvement practitioners to some of the key principles, concepts, and tools of implementation science. Over the years, the

BOX 3.4 Implementing an Evidence-Based Communication Protocol, Part 4

Using the Stages of Implementation Framework (Table 3.7)*:* In the exploration stage, the QI team continues to identify factors that might affect the quality of implementation and develops a package of strategies. In the installation stage, the team may begin conversations with early adopters who might serve as champions, and test and refine the messages that these champions should disseminate to other service providers. Once the messages have been finalized, the team may test the different methods for dissemination (e.g., face-to-face presentations at staff meetings, informational flyers, video presentations, and so forth). As more departments begin to use the protocol, the champions and other staff members involved in the implementation may organize local seminars and workshops where staff can share their experiences about the implementation process. Over time, as the protocol becomes part of everyday use, staff leaders in various departments may monitor its use and continue to provide support for implementation as required and training as new providers enter the system.

Using the Interactive Systems Framework: We can also use the Interactive Systems Framework to develop an implementation plan for the strategies in Table 3.6. The ISF helps to ensure that all aspects of the implementation are considered in a systematic way. As shown in Table 3.8, successful implementation of the communication protocol requires testing and adaptation of the strategies to ensure fit, (synthesis and translation system) requires hiring, training and utilizing leaders and champions to support the intervention (support systems) and needs a method to ensure that staff is motivated to use the protocol (delivery system). Both the Stages framework and the ISF present the same information in slightly different ways and QI teams can select on or the other, or both depending on their needs.

TABLE 3.7 Using the Stages of Implementation Framework for Implementation Planning

Implementation Stage	Implementation Strategy
Exploration	▪ Develop implementation strategies
Installation	▪ Select physician and nurse leaders who are enthusiastic about the protocol to champion the intervention ▪ Use these champions to present the details about the implementation of the protocol at staff meetings
Pre implementation	▪ Organize learning sessions where staff from different departments share their experiences with the implementation of the protocol
Final Implementation	▪ Link the implementation and use of the protocol to annual staff performance review

fields of quality improvement and implementation science have progressed side by side. QI methods have focused on the development of change packages and interventions with the assumption that someone else will take care of implementation or that implementation is the easy part if the intervention is sound. Implementation science has been concerned with the adaptation and implementation of evidence-based interventions, often without

TABLE 3.8 Using the Interactive Systems Framework for Implementation Planning

System	Implementation Strategy
Synthesis and Translation	▪ Test and adapt communication messages about the protocol and delivery methods to match the context and culture of the hospital
Support	▪ Select leaders from the doctor and nursing staff who are enthusiastic about the protocol to champion the intervention ▪ Use these champions to present the details about the implementation of the protocol at staff meetings ▪ Organize learning sessions where staff from different departments share their experiences with the implementation of the protocol
Delivery System	▪ Link the implementation and use of the protocol to annual staff performance review

a real understanding of what the intervention is and how it has been developed. As a result, improvement interventions are often poorly implemented, and implementation science has failed to benefit from the wealth of practical knowledge about theories of systems, processes, and variation that are cornerstones of good QI practice. The intent of this chapter is to bridge this gap. QI practitioners, armed with implementation science tools will be well equipped to realize the old adage: "*What is worth doing is worth doing well.*"

References

Bertram, R. M., Blase, K. A., & Fixsen, D. L. (2015). Improving programs and outcomes. *Research on Social Work Practice*, 25(4), 477–487. doi:10.1177/1049731514537687

Blanchard, C., Livet, M., Ward, C., Sorge, L., Sorensen, T. D., & McClurg, M. R. (2017). The Active Implementation Frameworks: A roadmap for advancing implementation of comprehensive medication management in primary care. *Research in Social & Administrative Pharmacy*, 13(5), 922–929. doi:10.1016/j.sapharm.2017.05.006

Breitenstein, S. M., Fogg, L., Garvey, C., Hill, C., Resnick, B., & Gross, D. (2010). Measuring implementation fidelity in a community-based parenting intervention. *Nursing Research*, 59(3), 158–165. doi:10.1097/NNR.0b013e3181dbb2e2

Carroll, C., Patterson, M., Wood, S., Booth, A., Rick, J., & Balain, S. (2007). A conceptual framework for implementation fidelity. *Implementation Science*, 2, 40. doi:10.1186/1748-5908-2-40

Chakravorty, S. S. (2010, January 25). Where process-improvement projects go wrong. *The Wall Street Journal*. Retrieved December 28, 2017, from https://www.wsj.com

Damschroder, L. J., Aron, D. C., Keith, R. E., Kirsh, S. R., Alexander, J. A., & Lowery, J. C. (2009). Fostering implementation of health services research findings into practice: a consolidated framework for advancing implementation science. *Implementation Science*, 4, 50. doi:10.1186/1748-5908-4-50

Di Fabio, A., & Gori, A. (2016). Developing a new instrument for assessing acceptance of change. *Frontiers in Psychology*, 7, 802. doi:10.3389/fpsyg.2016.00802

Dixon-Woods, M., & Martin, G. P. (2016). Does quality improvement improve quality? *Future Hospital Journal*, 3(3), 191–194.

Durlak, J. A., & DuPre, E. P. (2008). Implementation matters: a review of research on the influence of implementation on program outcomes and the factors affecting implementation. *American Journal of Community Psychology*, 41(3-4), 327–350. doi:10.1007/s10464-008-9165-0

Kirk, M. A., Kelley, C., Yankey, N., Birken, S. A., Abadie, B., & Damschroder, L. (2016). A systematic review of the use of the Consolidated Framework for Implementation Research. *Implementation Science*, 11, 72. doi:10.1186/s13012-016-0437-z

Leeman, J., Birken, S. A., Powell, B. J., Rohweder, C., & Shea, C. M. (2017). Beyond "implementation strategies": classifying the full range of strategies used in implementation science and practice. *Implementation Science, 12*(1), 125. doi:10.1186 /s13012-017-0657-x

Lewis, C. C., Fischer, S., Weiner, B. J., Stanick, C., Kim, M., & Martinez, R. G. (2015). Outcomes for implementation science: an enhanced systematic review of instruments using evidence-based rating criteria. *Implementation Science, 10*, 155. doi:10.1186/s13012-015-0342-x

Metz, A., & Bartley, L. (2012). Active implementation frameworks for program success: how to use implementation science to improve outcomes for children. *Zero to Three Journal, 34*(4), 11–18.

Michie, S., Richardson, M., Johnston, M., Abraham, C., Francis, J., ... Wood, C. E. (2013). The behavior change technique taxonomy (v1) of 93 hierarchically clustered techniques: Building an international consensus for the reporting of behavior change interventions, *Annals of Behavioral Medicine, 46*(1), 81–95. https://doi.org/10.1007/s12160-013-9486-6

Moraros, J., Lemstra, M., & Nwankwo, C. (2016). Lean interventions in healthcare: do they actually work? A systematic literature review. *International Journal for Quality in Health Care, 28*(2), 150–165. doi:10.1093 /intqhc/mzv123

National Implementation Research Network (NIRN). (2018). Implementation science defined. Retrieved May 13, 2018, from http://nirn.fpg.unc.edu

Nilsen, P. (2015). Making sense of implementation theories, models and frameworks. *Implementation Science, 10*, 53. doi:10.1186/s13012-015-0242-0

Powell, B. J., Waltz, T. J., Chinman, M. J., Damschroder, L. J., Smith, J. L., Matthieu, M. M., ... Kirchner, J. E. (2015). A refined compilation of implementation strategies: results from the Expert Recommendations for Implementing Change (ERIC) project. *Implementation Science, 10*, 21. doi:10.1186/s13012-015-0209-1

Proctor, E., Silmere, H., Raghavan, R., Hovmand, P., Aarons, G., Bunger, A., ... Hensley, M. (2011). Outcomes for implementation research: conceptual distinctions, measurement challenges, and research agenda. *Administration and Policy in Mental Health, 38*(2), 65–76. doi:10.1007/s10488-010-0319-7

Roberts, G., Becker, H., & Seay, P. (1997). A Process for Measuring Adoption of Innovation within the Supports Paradigm. *Journal of the Association for Persons with Severe Handicaps, 22*(2), 109–119. doi:10.1177/154079699702200210

Scaccia, J. P., Cook, B. S., Lamont, A., Wandersman, A., Castellow, J., Katz, J., & Beidas, R. S. (2015). A practical implementation science heuristic for organizational readiness: R = MC². *Journal of Community Psychology, 43*(4), 484–501. doi:10.1002/jcop.21698

Shea, C. M., Jacobs, S. R., Esserman, D. A., Bruce, K., & Weiner, B. J. (2014). Organizational readiness for implementing change: a psychometric assessment of a new measure. *Implementation Science, 9*, 7. doi:10.1186 /1748-5908-9-7

Waltz, T. J., Powell, B. J., Matthieu, M. M., Damschroder, L. J., Chinman, M. J., Smith, J. L., ... Kirchner, J. E. (2015). Use of concept mapping to characterize relationships among implementation strategies and assess their feasibility and importance: results from the Expert Recommendations for Implementing Change (ERIC) study. *Implementation Science, 10*, 109. doi:10.1186/s13012-015-0295-0

Wandersman, A., Duffy, J., Flaspohler, P., Noonan, R., Lubell, K., Stillman, L., ... Saul, J. (2008). Bridging the gap between prevention research and practice: the interactive systems framework for dissemination and implementation. *American Journal of Community Psychology, 41*(3–4), 171–181. doi:10.1007/s10464-008-9174-z

Weiner, B. J., Lewis, C. C., Stanick, C., Powell, B. J., Dorsey, C. N., Clary, A. S., ... Halko, H. (2017). Psychometric assessment of three newly developed implementation outcome measures. *Implementation Science, 12*(1), 108. doi:10.1186/s13012-017-0635-3

APPENDIX 3.1

Definitions of CFIR Constructs

Construct		Short Description
I. INTERVENTION CHARACTERISTICS		
A	Intervention Source	Perception of key stakeholders about whether the intervention is externally or internally developed.
B	Evidence Strength and Quality	Stakeholders' perceptions of the quality and validity of evidence supporting the belief that the intervention will have desired outcomes.
C	Relative Advantage	Stakeholders' perception of the advantage of implementing the intervention versus an alternative solution.
D	Adaptability	The degree to which an intervention can be adapted, tailored, refined, or reinvented to meet local needs.
E	Trialability	The ability to test the intervention on a small scale in the organization, and to be able to reverse course (undo implementation) if warranted.
F	Complexity	Perceived difficulty of implementation, reflected by duration, scope, radicalness, disruptiveness, centrality, and intricacy and number of steps required to implement.
G	Design Quality and Packaging	Perceived excellence in how the intervention is bundled, presented, and assembled.
H	Cost	Costs of the intervention and costs associated with implementing the intervention including investment, supply, and opportunity costs.

(continues)

Construct	Short Description
II. OUTER SETTING	
A Patient Needs and Resources	The extent to which patient needs, as well as barriers and facilitators to meet those needs, are accurately known and prioritized by the organization.
B Cosmopolitanism	The degree to which an organization is networked with other external organizations.
C Peer Pressure	Mimetic or competitive pressure to implement an intervention; typically because most or other key peer or competing organizations have already implemented or are in a bid for a competitive edge.
D External Policy and Incentives	A broad construct that includes external strategies to spread interventions, including policy and regulations (governmental or other central entity), external mandates, recommendations and guidelines, pay-for-performance, collaboratives, and public or benchmark reporting.
III. INNER SETTING	
A Structural Characteristics	The social architecture, age, maturity, and size of an organization.
B Networks and Communications	The nature and quality of webs of social networks and the nature and quality of formal and informal communications within an organization.
C Culture	Norms, values, and basic assumptions of a given organization.
D Implementation Climate	The absorptive capacity for change, shared receptivity of involved individuals to an intervention, and the extent to which use of that intervention will be rewarded, supported, and expected within their organization.
1 *Tension for change*	The degree to which stakeholders perceive the current situation as intolerable or needing change.
2 *Compatibility*	The degree of tangible fit between meaning and values attached to the intervention by involved individuals, how those align with individuals' own norms, values, and perceived risks and needs, and how the intervention fits with existing workflows and systems.

3	*Relative priority*	Individuals' shared perception of the importance of the implementation within the organization.
4	*Organizational incentives and rewards*	Extrinsic incentives such as goal-sharing awards, performance reviews, promotions, and raises in salary, and less tangible incentives such as increased stature or respect.
5	*Goals and feedback*	The degree to which goals are clearly communicated, acted upon, and fed back to staff, and alignment of that feedback with goals.
6	*Learning climate*	A climate in which: a) leaders express their own fallibility and need for team members' assistance and input; b) team members feel that they are essential, valued, and knowledgeable partners in the change process; c) individuals feel psychologically safe to try new methods; and d) there is sufficient time and space for reflective thinking and evaluation.
E	Readiness for Implementation	Tangible and immediate indicators of organizational commitment to its decision to implement an intervention.
1	*Leadership engagement*	Commitment, involvement, and accountability of leaders and managers with the implementation.
2	*Available resources*	The level of resources dedicated for implementation and on-going operations, including money, training, education, physical space, and time.
3	*Access to knowledge and information*	Ease of access to digestible information and knowledge about the intervention and how to incorporate it into work tasks.

IV. CHARACTERISTICS OF INDIVIDUALS

A	Knowledge and Beliefs About the Intervention	Individuals' attitudes toward and value placed on the intervention as well as familiarity with facts, truths, and principles related to the intervention.
B	Self-efficacy	Individual belief in their own capabilities to execute courses of action to achieve implementation goals.
C	Individual Stage of Change	Characterization of the phase an individual is in, as he or she progresses toward skilled, enthusiastic, and sustained use of the intervention.

(continues)

Construct		Short Description
D	Individual Identification with Organization	A broad construct related to how individuals perceive the organization, and their relationship and degree of commitment with that organization.
E	Other Personal Attributes	A broad construct to include other personal traits such as tolerance of ambiguity, intellectual ability, motivation, values, competence, capacity, and learning style.
V. PROCESS		
A	Planning	The degree to which a scheme or method of behavior and tasks for implementing an intervention are developed in advance, and the quality of those schemes or methods.
B	Engaging	Attracting and involving appropriate individuals in the implementation and use of the intervention through a combined strategy of social marketing, education, role modeling, training, and other similar activities.
	1 Opinion leaders	Individuals in an organization who have formal or informal influence on the attitudes and beliefs of their colleagues with respect to implementing the intervention.
	2 Formally appointed internal implementation leaders	Individuals from within the organization who have been formally appointed with responsibility for implementing an intervention as coordinator, project manager, team leader, or other similar role.
	3 Champions	Individuals who dedicate themselves to supporting, marketing, and 'driving through' the implementation of an intervention, overcoming indifference or resistance that the intervention may provoke in an organization.
	4 External change agents	Individuals who are affiliated with an outside entity who formally influence or facilitate intervention decisions in a desirable direction.
C	Executing	Carrying out or accomplishing the implementation according to plan.
D	Reflecting and Evaluating	Quantitative and qualitative feedback about the progress and quality of implementation accompanied with regular personal and team debriefing about progress and experience.

APPENDIX 3.2

Implementation Strategies and Definitions

Strategy	Definitions
Access new funding	Access new or existing money to facilitate the implementation.
Alter incentive/allowance structures	Work to incentivize the adoption and implementation of the clinical innovation.
Alter patient/consumer fees	Create fee structures where patients/consumers pay less for preferred treatments (the clinical innovation) and more for less-preferred treatments.
Assess for readiness and identify barriers and facilitators	Assess various aspects of an organization to determine its degree of readiness to implement, barriers that may impede implementation, and strengths that can be used in the implementation effort.
Audit and provide feedback	Collect and summarize clinical performance data over a specified time period and give it to clinicians and administrators to monitor, evaluate, and modify provider behavior.
Build a coalition	Recruit and cultivate relationships with partners in the implementation effort.
Capture and share local knowledge	Capture local knowledge from implementation sites on how implementers and clinicians made something work in their setting and then share it with other sites.
Centralize technical assistance	Develop and use a centralized system to deliver technical assistance focused on implementation issues.

(continues)

Strategy	Definitions
Change accreditation or membership requirements	Strive to alter accreditation standards so that they require or encourage use of the clinical innovation. Work to alter membership organization requirements so that those who want to affiliate with the organization are encouraged or required to use the clinical innovation.
Change liability laws	Participate in liability reform efforts that make clinicians more willing to deliver the clinical innovation.
Change physical structure and equipment	Evaluate current configurations and adapt, as needed, the physical structure and/or equipment (e.g., changing the layout of a room, adding equipment) to best accommodate the targeted innovation.
Change record systems	Change records systems to allow better assessment of implementation or clinical outcomes.
Change service sites	Change the location of clinical service sites to increase access.
Conduct cyclical small tests of change	Implement changes in a cyclical fashion using small tests of change before taking changes system-wide. Tests of change benefit from systematic measurement, and results of the tests of change are studied for insights on how to do better. This process continues serially over time, and refinement is added with each cycle.
Conduct educational meetings	Hold meetings targeted toward different stakeholder groups (e.g., providers, administrators, other organizational stakeholders, and community, patient/consumer, and family stakeholders) to teach them about the clinical innovation.
Conduct educational outreach visits	Have a trained person meet with providers in their practice settings to educate providers about the clinical innovation with the intent of changing the provider's practice.
Conduct local consensus discussions	Include local providers and other stakeholders in discussions that address whether the chosen problem is important and whether the clinical innovation to address it is appropriate.
Conduct local needs assessment	Collect and analyze data related to the need for the innovation.
Conduct ongoing training	Plan for and conduct training in the clinical innovation in an ongoing way.
Create a learning collaborative	Facilitate the formation of groups of providers or provider organizations and foster a collaborative learning environment to improve implementation of the clinical innovation.

Create new clinical teams	Change who serves on the clinical team, adding different disciplines and different skills to make it more likely that the clinical innovation is delivered (or is more successfully delivered).
Create or change credentialing and/or licensure standards	Create an organization that certifies clinicians in the innovation or encourage an existing organization to do so. Change governmental professional certification or licensure requirements to include delivering the innovation. Work to alter continuing education requirements to shape professional practice toward the innovation.
Develop a formal implementation blueprint	Develop a formal implementation blueprint that includes all goals and strategies. The blueprint should include the following: (1) aim/purpose of the implementation; (2) scope of the change (e.g., what organizational units are affected); (3) timeframe and milestones; and (4) appropriate performance/progress measures. Use and update this plan to guide the implementation effort over time.
Develop academic partnerships	Partner with a university or academic unit for the purposes of shared training and bringing research skills to an implementation project.
Develop an implementation glossary	Develop and distribute a list of terms describing the innovation, implementation, and stakeholders in the organizational change.
Develop and implement tools for quality monitoring	Develop, test, and introduce into quality-monitoring systems the right input—the appropriate language, protocols, algorithms, standards, and measures (of processes, patient/consumer outcomes, and implementation outcomes) that are often specific to the innovation being implemented.
Develop and organize quality monitoring systems	Develop and organize systems and procedures that monitor clinical processes and/or outcomes for the purpose of quality assurance and improvement.
Develop disincentives	Provide financial disincentives for failure to implement or use the clinical innovations.
Develop educational materials	Develop and format manuals, toolkits, and other supporting materials in ways that make it easier for stakeholders to learn about the innovation and for clinicians to learn how to deliver the clinical innovation.
Develop resource-sharing agreements	Develop partnerships with organizations that have resources needed to implement the innovation.
Distribute educational materials	Distribute educational materials (including guidelines, manuals, and toolkits) in person, by mail, and/or electronically.

(continues)

Strategy	Definitions
Facilitate relay of clinical data to providers	Provide as close to real-time data as possible about key measures of process/outcomes using integrated modes/channels of communication in a way that promotes use of the targeted innovation.
Facilitation	A process of interactive problem solving and support that occurs in a context of a recognized need for improvement and a supportive interpersonal relationship.
Fund and contract for the clinical innovation	Governments and other payers of services issue requests for proposals to deliver the innovation, use contracting processes to motivate providers to deliver the clinical innovation, and develop new funding formulas that make it more likely that providers will deliver the innovation.
Identify and prepare champions	Identify and prepare individuals who dedicate themselves to supporting, marketing, and driving through an implementation, overcoming indifference or resistance that the intervention may provoke in an organization.
Identify early adopters	Identify early adopters at the local site to learn from their experiences with the practice innovation.
Increase demand	Attempt to influence the market for the clinical innovation to increase competition intensity and to increase the maturity of the market for the clinical innovation.
Inform local opinion leaders	Inform providers identified by colleagues as opinion leaders or "educationally influential" about the clinical innovation in the hopes that they will influence colleagues to adopt it.
Intervene with patients/consumers to enhance uptake and adherence	Develop strategies with patients to encourage and problem solve around adherence.
Involve executive boards	Involve existing governing structures (e.g., boards of directors, medical staff boards of governance) in the implementation effort, including the review of data on implementation processes.
Involve patients/consumers and family members	Engage or include patients/consumers and families in the implementation effort.
Make billing easier	Make it easier to bill for the clinical innovation.

Make training dynamic	Vary the information delivery methods to cater to different learning styles and work contexts and shape the training in the innovation to be interactive.
Mandate change	Have leadership declare the priority of the innovation and their determination to have it implemented.
Model and simulate change	Model or simulate the change that will be implemented prior to implementation.
Obtain and use patients/consumers and family feedback	Develop strategies to increase patient/consumer and family feedback on the implementation effort.
Obtain formal commitments	Obtain written commitments from key partners that state what they will do to implement the innovation.
Organize clinician implementation team meetings	Develop and support teams of clinicians who are implementing the innovation and give them protected time to reflect on the implementation effort, share lessons learned, and support one another's learning.
Place innovation on fee-for-service lists or formularies	Work to place the clinical innovation on lists of actions for which providers can be reimbursed (e.g., a drug is placed on a formulary, a procedure is now reimbursable).
Prepare patients/consumers to be active participants	Prepare patients/consumers to be active in their care, to ask questions, and specifically to inquire about care guidelines, the evidence behind clinical decisions, or about available evidence-supported treatments.
Promote adaptability	Identify the ways a clinical innovation can be tailored to meet local needs and clarify which elements of the innovation must be maintained to preserve fidelity.
Promote network weaving	Identify and build on existing high-quality working relationships and networks within and outside the organization, organizational units, teams, etc. to promote information sharing, collaborative problem-solving, and a shared vision/goal related to implementing the innovation.
Provide clinical supervision	Provide clinicians with ongoing supervision focusing on the innovation. Provide training for clinical supervisors who will supervise clinicians who provide the innovation.
Provide local technical assistance	Develop and use a system to deliver technical assistance focused on implementation issues using local personnel.

(continues)

Strategy	Definitions
Provide ongoing consultation	Provide ongoing consultation with one or more experts in the strategies used to support implementing the innovation.
Purposely reexamine the implementation	Monitor progress and adjust clinical practices and implementation strategies to continuously improve the quality of care.
Recruit, designate, and train for leadership	Recruit, designate, and train leaders for the change effort.
Remind clinicians	Develop reminder systems designed to help clinicians to recall information and/or prompt them to use the clinical innovation.
Revise professional roles	Shift and revise roles among professionals who provide care and redesign job characteristics.
Shadow other experts	Provide ways for key individuals to directly observe experienced people engage with or use the targeted practice change/innovation.
Stage implementation scale up	Phase implementation efforts by starting with small pilots or demonstration projects and gradually move to a system wide rollout.
Start a dissemination organization	Identify or start a separate organization that is responsible for disseminating the clinical innovation. It could be a for-profit or non-profit organization.
Tailor strategies	Tailor the implementation strategies to address barriers and leverage facilitators that were identified through earlier data collection.
Use advisory boards and work groups	Create and engage a formal group of multiple kinds of stakeholders to provide input and advice on implementation efforts and to elicit recommendations for improvements.
Use an implementation advisor	Seek guidance from experts in implementation.
Use capitated payments	Pay providers or care systems a set amount per patient/consumer for delivering clinical care.
Use data experts	Involve, hire, and/or consult experts to inform management on the use of data generated by implementation efforts.
Use data warehousing techniques	Integrate clinical records across facilities and organizations to facilitate implementation across systems.

Use mass media	Use media to reach large numbers of people to spread the word about the clinical innovation.
Use other payment schemes	Introduce payment approaches (in a catch-all category).
Use train-the-trainer strategies	Train designated clinicians or organizations to train others in the clinical innovation.
Visit other sites	Visit sites where a similar implementation effort has been considered successful.
Work with educational institutions	Encourage educational institutions to train clinicians in the innovation.

Based on Laura J Damschroder, David C Aron, Rosalind E Keith, Susan R Kirsh, Jeffery A Alexander and Julie C Lowery, "Fostering implementation of health services research findings into practice: a consolidated framework for advancing implementation science", © Damschroder et al., licensee BioMed Central Ltd. 2009.

APPENDIX 3.3

Categories and Strategies

Category	Discrete Strategy
Engage customers	▪ Increase demand. ▪ Intervene with patients/consumers to enhance uptake and adherence. ▪ Involve patients/consumers and family members. ▪ Prepare patients/consumers to be active participants. ▪ Use mass media.
Use evaluative and iterative strategies	▪ Assess for readiness and identify barriers and facilitators. ▪ Audit and provide feedback. ▪ Conduct cyclical small tests of change. ▪ Conduct local needs assessment. ▪ Develop a formal implementation blueprint. ▪ Stage implementation scale up. ▪ Develop and implement tools for quality monitoring. ▪ Develop and organize quality monitoring systems. ▪ Obtain and use patients/consumers and family feedback. ▪ Purposefully reexamine the implementation.
Provide technical assistance	▪ Centralize technical assistance. ▪ Provide local technical assistance.
Adapt and tailor to the context	▪ Promote adaptability. ▪ Tailor strategies. ▪ Use data experts. ▪ Use data warehousing techniques.
Develop stakeholder relationships	▪ Build a coalition. ▪ Conduct local consensus discussions. ▪ Involve executive boards. ▪ Obtain formal commitments. ▪ Promote network weaving.

- Use advisory boards and workgroup.
- Develop academic partnerships.
- Develop an implementation glossary.
- Identify early adopters.
- Inform local opinion leaders.
- Identify and prepare champion.
- Model and simulate change.
- Organize clinician implementation team meetings.
- Recruit, designate, and train for leadership.
- Use an implementation advisor.
- Visit other sites.

Train and educate stakeholders

- Conduct educational meetings.
- Conduct educational outreach visits.
- Develop educational materials.
- Shadow other experts.
- Conduct ongoing training.
- Create a learning collaborative.
- Distribute educational materials.
- Make training dynamic.
- Provide ongoing consultation.
- Use train-the-trainer strategies.
- Work with educational institutions.

Support clinicians

- Create new clinical teams.
- Develop resource sharing agreements.
- Facilitate relay of clinical data to providers.
- Revise professional roles.

Utilize financial strategies

- Access new funding.
- Alter incentive/allowance structures.
- Alter patient/consumer fees.
- Develop disincentives.
- Fund and contract for the clinical innovation.
- Make billing easier.
- Place innovation on fee-for-service lists or formularies.
- Use capitated payments.
- Use other payment scheme.

Change infrastructure

- Change accreditation or membership requirements.
- Change liability laws.
- Change physical structure and equipment.
- Change record systems.
- Change service sites.
- Create or change credentialing and/or licensure standards.
- Mandate change.
- Start a dissemination organization.

Based on Waltz, T. J., Powell, B. J., Matthieu, M. M., Damschroder, L. J., Chinman, M. J., Smith, J. L., Kirchner, J. E. (2015). Use of concept mapping to characterize relationships among implementation strategies and assess their feasibility and importance: results from the Expert Recommendations for Implementing Change (ERIC) study. © Waltz et al. 2015.

APPENDIX 3.4

List of Behavioral Change Techniques

No.	Label	Definition	Examples
1. Goals and planning			
1.1	***Goal setting (behavior)***	Set or agree on a goal defined in terms of the behavior to be achieved. *Note: only code goal-setting if there is sufficient evidence that goal set as part of intervention; if goal unspecified or a behavioral outcome, code **1.3, Goal setting (outcome)**; if the goal defines a specific context, frequency, duration or intensity for the behavior, also code **1.4, Action planning**.*	Agree on a daily walking goal (e.g., 3 miles) with the person and reach agreement about the goal. Set the goal of eating 5 pieces of fruit per day as specified in public health guidelines.
1.2	***Problem solving***	Analyze, or prompt the person to analyze, factors influencing the behavior and generate or select strategies that include overcoming barriers and/or increasing facilitators (includes **Relapse Prevention** and **Coping Planning**).	Identify specific triggers (e.g., being in a pub, feeling anxious) that generate the urge/want/ need to drink and develop strategies for avoiding environmental triggers or for managing negative emotions, such as anxiety, that motivate drinking.

		Note: barrier identification without solutions is not sufficient. If the BCT does not include analyzing the behavioral problem, consider 12.3, Avoidance/changing exposure to cues for the behavior, 12.1, Restructuring the physical environment, 12.2, Restructuring the social environment, or 11.2, Reduce negative emotions	Prompt the patient to identify barriers preventing them from starting a new exercise regimen (e.g., lack of motivation), and discuss ways in which they could help overcome them (e.g., going to the gym with a buddy).
1.3	*Goal setting (outcome)*	Set or agree on a goal defined in terms of a positive outcome of wanted behavior. *Note: only code guidelines if set as a goal in an intervention context; if goal is a behavior, code 1.1, Goal setting (behavior); if goal unspecified, code 1.3, Goal setting (outcome).*	Set a weight loss goal (e.g., 0.5 kilogram over one week) as an outcome of changed eating patterns.
1.4	*Action planning*	Prompt detailed planning of performance of the behavior (must include at least one of context, frequency, duration and intensity). Context may be environmental (physical or social) or internal (physical, emotional or cognitive) (includes **Implementation Intentions**). *Note: evidence of action planning does not necessarily imply goal setting, only code latter if sufficient evidence.*	Encourage a plan to carry condoms when going out socially at weekends. Prompt planning the performance of a particular physical activity (e.g., running) at a particular time (e.g., before work) on certain days of the week.
1.5	*Review behavior goal(s)*	Review behavior goal(s) jointly with the person and consider modifying goal(s) or behavior change strategy in light of achievement. This may lead to re-setting the same goal, a small change in that goal or setting a new goal instead of (or in addition to) the first, or no change. *Note: if goal specified in terms of behavior, code 1.5, Review behavior goal(s), if goal unspecified, code 1.7, Review outcome goal(s); if discrepancy created consider also 1.6, Discrepancy between current behavior and goal.*	Examine how well a person's performance corresponds to agreed goals (e.g., whether they consumed less than one unit of alcohol per day), and consider modifying future behavioral goals accordingly (e.g., by increasing or decreasing alcohol target or changing type of alcohol consumed).

(continues)

No.	Label	Definition	Examples
1.6	*Discrepancy between current behavior and goal*	Draw attention to discrepancies between a person's current behavior (in terms of the *form, frequency, duration, or intensity* of that behavior) and the person's previously set outcome goals, behavioral goals or action plans (goes beyond self-monitoring of behavior). *Note: if discomfort is created only code* **13.3, Incompatible beliefs** *and* <u>not</u> **1.6, Discrepancy between current behavior and goal***; if goals are modified, also code* **1.5, Review behavior goal(s)** *and/or* **1.7, Review outcome goal(s)***; if feedback is provided,* <u>also</u> *code* **2.2, Feedback on behavior***.*	Point out that the recorded exercise fell short of the goal set.
1.7	*Review outcome goal(s)*	Review outcome goal(s) jointly with the person and consider modifying goal(s) in light of achievement. This may lead to re-setting the same goal, a small change in that goal or setting a new goal instead of, or in addition to the first. *Note: if goal specified in terms of behavior, code* **1.5, Review behavior goal(s)***, if goal unspecified, code* **1.7, Review outcome goal(s)***; if discrepancy created consider also* **1.6, Discrepancy between current behavior and goal***.*	Examine how much weight has been lost and consider modifying outcome goal(s) accordingly (e.g., by increasing or decreasing subsequent weight-loss targets).
1.8	*Behavioral contract*	Create a written specification of the behavior to be performed, agreed on by the person, and witnessed by another *Note:* <u>also</u> *code* **1.1, Goal setting (behavior)***.*	Sign a contract with the person (e.g., specifying that they will not drink alcohol for 1 week).

| 1.9 | *Commitment* | Ask the person to affirm or reaffirm statements indicating commitment to change the behavior
    *Note: if defined in terms of the behavior to be achieved <u>also</u> code **1.1, Goal setting (behavior)**.* | Ask the person to use an "I will" statement to affirm or reaffirm a strong commitment (i.e., using the words "strongly", "committed" or "high priority") to start, continue or restart the attempt to take medication as prescribed. |

2. Feedback and monitoring

| 2.1 | *Monitoring of behavior by others without feedback* | Observe or record behavior with the person's knowledge as part of a behavior change strategy
    *Note: if monitoring is part of a data collection procedure rather than a strategy aimed at changing behavior, do not code; if feedback given, code only **2.2, Feedback on behavior**, and <u>not</u> **2.1, Monitoring of behavior by others without feedback**; if monitoring outcome(s) code **2.5, Monitoring outcome(s) of behavior by others without feedback**; if self-monitoring behavior, code **2.3, Self-monitoring of behavior**.* | Watch hand washing behaviors among health care staff and make notes on context, frequency and technique used. |
| 2.2 | *Feedback on behavior* | Monitor and provide informative or evaluative feedback on performance of the behavior *(e.g., form, frequency, duration, intensity)*.
    *Note: if Biofeedback, code only **2.6, Biofeedback** and <u>not</u> **2.2, Feedback on behavior**; if feedback is on **outcome(s)** of behavior, code **2.7, Feedback on outcome(s) of behavior**; if there is no clear evidence that feedback was given, code **2.1, Monitoring of behavior by others without feedback**; if feedback on behavior is evaluative e.g., praise, also code **10.4, Social reward**.* | Inform the person of how many steps they walked each day (as recorded on a pedometer) or how many calories they ate each day (based on a food consumption questionnaire). |

(continues)

No.	Label	Definition	Examples
2.3	***Self-monitoring of behavior***	Establish a method for the person to monitor and record their behavior(s) as part of a behavior change strategy. *Note: if monitoring is part of a data collection procedure rather than a strategy aimed at changing behavior, do not code; if monitoring of outcome of behavior, code **2.4, Self-monitoring of outcome(s) of behavior**; if monitoring is by someone else (without feedback), code **2.1, Monitoring of behavior by others without feedback**.*	Ask the person to record daily, in a diary, whether they have brushed their teeth for at least two minutes before going to bed. Give patient a pedometer and a form for recording daily total number of steps.
2.4	***Self-monitoring of outcome(s) of behavior***	Establish a method for the person to monitor and record the **outcome(s)** of their behavior as part of a behavior change strategy. *Note: if monitoring is part of a data collection procedure rather than a strategy aimed at changing behavior, do not code; if monitoring behavior, code **2.3, Self-monitoring of behavior**; if monitoring is by someone else (without feedback), code **2.5, Monitoring outcome(s) of behavior by others without feedback**.*	Ask the person to weigh themselves at the end of each day, over a 2-week period, and record their daily weight on a graph to increase exercise behaviors.
2.5	***Monitoring outcome(s) of behavior by others without feedback***	Observe or record outcomes of behavior with the person's knowledge as part of a behavior change strategy. *Note: if monitoring is part of a data collection procedure rather than a strategy aimed at changing behavior, do not code; if feedback given, code only **2.7, Feedback on outcome(s) of behavior**; if monitoring behavior code **2.1, Monitoring of behavior by others without feedback**; if self-monitoring outcome(s), code **2.4, Self-monitoring of outcome(s) of behavior**.*	Record blood pressure, blood glucose, weight loss, or physical fitness.

2.6	*Biofeedback*	Provide feedback about the body *(e.g., physiological or biochemical state)* using an external monitoring device as part of a behavior change strategy. *Note: if Biofeedback, code only **2.6, Biofeedback** and <u>not</u> **2.2, Feedback on behavior** or **2.7, Feedback on outcome(s) of behavior**.*	Inform the person of their blood pressure reading to improve adoption of health behaviors.
2.7	*Feedback on outcome(s) of behavior*	Monitor and provide feedback on the outcome of performance of the behavior. *Note: if Biofeedback, code only **2.6, Biofeedback** and <u>not</u> **2.7, Feedback on outcome(s) of behavior**; if feedback is on **behavior** code **2.2, Feedback on behavior**; if there is no clear evidence that feedback was given code **2.5, Monitoring outcome(s) of behavior by others without feedback**; if feedback on behavior is evaluative e.g., praise, also code **10.4, Social reward**.*	Inform the person of how much weight they have lost following the implementation of a new exercise regimen.

3. Social support

| 3.1 | *Social support (unspecified)* | Advise on, arrange or provide social support (e.g., from friends, relatives, colleagues, buddies, or staff) or non-contingent praise or reward for performance of the behavior. It includes encouragement and counselling, but only when it is directed at the **behavior**.
*Note: attending a group class and/or mention of "follow-up" does not necessarily apply this BCT, support must be explicitly mentioned; if practical, code **3.2, Social support (practical)**; if emotional, code **3.3, Social support (emotional)** (includes **<u>Motivational interviewing</u>** and **<u>Cognitive Behavioral Therapy</u>**).* | Advise the person to call a "buddy" when they experience an urge to smoke.
Arrange for a housemate to encourage continuation with the behavior change program.
Give information about a self-help group that offers support for the behavior. |

(continues)

No.	Label	Definition	Examples
3.2	***Social support (practical)***	Advise on, arrange, or provide **practical** help *(e.g., from friends, relatives, colleagues, "buddies" or staff)* for performance of the behavior. *Note: if emotional, code **3.3, Social support (emotional)**; if general or unspecified, code **3.1, Social support (unspecified)** If only restructuring the physical environment or adding objects to the environment, code **12.1, Restructuring the physical environment** or **12.5, Adding objects to the environment;** attending a group or class and/or mention of "follow-up" does not necessarily apply this BCT, support must be explicitly mentioned.*	Ask the partner of the patient to put their tablet on the breakfast tray so that the patient remembers to take it.
3.3	***Social support (emotional)***	Advise on, arrange, or provide **emotional** social support *(e.g., from friends, relatives, colleagues, "buddies" or staff)* for performance of the behavior. *Note: if practical, code **3.2, Social support (practical)**; if unspecified, code **3.1, Social support (unspecified)**.*	Ask the patient to take a partner or friend with them to their colonoscopy appointment.
4. Shaping knowledge			
4.1	***Instruction on how to perform a behavior***	Advise or agree on how to perform the behavior (includes **Skills training**) *Note: when the person attends classes such as exercise or cookery, code **4.1, Instruction on how to perform the behavior, 8.1, Behavioral practice/rehearsal** <u>and</u> **6.1, Demonstration of the behavior**.*	Advise the person how to put a condom on a model of a penis correctly.
4.2	***Information about antecedents***	Provide information about antecedents *(e.g., social and environmental situations and events, emotions, cognitions)* that reliably predict performance of the behavior.	Advise to keep a record of snacking and of situations or events occurring prior to snacking.

| 4.3 | **Re-attribution** | Elicit perceived causes of behavior and suggest alternative explanations (*e.g., external or internal and stable or unstable*). | If the person attributes their overeating to the frequent presence of delicious food, suggest that the "real" cause may be the person's inattention to bodily signals of hunger and satiety. |
| 4.4 | **Behavioral experiments** | Advise on how to identify and test hypotheses about the behavior, its causes and consequences, by collecting and interpreting data. | Ask a family physician to give evidence-based advice rather than prescribe antibiotics and to note whether the patients are grateful or annoyed. |

5. Natural consequences

| 5.1 | **Information about health consequences** | Provide information (e.g., written, verbal, visual) about health consequences of performing the behavior.
   Note: consequences can be for any target, not just the recipient(s) of the intervention; emphasizing importance of consequences is not sufficient; if information about emotional consequences, code **5.6, Information about emotional consequences**; *if about social, environmental or unspecified consequences code* **5.3, Information about social and environmental consequences**. | Explain that not finishing a course of antibiotics can increase susceptibility to future infection.
   Present the likelihood of contracting a sexually transmitted infection following unprotected sexual behavior. |
| 5.2 | **Salience of consequences** | Use methods specifically designed to **emphasize** the consequences of performing the behavior with the aim of making them more memorable (goes beyond informing about consequences).
   Note: if information about consequences, also code **5.1, Information about health consequences, 5.6, Information about emotional consequences** or **5.3, Information about social and environmental consequences.** | Produce cigarette packets showing pictures of health consequences (e.g., diseased lungs), to highlight the dangers of continuing to smoke. |

(continues)

No.	Label	Definition	Examples
5.3	*Information about social and environmental consequences*	Provide information (e.g., written, verbal, visual) about social and environmental consequences of performing the behavior. 　*Note: consequences can be for any target, not just the recipient(s) of the intervention; if information about health or consequences, code **5.1, Information about health consequences**; if about emotional consequences, code **5.6, Information about emotional consequences**; if unspecified, code **5.3, Information about social and environmental consequences**.*	Tell family physician about financial remuneration for conducting health screening. 　Inform a smoker that the majority of people disapprove of smoking in public places.
5.4	*Monitoring of emotional consequences*	Prompt assessment of **feelings** after attempts at performing the behavior.	Agree that the person will record how they feel after taking their daily walk.
5.5	*Anticipated regret*	Induce or raise awareness of expectations of future regret about performance of the unwanted behavior. 　*Note: not including **5.6, Information about emotional consequences**. if suggests adoption of a perspective or new perspective in order to change cognitions also code **13.2, Framing/reframing**.*	Ask the person to assess the degree of regret they will feel if they do not quit smoking.
5.6	*Information about emotional consequences*	Provide information (e.g., written, verbal, visual) about emotional consequences of performing the behavior. 　*Note: consequences can be related to emotional health disorders (e.g., depression, anxiety) and/or states of mind (e.g., low mood, stress); not including **5.5, Anticipated regret**; consequences can be for any target, not just the recipient(s) of the intervention; if information about health consequences code **5.1, Information about health consequences**; if about social, environmental or unspecified code **5.3, Information about social and environmental consequences**.*	Explain that quitting smoking increases happiness and life satisfaction.

6. Comparison of behavior

6.1	**Demonstration of the behavior**	Provide an observable sample of the performance of the behavior, directly in person or indirectly e.g., via film, pictures, for the person to aspire to or imitate (includes **Modeling**). *Note:* if advised to practice, *also* code, **8.1, Behavioral practice and rehearsal**; *If provided with instructions on how to perform,* *also* code **4.1, Instruction on how to perform the behavior**.	Demonstrate to nurses how to raise the issue of excessive drinking with patients via a role-play exercise.
6.2	**Social comparison**	Draw attention to others' performance to allow comparison with the person's own performance *Note: being in a group setting does not necessarily mean that social comparison is actually taking place.*	Show the doctor the proportion of patients who were prescribed antibiotics for a common cold by other doctors and compare with their own data.
6.3	**Information about others' approval**	Provide information about what other people think about the behavior. The information clarifies whether others will like, approve or disapprove of what the person is doing or will do.	Tell the staff at the hospital ward that staff at all other wards approve of washing their hands according to the guidelines.

7. Associations

| 7.1 | **Prompts/cues** | Introduce or define environmental or social stimulus with the purpose of prompting or cueing the behavior. The prompt or cue would normally occur at the time or place of performance *Note: when a stimulus is linked to a specific action in an if-then plan including one or more of frequency, duration or intensity also code **1.4, Action planning**.* | Put a sticker on the bathroom mirror to remind people to brush their teeth. |

(continues)

No.	Label	Definition	Examples
7.2	*Cue signaling reward*	Identify an environmental stimulus that reliably predicts that reward will follow. the behavior (includes **Discriminative cue**).	Advise that a fee will be paid to dentists for a particular dental treatment of 6- to 8-year-old, but not older, children to encourage delivery of that treatment (the 6- to 8-year-old children are the environmental stimulus).
7.3	*Reduce prompts/cues*	Withdraw gradually prompts to perform the behavior (includes **"Fading"**).	Reduce gradually the number of reminders used to take medication.
7.4	*Remove access to the reward*	Advise or arrange for the person to be separated from situations in which unwanted behavior can be rewarded in order to reduce the behavior (includes **"Time out"**).	Arrange for cupboard containing high calorie snacks to be locked for a specified period to reduce the consumption of sugary foods in between meals.
7.5	*Remove aversive stimulus*	Advise or arrange for the removal of an aversive stimulus to facilitate behavior change (includes **Escape learning**).	Arrange for a gym buddy to stop nagging the person to do more exercise in order to increase the desired exercise behavior.
7.6	*Satiation*	Advise or arrange repeated exposure to a stimulus that reduces or extinguishes a drive for the unwanted behavior.	Arrange for the person to eat large quantities of chocolate, in order to reduce the person's appetite for sweet foods.
7.7	*Exposure*	Provide systematic confrontation with a feared stimulus to reduce the response to a later encounter.	Agree a schedule by which the person who is frightened of surgery will visit the hospital where they are scheduled to have surgery.
7.8	*Associative learning*	Present a neutral stimulus jointly with a stimulus that already elicits the behavior repeatedly until the neutral stimulus elicits that behavior (includes **Classical/Pavlovian Conditioning**).	Repeatedly present fatty foods with a disliked sauce to discourage the consumption of fatty foods.

Note: when a BCT involves reward or punishment, code one or more of: **10.2, Material reward (behavior); 10.3, Non-specific reward; 10.4, Social reward, 10.9, Self-reward; 10.10, Reward (outcome)**.

8. Repetition and substitution

8.1	**Behavioral practice/ rehearsal**	Prompt practice or rehearsal of the performance of the behavior one or more times in a context or at a time when the performance may not be necessary, in order to increase habit and skill. *Note: if aiming to associate performance with the context, also code* **8.3, Habit formation**.	Prompt asthma patients to practice measuring their peak flow in the nurse's consulting room.
8.2	**Behavior substitution**	Prompt substitution of the unwanted behavior with a wanted or neutral behavior. *Note: if this occurs regularly, also code* **8.4, Habit reversal**.	Suggest that the person goes for a walk rather than watch television.
8.3	**Habit formation**	Prompt rehearsal and repetition of the behavior in the same context repeatedly so that the context elicits the behavior. *Note: also code* **8.1, Behavioral practice/rehearsal**.	Prompt patients to take their statin tablet before brushing their teeth every evening.
8.4	**Habit reversal**	Prompt rehearsal and repetition of an alternative behavior to **replace** an unwanted habitual behavior. *Note: also code* **8.2, Behavior substitution**.	Ask the person to walk up stairs at work where they previously always took the elevator.
8.5	**Overcorrection**	Ask to repeat the wanted behavior in an exaggerated way following an unwanted behavior.	Ask to eat only fruit and vegetables the day after a poor diet.
8.6	**Generalisation of a target behavior**	Advise to perform the wanted behavior, which is already performed in a particular situation, in another situation.	Advise to repeat toning exercises learned in the gym when at home.

(continues)

No.	Label	Definition	Examples
8.7	*Graded tasks*	Set easy-to-perform tasks, making them increasingly difficult, but achievable, until behavior is performed.	Ask the person to walk for 100 yards a day for the first week, then half a mile a day after they have successfully achieved 100 yards, then 2 miles a day after they have successfully achieved 1 mile.

9. Comparison of outcomes

No.	Label	Definition	Examples
9.1	*Credible source*	Present verbal or visual communication from a credible source **in favor of or against the behavior**. *Note: code this BCT if source generally agreed on as credible, e.g., health professionals, celebrities or words used to indicate expertise or leader in field and if the communication has the aim of persuading; if information about health consequences, also code* **5.1, Information about health consequences**, *if about emotional consequences, also code* **5.6, Information about emotional consequences**; *if about social, environmental or unspecified consequences also code* **5.3, Information about social and environmental consequences**.	Present a speech given by a high-status professional to emphasize the importance of not exposing patients to unnecessary radiation by ordering x-rays for back pain.
9.2	*Pros and cons*	Advise the person to identify and compare reasons for wanting (pros) and not wanting to (cons) change the behavior (includes **Decisional balance**).	Advise the person to list and compare the advantages and disadvantages of prescribing antibiotics for upper respiratory tract infections.

*Note: if providing information about health consequences, <u>also</u> code **5.1, Information about health consequences**; if providing information about emotional consequences, <u>also</u> code **5.6, Information about emotional consequences**; if providing information about social, environmental or unspecified consequences <u>also</u> code **5.3, Information about social and environmental consequences***

| 9.3 | ***Comparative imagining of future outcomes*** | Prompt or advise the imagining and comparing of future outcomes of changed versus unchanged behavior. | Prompt the person to imagine and compare likely or possible outcomes following attending versus not attending a screening appointment. |

10. Reward and threat

| 10.1 | ***Material incentive (behavior)*** | Inform that money, vouchers or other valued objects **will be** delivered if and only if there has been effort and/or progress in performing the behavior (includes **Positive reinforcement**). *Note: if incentive is social, code* **10.5, Social incentive** *if unspecified code* **10.6, Non-specific incentive,** *and <u>not</u>* **10.1, Material incentive (behavior)**; *if incentive is for* **outcome,** *code* **10.8, Incentive (outcome).** *If reward is delivered also code one of:* **10.2, Material reward (behavior); 10.3, Non-specific reward; 10.4, Social reward, 10.9, Self-reward; 10.10, Reward (outcome)**. | Inform that a financial payment will be made each month in pregnancy that the woman has not smoked. |

(continues)

No.	Label	Definition	Examples
10.2	*Material reward (behavior)*	Arrange for the delivery of money, vouchers or other valued objects if and only if there **has been** effort and/or progress in performing the behavior (includes **Positive reinforcement**). *Note: If reward is social, code* **10.4, Social reward**, *if unspecified code* **10.3, Non-specific reward**, *and not* **10.1, Material reward (behavior)**; *if reward is for* **outcome**, *code* **10.10, Reward (outcome)**. *If informed of reward in advance of rewarded behavior, also code one of:* **10.1, Material incentive (behavior); 10.5, Social incentive; 10.6, Non-specific incentive; 10.7, Self-incentive; 10.8, Incentive (outcome)**.	Arrange for the person to receive money that would have been spent on cigarettes if and only if the smoker has not smoked for 1 month.
10.3	*Non-specific reward*	Arrange delivery of a reward if and only if there **has been** effort and/or progress in performing the behavior (includes **Positive reinforcement**). *Note: if reward is material, code* **10.2, Material reward (behavior)**, *if social, code* **10.4, Social reward**, *and not* **10.3, Non-specific reward**; *if reward is for* **outcome** *code* **10.10, Reward (outcome)**. *If informed of reward in advance of rewarded behavior, also code one of:* **10.1, Material incentive (behavior); 10.5, Social incentive; 10.6, Non-specific incentive; 10.7, Self-incentive; 10.8, Incentive (outcome)**	Identify something (e.g., an activity such as a visit to the cinema) that the person values and arrange for this to be delivered if and only if they attend for health screening.
10.4	*Social reward*	Arrange verbal or non-verbal reward if and only if there **has been** effort and/or progress in performing the behavior (includes Positive **reinforcement**).	Congratulate the person for each day they eat a reduced-fat diet.

Note: if reward is material, code
10.2, Material reward (behavior), *if unspecified code* **10.3, Non-specific reward,** *and* <u>not</u> **10.4, Social reward**; *if reward is for* **outcome** *code* **10.10, Reward (outcome).** *If informed of reward in advance of rewarded behavior, also code one of:* **10.1, Material incentive (behavior); 10.5, Social incentive; 10.6, Non-specific incentive; 10.7, Self-incentive; 10.8, Incentive (outcome).**

| 10.5 | **Social incentive** | Inform that a verbal or non-verbal reward **will be** delivered if and only if there has been effort and/or progress in performing the behavior (includes "Positive **reinforcement**").
Note: if incentive is material, code **10.1, Material incentive (behavior),** *if unspecified code* **10.6, Non-specific incentive,** *and* <u>not</u> **10.5, Social incentive**; *if incentive is for* **outcome** *code* **10.8, Incentive (outcome).** *If reward is delivered also code one of:* **10.2, Material reward (behavior); 10.3, Non-specific reward; 10.4, Social reward, 10.9, Self-reward; 10.10, Reward (outcome).** | Inform that they will be congratulated for each day they eat a reduced-fat diet. |
| 10.6 | **Non-specific incentive** | Inform that a reward **will be** delivered if and only if there has been effort and/or progress in performing the behavior (includes Positive **reinforcement**).
Note: if incentive is material, code **10.1, Material incentive (behavior),** *if social, code* **10.5, Social incentive** *and* <u>not</u> **10.6, Non-specific incentive**; *if incentive is for* **outcome** *code* **10.8, Incentive (outcome).** *If reward is delivered also code one of:* **10.2, Material reward (behavior); 10.3, Non-specific reward; 10.4, Social reward, 10.9, Self-reward; 10.10, Reward (outcome).** | Identify an activity that the person values and inform them that this will happen if and only if they attend for health screening. |

(continues)

No.	Label	Definition	Examples
10.7	*Self-incentive*	Plan to reward self in future if and only if there has been effort and/or progress in performing the behavior. *Note: if self-reward is material, also code **10.1, Material incentive (behavior)**, if social, also code **10.5, Social incentive**, if unspecified, also code **10.6, Non-specific incentive**; if incentive is for **outcome** code **10.8, Incentive (outcome)**. If reward is delivered also code one of: **10.2, Material reward (behavior); 10.3, Non-specific reward; 10.4, Social reward, 10.9, Self-reward; 10.10, Reward (outcome)**.*	Encourage to provide self with material (e.g., new clothes) or other valued objects if and only if they have adhered to a healthy diet.
10.8	*Incentive (outcome)*	Inform that a reward **will be** delivered if and only if there has been effort and/or progress in achieving the behavioral **outcome** (*includes **Positive reinforcement**). *Note: this includes social, material, self- and non-specific incentives for outcome; if incentive is for the **behavior** code **10.5, Social incentive, 10.1, Material incentive (behavior), 10.6, Non-specific incentive** or **10.7, Self-incentive** and not **10.8, Incentive (outcome)**. If reward is delivered also code one of: **10.2, Material reward (behavior); 10.3, Non-specific reward; 10.4, Social reward, 10.9, Self-reward; 10.10, Reward (outcome)**.*	Inform the person that they will receive money if and only if a certain amount of weight is lost.
10.9	*Self-reward*	Prompt self-praise or self-reward if and only if there **has been** effort and/or progress in performing the behavior.	Encourage to reward self with material (e.g., new clothes) or other valued objects if and only if they have adhered to a healthy diet.

*Note: if self-reward is material, <u>also</u> code **10.2, Material reward (behavior)**, if social, <u>also</u> code **10.4, Social reward**, if unspecified, <u>also</u> code **10.3, Non-specific reward**; if reward is for **outcome** code **10.10, Reward (outcome)**. If informed of reward in advance of rewarded behavior, also code one of: **10.1, Material incentive (behavior); 10.5, Social incentive; 10.6, Non-specific incentive; 10.7, Self-incentive; 10.8, Incentive (outcome)**.*

10.10	*Reward (outcome)*	Arrange for the delivery of a reward if and only if there **has been** effort and/or progress in achieving the behavioral **outcome** (includes Positive **reinforcement**). *Note: this includes social, material, self- and non-specific rewards for outcome; if reward is for the **behavior** code **10.4, Social reward, 10.2, Material reward (behavior), 10.3, Non-specific reward** or **10.9, Self-reward** and <u>not</u> **10.10, Reward (outcome)**. If informed of reward in advance of rewarded behavior, also code one of: **10.1, Material incentive (behavior); 10.5, Social incentive; 10.6, Non-specific incentive; 10.7, Self-incentive; 10.8, Incentive (outcome)**.*	Arrange for the person to receive money if and only if a certain amount of weight is lost.
10.11	*Future punishment*	Inform that future punishment or removal of reward will be a consequence of performance of an unwanted behavior (may include fear arousal) (includes **Threat**).	Inform that continuing to consume 30 units of alcohol per day is likely to result in loss of employment if the person continues.

(continues)

No.	Label	Definition	Examples
11. Regulation			
11.1	**Pharmacological support**	Provide, or encourage the use of or adherence to, drugs to facilitate behavior change. *Note: if pharmacological support to reduce negative emotions (i.e. anxiety) then also code* **11.2, Reduce negative emotions**.	Suggest the patient asks the family physician for nicotine replacement therapy to facilitate smoking cessation.
11.2	**Reduce negative emotions b**	Advise on ways of reducing negative emotions to facilitate performance of the behavior (includes **Stress Management**). *Note: if includes analysing the behavioral problem, also code* **1.2, Problem solving**.	Advise on the use of stress management skills, (e.g., to reduce anxiety) about joining Alcoholics Anonymous.
11.3	**Conserving mental resources**	Advise on ways of minimizing demands on mental resources to facilitate behavior change.	Advise to carry food calorie content information to reduce the burden on memory in making food choices.
11.4	**Paradoxical instructions**	Advise to engage in some form of the unwanted behavior with the aim of reducing motivation to engage in that behavior.	Advise a smoker to smoke twice as many cigarettes a day as they usually do. Tell the person to stay awake as long as possible in order to reduce insomnia.
12. Antecedents			
12.1	**Restructuring the physical environment**	Change, or advise to change the **physical** environment in order to facilitate performance of the wanted behavior or create barriers to the unwanted behavior (other than prompts/cues, rewards and punishments). *Note: this may also involve* **12.3, Avoidance/reducing exposure to cues for the behavior**; *if restructuring of the social environment code* **12.2, Restructuring the social environment**;	Advise to keep sweets and snacks in a cupboard that is inconvenient to get to. Arrange to move vending machine out of the school.

		If only adding objects to the environment, code **12.5, Adding objects to the environment**.	
12.2	*Restructuring the social environment*	Change, or advise to change the **social** environment in order to facilitate performance of the wanted behavior or create barriers to the unwanted behavior (other than prompts/cues, rewards and punishments). Note: this may also involve **12.3, Avoidance/reducing exposure to cues for the behavior**; if also restructuring of the physical environment also code **12.1, Restructuring the physical environment**.	Advise to minimize time spent with friends who drink heavily to reduce alcohol consumption.
12.3	*Avoidance/ reducing exposure to cues for the behavior*	Advise on how to avoid exposure to specific social and contextual/physical cues for the behavior, including changing daily or weekly routines. Note: this may also involve **12.1, Restructuring the physical environment** and/or **12.2, Restructuring the social environment**; if the BCT includes analysing the behavioral problem, only code **1.2, Problem solving**.	Suggest to a person who wants to quit smoking that their social life focus on activities other than pubs and bars which have been associated with smoking.
12.4	*Distraction*	Advise or arrange to use an alternative focus for attention to avoid triggers for unwanted behavior.	Suggest to a person who is trying to avoid between-meal snacking to focus on a topic they enjoy (e.g., holiday plans) instead of focusing on food.
12.5	*Adding objects to the environment*	Add objects to the environment in order to facilitate performance of the behavior.	Provide free condoms to facilitate safe sex. Provide attractive toothbrush to improve tooth brushing technique.

(continues)

No.	Label	Definition	Examples
		*Note: Provision of information (e.g., written, verbal, visual) in a booklet or leaflet is insufficient. If this is accompanied by social support, also code **3.2, Social support (practical)**; if the environment is changed beyond the addition of objects, also code **12.1, Restructuring the physical environment**.*	
12.6	*Body changes*	Alter body structure, functioning or support **directly** to facilitate behavior change.	Prompt strength training, relaxation training or provide assistive aids (e.g., a hearing aid).

13. Identity

No.	Label	Definition	Examples
13.1	*Identification of self as role model*	Inform that one's own behavior may be an example to others.	Inform the person that if they eat healthily, that may be a good example for their children.
13.2	*Framing/ reframing*	Suggest the deliberate adoption of a perspective or new perspective on behavior (e.g., its purpose) in order to change cognitions or emotions about performing the behavior (includes '**Cognitive structuring**'). *Note: If information about consequences then code **5.1, Information about health consequences, 5.6, Information about emotional consequences** or **5.3, Information about social and environmental consequences** instead of **13.2, Framing/reframing**.*	Suggest that the person might think of the tasks as reducing sedentary behavior (rather than increasing activity).
13.3	*Incompatible beliefs*	Draw attention to discrepancies between current or past behavior and self-image, in order to create discomfort (includes **Cognitive dissonance**).	Draw attention to a doctor's liberal use of blood transfusion and their self-identification as a proponent of evidence-based medical practice.

13.4	**Valued self-identity**	Advise the person to write or complete rating scales about a cherished value or personal strength as a means of affirming the person's identity as part of a behavior change strategy (includes **Self-affirmation**).	Advise the person to write about their personal strengths before they receive a message advocating the behavior change.
13.5	**Identity associated with changed behavior**	Advise the person to construct a new self-identity as someone who "used to engage with the unwanted behavior."	Ask the person to articulate their new identity as an "ex-smoker."

14. Scheduled consequences

14.1	**Behavior cost**	Arrange for withdrawal of something valued if and only if an unwanted behavior is performed (includes **Response cost**). Note if withdrawal of contingent reward code, *14.3, Remove reward*.	Subtract money from a prepaid refundable deposit when a cigarette is smoked.
14.2	**Punishment**	Arrange for aversive consequence contingent on the performance of the unwanted behavior.	Arrange for the person to wear unattractive clothes following consumption of fatty foods.
14.3	**Remove reward**	Arrange for discontinuation of contingent reward following performance of the unwanted behavior (includes **Extinction**).	Arrange for the other people in the household to ignore the person every time they eat chocolate (rather than attending to them by criticizing or persuading).
14.4	**Reward approximation**	Arrange for reward following any approximation to the target behavior, gradually rewarding only performance closer to the wanted behavior (includes **Shaping**). *Note: also code one of **59-63**.*	Arrange reward for any reduction in daily calories, gradually requiring the daily calorie count to become closer to the planned calorie intake.

(continues)

No.	Label	Definition	Examples
14.5	*Rewarding completion*	Build up behavior by arranging reward following final component of the behavior; gradually add the components of the behavior that occur earlier in the behavioral sequence (includes **Backward chaining**). *Note: also, code one of **10.2, Material reward (behavior); 10.3, Non-specific reward; 10.4, Social reward, 10.9, Self-reward; 10.10, Reward (outcome)**	Reward eating a supplied low-calorie meal; then make reward contingent on cooking and eating the meal; then make reward contingent on purchasing, cooking, and eating the meal.
14.6	*Situation-specific reward*	Arrange for reward following the behavior in one situation but not in another (includes **Discrimination training**). *Note: also code one of **10.2, Material reward (behavior); 10.3, Non-specific reward; 10.4, Social reward, 10.9, Self-reward; 10.10, Reward (outcome)**	Arrange reward for eating at mealtimes but not between meals.
14.7	*Reward incompatible behavior*	Arrange reward for responding in a manner that is incompatible with a previous response to that situation (includes **Counter-conditioning**). *Note: also code one of **10.2, Material reward (behavior); 10.3, Non-specific reward; 10.4, Social reward, 10.9, Self-reward; 10.10, Reward (outcome)**.	Arrange reward for ordering a soft drink at the bar rather than an alcoholic beverage.
14.8	*Reward alternative behavior*	Arrange reward for performance of an alternative to the unwanted behavior (includes **Differential reinforcement**). *Note: also code one of **10.2, Material reward (behavior); 10.3, Non-specific reward; 10.4, Social reward, 10.9, Self-reward; 10.10, Reward (outcome)**; consider also coding **1.2, Problem solving**.	Reward for consumption of low fat foods but not consumption of high fat foods.

14.9	**Reduce reward frequency**	Arrange for rewards to be made contingent on increasing duration or frequency of the behavior (includes **Thinning**). *Note: also code one of **10.2, Material reward (behavior); 10.3, Non-specific reward; 10.4, Social reward, 10.9, Self-reward; 10.10, Reward (outcome)**.*	Arrange reward for each day without smoking, then each week, then each month, then every 2 months and so on.
14.10	**Remove punishment**	Arrange for removal of an unpleasant consequence contingent on performance of the wanted behavior (includes **Negative reinforcement)**.	Arrange for someone else to do housecleaning only if the person has adhered to the medication regimen for a week.

15. Self-belief

15.1	**Verbal persuasion about capability**	Tell the person that they can successfully perform the wanted behavior, arguing against self-doubts and asserting that they can and will succeed.	Tell the person that they can successfully increase their physical activity, despite their recent heart attack.
15.2	**Mental rehearsal of successful performance**	Advise to practice imagining performing the behavior successfully in relevant contexts.	Advise to imagine eating and enjoying a salad in a work canteen.
15.3	**Focus on past success**	Advise to think about or list previous successes in performing the behavior (or parts of it).	Advise to describe or list the occasions on which the person had ordered a non-alcoholic drink in a bar.
15.4	**Self-talk**	Prompt positive self-talk (aloud or silently) before and during the behavior.	Prompt the person to tell themselves that a walk will be energizing.

16. Covert learning

16.1	**Imaginary punishment**	Advise to imagine performing the **unwanted** behavior in a real-life situation followed by imagining an unpleasant consequence (includes **Covert sensitization**).	Advise to imagine overeating and then vomiting.

(continues)

16.2	*Imaginary reward*	Advise to imagine performing the **wanted** behavior in a real-life situation followed by imagining a pleasant consequence (includes **Covert conditioning**).	Advise the health professional to imagine giving dietary advice followed by the patient losing weight and no longer being diabetic.
16.3	*Vicarious consequences*	Prompt observation of the consequences (including rewards and punishments) for others when they perform the behavior *Note: if observation of health consequences, also code **5.1, Information about health consequences**; if of emotional consequences, <u>also</u> code **5.6, Information about emotional consequences**, if social, environmental or unspecified consequences, <u>also</u> code **5.3, Information about social and environmental consequences**.*	Draw attention to the positive comments other staff get when they disinfect their hands regularly.

Reproduced from Michie, Annals of Behavioral Medicine. The behavior change technique taxonomy (v1) of 93 hierarchically clustered techniques: building an international consensus for the reporting of behavior change techniques. 2013 Aug;46(1):81-95. doi: 10.1007/s12160-013-9486-6.

CHAPTER 4

Understanding Variation, Tools, and Data Sources for CQI in Health Care

William A. Sollecito and David Hardison

Information is random and miscellaneous, but knowledge is orderly and cumulative.

—**Daniel Boorstin**

Continuous quality improvement (CQI) requires knowledge about the behavior of systems and processes, which is most often obtained from data and other sources of information collected for that specific purpose and through the application of tools and techniques that have proven to be effective throughout the evolution of CQI as described earlier in this text. The use of data and tools is part of the concept of statistical thinking, which is a key component of both the philosophy and processes of CQI. Central to decisions about innovations and especially CQI in health care is the need to improve our knowledge about health care process performance through an understanding of the context in which processes behave, asking the right questions, and then the collecting and analyzing appropriate data.

The goal is not simply to analyze data, but to gain knowledge by utilizing data to understand processes, sources of variation, and the impact of improvements. Most important in CQI applications is the requirement to understand variability and the predictability of health care processes. As described in Chapters 1 and 2, CQI requires a systems approach that analyzes assumptions and focuses on customers/patients, processes, and interdependencies based on knowledge. This approach is most efficiently accomplished using stepwise, yet cyclical, procedures that span planning, implementation, and an assessment of the impact of the decisions made in identifying and applying changes—including how to determine when a change is needed and whether it leads to an improvement (Langley et al., 2009). Although many different methods can be applied to carry out these steps, CQI efforts in the past have spawned methods that have proven to be robust and efficient when focused on listening to the "voice of the process" underpinned with an understanding of variation (Wheeler & Chambers, 2010). These methods include a continuous assessment of process performance, including an understanding of sources of variation, followed by decision making based on the application of knowledge about systems and measurements. Over the years, a set of tools have been developed to carry out these steps in the most efficient manner; as with CQI itself, these tools have undergone a continuous improvement process that enhances our learning about how to apply them, and when to introduce new tools. Especially in health care, which itself has undergone an evolutionary process rooted in new knowledge and the greater use of technology, new tools and data sources have been developed to ensure that the "Quadruple Aim" of health care—improving the experience of care, improving the health of populations, and reducing the per capita costs of health care while improving the work life of clinicians and health care staff (discussed in Chapter 2)—has been met (Bodenheimer & Sinsky, 2014; Sikka, Morath, & Leape, 2015). At the heart of these procedures is the use of evidence-based approaches that rely on health information technology that provides high-quality data to ensure that correct decisions are made in the efficient application of the "data-to-decision cycle" (McLaughlin & Kibbe, 2013). The greater use of technology to collect and analyze health care data presents greater opportunities for both converting data into information or knowledge and applying powerful methodologies for implementing improvement, but it also presents challenges to ensure the most appropriate application of tools and techniques to carry out CQI initiatives.

Many valuable texts are available that explain the mechanics of CQI analysis methods and tools (e.g., Balestracci, 2009; Bialek, Duffy, & Moran, 2009; Carey & Lloyd, 2001; Langley et al., 2009; Lighter & Fair, 2004; Lloyd, 2019; Streibel, Sholtes, & Joiner, 2003). This chapter will not duplicate the information provided in those texts. Rather, the purpose of this chapter is to assist in understanding

the role of variation in quality improvement, why measurement and statistical thinking are vital to quality improvement efforts, and to illustrate a few fundamental CQI tools that are particularly useful in health care to enhance our learning about process changes and facilitate improvement in health care processes. A minimum, but sufficient amount of detail, with relevant examples, will be provided to enhance understanding and enable the reader to develop and apply these tools. Finally, the chapter presents a brief overview of the strengths and weaknesses of various forms of health information data sources that are currently being used to carry out CQI initiatives.

▶ Health Care Systems and Processes

The early work of Donabedian is foundational in understanding health care systems and processes (Donabedian, 1980). He described the process of care as a system involving three components: structure, process and outcomes that comprise a set of activities requiring interaction between patients and providers. More recently, there has been greater attention paid to patient centered care and the Donabedian model has been expanded to include greater emphasis on the patient experience (Spath & Kelly, 2017). This is reflected to some degree in the greater emphasis on patient satisfaction data and its role in measuring quality of care; this source of data and information has strengths and weaknesses in CQI, which will be discussed in greater detail later in this chapter. The main emphasis of this section is the central role of concepts such as the Donabedian Model in understanding health care processes and outcomes.

Process Capability

To understand the expected output of a process relative to a particular outcome or quality characteristic, or process capability, the process must be stable, and, hence, predictable within limits. Benefits of a stable process (Deming, 1986) include:

- The process has an identity (capability); it is predictable. Therefore, there is a rational basis for planning.
- Costs and quality are predictable.
- Productivity is at a maximum and costs at a minimum under the present system.
- The effect of changes in the process can be assessed with greater speed and reliability. In an unstable process, it is difficult to separate changes to the process from special causes of variation. Therefore, it is more difficult to know when a change results in improvement.

Interpreting Process Requirements and Performance

Variation exists in every process and always will. It is the manager's job to understand variation and continuously improve the processes so that they manage to meet the needs of the customers who depend upon their processes. The customer of each process has requirements which specify the level of performance that is needed. A provider working in the emergency department (ED) would require more rapid turnaround time (TAT) of laboratory results than a provider working in a primary care office. A 30-minute TAT in the ED may be unacceptable, whereas a 24-hour TAT may be acceptable for a primary care office. There may also be specific requirements for analyzing the laboratory specimen. Technology used for one type of test may require 30 minutes to be processed, while a different type of test can be completed within seconds. Customer and technical requirements must both be taken into account in order to interpret whether the performance of the process is acceptable or whether the process needs to be improved. That said, every process can be improved in the spirit of CQI.

Process requirements may be thought of as the criteria from which the effectiveness of a process may be evaluated from the process customer's perspective. They function as both inputs to designing a process and outputs from executing a process. It is essential to first identify the customers of a process. Chapter 7 provides an in-depth discussion of customers of health care organizations (i.e., the role of patients in CQI). Brief definitions, using a systems perspective, are provided here. A customer is defined as anyone who has expectations regarding a process operation or outputs. In health care delivery organizations, the primary customer is the patient, while the community may be the primary customer for a public health agency. Internal customers are those within the organizations and are sometimes thought of as those departments or coworkers "downstream" from the process. In other words, who the customers of a process are depends on the outputs of a process. For example, the recovery room or postanesthesia care unit may be thought of as the customer of the operating room. Patient care units may be thought of as customers of diagnostic departments (e.g., laboratory, radiology). Payers may be considered as external customers—those outside the provider organization. A stakeholder is anyone with an interest in or affected by the work you do. Regulatory bodies such as The Joint Commission (TJC), formerly known as the Joint Commission on Accreditation of Healthcare Organizations, or the National Commission on Quality Assurance (NCQA) would be considered stakeholders for hospitals and health insurance companies, respectively. Professional societies that define practice standards may also be thought of as stakeholders. The market refers to the environment in which you operate and do business and may include socioeconomic, demographic, geographic, and competitive considerations.

Once customers, stakeholders, and markets have been identified, it is essential to identify and understand what they require of your services. For example, patients may require access and competent, courteous providers; payers may require a certain level of clinical results delivered in a cost-effective manner; regulatory bodies require compliance; and markets may require a culturally diverse approach to delivering services.

These requirements are vital to determining what services are needed and how the processes comprising the services are designed and improved. These requirements also provide the basis for selecting variables or attributes that will measure the process performance from the perspective of the customer.

TABLE 4.1 illustrates how one health-services organization operationalizes the links between customer requirements, process design, measurement, and goals.

TABLE 4.2 illustrates the core processes for each phase of the continuum of inpatient care. The patients' interface with this organization follows the following path:

Admission → Assessment → Care Delivery/ Treatment → Discharge

The core process(es) for each phase of care are shown in the first column. The second column lists the key requirements for the process, derived from a variety of methods targeted toward understanding requirements of patients, internal customers, stakeholders, and the market in which the organization operates. The third column lists the attributes or variables that the organization measures to understand the degree to which its processes are meeting stakeholder requirements.

It is management's job to ensure that the process requirements (also referred to as the Voice of the Customer) and the process performance (also referred to as the Voice of the Process) are aligned (Carey & Lloyd, 2001; Wheeler, 2000; Wheeler & Chambers, 2010). If the two are not in alignment, then the process must be improved. The analysis of process performance must be based upon knowledge of the sources of variation in the process (i.e., common and special causes). This process analysis

TABLE 4.1 Links Between Customer Requirements, Process Design, and Measurement

Requirements	Key Processes	Measures	Goals
Regulatory–legal	■ Corporate responsibility process	■ Number of government investigations	■ 0
	■ Contract review	■ Turnaround time	■ 24–48 hours
	■ Licensure	■ Licensure	■ Licensure
Accreditation	■ TJC survey	■ Scores	■ 100%
Risk management	■ Public safety	■ Infection rates	■ 0
		■ Dangerous abbreviations	■ 0
		■ Restraints	■ 0
		■ Patient falls	■ 0
Community health	■ Charity care	■ Cost of charity care	■ 25% prior year's operating margin
	■ Healthy communities programs	■ Health status in selected populations for individual projects	■ Project specific

TABLE 4.2 Links Between Process Stages, Requirements, and Measures

Process	Key Requirements	Key Measures
Admit Admitting–registration	Timeliness	▪ Time to admit patients to the setting of care ▪ Timeliness in admitting–registration rate on patient satisfaction survey questions
Assess Patient assessment	Timeliness	▪ Percentage of histories and physicals charted within 24 hours and/or prior to surgery ▪ Pain assessed at appropriate intervals per hospital policy
Clinical laboratory and radiology services	Accuracy and timeliness	▪ Quality control results–repeat rates ▪ Turnaround time ▪ Response rate on medical staff satisfaction survey
Care delivery–treatment Provision of clinical care	Nurse responsiveness, pain management, successful clinical outcomes	▪ Response rate on patient satisfaction and medical staff survey questions ▪ Wait time for pain medications ▪ Percentage of CHF patients received medication instruction–weighing ▪ Percentage of ischemic heart patients discharged on proven therapies ▪ Unplanned readmissions–return to ER or operating room mortality
Pharmacy–medication use	Accuracy	▪ Use of dangerous abbreviations in medication orders ▪ Medication error rate of adverse drug events resulting from medication errors
Surgical services–anesthesia	Professional skill, competences, communication	▪ Clear documentation of informed surgical and anesthesia consent ▪ Peri-operative mortality ▪ Surgical site infection rates
Discharge Case management	Appropriate utilization	▪ Average length of stay (ALOS) ▪ Payment denials ▪ Unplanned re-admits
Discharge from setting of care	Assistance and clear directions	▪ Discharge instructions documented and provided to patient ▪ Response rate on patient satisfaction survey

which will be described in detail later in this chapter, is accomplished by collecting data on process outcomes, plotting that data over time, constructing process behavior (also known as control) charts, and interpreting them based upon an understanding of variation. This is essentially converting those data into information and knowledge (Ross, 2014). Other considerations, to be discussed later in this chapter, include choosing the optimal sources of data with consideration of data quality and choosing appropriate tools and techniques that are useful for carrying out these analyses.

Each of these methods has a common approach to be successful in analyzing process performance; that is the need for careful measurement and an understanding of sources of variation, which will be covered in the next sections.

▶ Gaining Knowledge Through Measurement

In order to convert data into knowledge and make appropriate decisions about process improvements, critical and statistical thinking is required. This sounds very simple, but in our modern age of high-speed computing, it is all too easy to apply statistical methods and focus on results without the necessary step of thinking critically and understanding what our data tell us about the system we are trying to improve. This point was emphasized in 1996 by Dr. Donald Berwick, among others, when he noted that "measurement is only a handmaiden to improvement, but improvement cannot act without it. We speak here not of measurement for the purpose of judgment (for deciding whether or not to buy, accept, or reject or who to blame) but for the purpose of learning" (Berwick, 1996, p. 621). Not only is this view consistent with the guidelines for improvement spelled out in the earliest applications of CQI—for example, by W. Edwards Deming in his well-known 14 points (1986)—this view is also well understood and espoused in recent statistical literature (Balestracci, 2009; Langley et al., 2009). With this cautionary note in mind, we will address the important concept of understanding process variation.

The Critical Role of Understanding Variation

It has long been established that a starting point for any quality improvement effort is understanding variation (Deming, 1986, 1993; Nolan & Provost, 1990; Nolan, Perla, & Provost, 2016; Wheeler, 2000; Wheeler & Chambers, 2010). It was Shewhart's idea (1931) that statistically controlled variation of processes (also called statistical process control) is the foundation of all empirical CQI activities. In fact, listening to the voice of the process with knowledge of variation will lead to the appropriate actions to take for improvement and is fundamental to CQI (Deming, 1986, 1993; Nolan, Perla, & Provost, 2016; Nolan & Provost, 1990; Wheeler, 2000; Wheeler & Chambers, 2010).

One of the key elements of the system of profound knowledge proposed by Deming (1993) is knowledge about variation and how it interacts with other elements of knowledge to lead to a transformation based on CQI. As quality improvement has evolved over the years from business applications to health care, the concepts related to understanding variation have also been applied specifically to health care with many examples and how the action required for improvement is dependent on this understanding (Carey & Lloyd, 2001; McLaughlin & Kaluzny, 2006; Nelson, Splaine, Batalden, & Plume, 1998).

This section introduces the general concept of variation, discusses variation in relation to processes, and begins to describe why measurement and appropriate analysis are vital to guiding actions for improvement. Its emphasis is on health care applications, with numerous examples presented.

Variation: What Is It and Why Study It?

Variation is everywhere—a diabetic's glucose level, the waiting time in a physician's office, blood pressure, the balance of trade, the behavior of people, the incidence of cancer, and the price of eggs all vary over time. In order to understand variation, two definitions are important. *Common causes of variation* are the causes and conditions inherently present that impact every outcome of a process. *Special causes of variation* are not a part of the process all of the time and do not affect every outcome but arise because of specific circumstances (Deming, 1986). For the sake of completeness and clarity, it should also be noted that some authors refer to these two causes in process analysis as *noise* and *signals*, respectively (Wheeler, 2000). The appropriate action for improvement depends upon the correct interpretation of patterns in the variation observed. Is the variation random and attributable to the materials, methods, environment, people, etc. that are common to every outcome, or was there a signal of a trend or another discernable pattern in the data indicating that a special cause is present in the process? As will be described shortly in our discussion of process behavior charts, variation in a process over time can be measured, analyzed, and displayed in a manner that helps to distinguish its source (i.e., special vs. common cause). The importance of understanding this classification of causes directly relates to predictability of the outcomes of a process, and where special causes of variation are detected, outcomes are not predictable with any reasonable degree of belief (Deming, 1986; Langley et al., 2009; Shewhart, 1931; Wheeler, 2000; Wheeler & Chambers, 2010). This is of critical importance in health care.

Berwick (1991) describes the role of variation and predictability in processes carried out daily in health care organizations:

Those who prepare [patients] for [cardiac] surgery rely . . . upon the predictability of the systems . . . that affect [their] care and outcome. The surgeon knows that coagulation test reports will be returned within 20 and 25 minutes of their being sent; the anesthesiologist knows that blood gas values will be back in 4 to 8 minutes; the pump technician knows that tubing connections will tolerate pressures within a certain range. Each makes plans in accordance with those predictions, and each bases those predictions on prior experience, which is judged to be informative. Sudden, unpredicted variation is experienced as trouble. (p. 1217)

From the national, organizational, or individual perspective, one cannot escape the role and influence of variation on health care quality (Gold, 2004). Understanding causes of variation and using that knowledge to determine when and how to make process improvements involves the use of tools and procedures designed for these purposes. A key point to remember is that these tools can be used together in a complementary cyclical manner to identify the need for process improvement, decide on what improvements are needed, measure the impact of those changes and assess what further improvements are needed. For example, the use of process behavior charts may lead to the identification of special causes of variation, which will require process improvement; the determination of specific steps needed to make improvements can be accomplished through involvement of team members in a brainstorming exercise or other analyses to identify process changes, and implementation and measurement of the impact of changes will require methods such as the PDSA cycle described throughout this text; then followed by use of process behavior charts to assess the need for further improvements and this improvement cycle will then be repeated (Langley et al., 2009).

Nature of Process Variation and Actions for Improvement

A couple of other definitions are important to help clarify why understanding variation is vital to CQI. A process is said to be stable and "in statistical control" if only common causes are affecting the outcomes over time. This does not mean that the outcomes are good or bad or that there is no variation. It means that the outcomes are predictable within statistically determined limits. Similarly, an unstable process is a process in which outcomes are affected by both common and special causes, and the outcomes are unpredictable. The appropriate actions for improvement of a process depend upon whether the process is stable or unstable. If the process is unstable, then variation is produced by both common and special causes so the appropriate action for improvement is to investigate and prevent the special causes from happening again. Once the process is stable, then the appropriate action for improvement is to make a change which reduces or removes some of the common causes. Luckily, Shewhart (1931) provided a method to operationally define a stable process using a control chart.

Control Charts/Process Behavior Charts

The control chart, which is often described as one of many CQI tools (Bialek, Duffy, & Moran, 2009; Langley et al., 2009) is arguably the most important since it represents a powerful methodology for explaining concepts of process variation. It was first developed by Shewhart as a methodology for analyzing and understanding process variability and predictability (Shewhart, 1931; Wheeler, 2000, Wheeler & Chambers, 2010). In the evolution of CQI that was described in Chapter 1, this "tool" has been found to be very useful in many settings and has been called by several names, including Shewhart control charts and most recently, process behavior charts, which

is derived from its broad use as a descriptor of process variability. We will use *control chart* and *process behavior chart* interchangeably throughout this chapter and this text.

A control chart is a plot of process measurements over time overlaid by three statistically computed lines: a center line, an upper control limit, and a lower control limit. The vertical axis of a control chart represents the actual value of the measure we are studying to assess process performance and variability; the horizontal axis represents the time scale over which we have collected process measures. One important goal of a control chart is to display individual process data in a time series, which is much more useful than simply analyzing measures of central tendency alone (e.g., an arithmetic average), when carrying out a process behavior analysis in CQI. In this way, a control chart illustrates and concentrates on the behavior of the underlying process. The upper and lower control limits of a process behavior chart define the Natural Process Limits (i.e., what the process will deliver as long as it continues to operate as consistently as possible), thus describing what Wheeler (2000) defines as the voice of the process. While the Run Chart, which will be described later in this chapter, is also an extremely useful CQI tool for displaying time series summaries of process measures, the control chart has one very important unique capability and purpose: it is the most powerful tool for distinguishing between common and special causes of variation and predicting future performance of a stable process within a range (Langley et al., 2009). Further increasing the usefulness of this tool, but also adding some level of confusion, especially to novices in CQI, is that there have been many types of control charts described in the CQI literature over many years. These differ according to their application to various types of data with different measurement scales (Langley et al., 2009):

1. Classification data/nominal data: p chart or np chart
2. Count data: c chart or u chart

3. Continuous data: I chart (X chart/ XmR chart), Xbar chart (with R chart or S chart)

Other differences among these charts relate to the number of observations per time point; for example, for continuous data, the Xbar chart is useful when there are multiple observations per time point and individual, or XmR charts are used when there is one observation per time point. Before describing details about how to produce control charts, it is useful to review the interpretive concepts that are common to all forms of control charts.

FIGURE 4.1 shows a series of X-bar charts, including a solid center line (mean, i.e., arithmetic average) and two dashed lines, representing lower and upper control limits. These three charts illustrate the following: Segment (A) represents a situation when the data are considered to be stable; the points do not go outside of the control limits and there are no discernable patterns within the limits. This process will continue to produce predictable outcomes within these limits as long as the conditions that produced all of these results continue. The latter is a subject matter judgment, not a statistical one. Improvement will come from changing the process that impacts every output of the process (i.e., the common causes). In segment (B) there are values outside the control limits; thus, the process is unstable due to special causes of variation. The appropriate action is to investigate the special causes and determine how to remove them. Finally, segment (C) describes the situation when there is a discernable pattern within the control limits. In this case, there are too many values in a row below the center line. The exact definition of how many is too many varies by several factors, including sample size and number of time points. These are discussed by several authors along with other rules that define patterns which may signal special cause variation (Balestracci, 2009; Perla, Provost, & Murray, 2011; Wheeler, 2000).

In addition to measuring process behavior to determine common vs. special causes

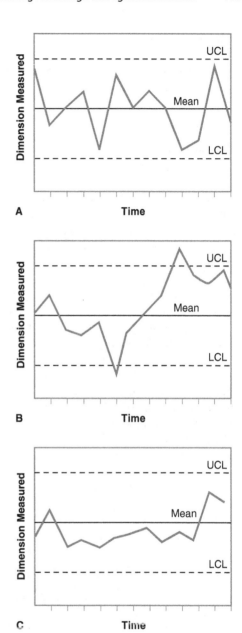

FIGURE 4.1 Three Examples of Control Charts

of variation, control charts are also used to assess the impact of an improvement effort by continuing to plot the process outcomes after a change is made to the process. The change should show up as a special cause signal in the chart and should settle down to a new center line over time unless unplanned special causes impact the process. The process should continue to be monitored and the same diagnostics and actions for improvement as described previously should be employed.

XmR Charts

"Individual values" charts, also called XmR charts, have proven to be the very useful in health care and have the advantage of being "non-parametric," thereby being applicable to a multiple types of measurement scales. Wheeler points out that when measurements are based on counts or percentages and data are displayed in p charts, for example, assumptions are necessary about the specific probability models (e.g., binomial or Poisson) in order to compute theoretical limits; however, XmR charts are based on empirical limits and no assumptions are needed (Wheeler, 2000, p. 140).

XmR charts are actually two charts: (1) a plot of the individual process outcomes, or X values, over time; and (2) a plot of the absolute differences from one X to the next X over time, or the Moving Ranges—designated mR (Wheeler, 2000). The center line of the X chart is typically the average (mean) of the individual X values and the Upper Control Limit or UCL is the average(of X values) +2.66 times the average of the Moving Ranges. The Lower Control Limit or LCL is the average(of X values) −2.66 times the average of the Moving

Ranges. Similarly, the center line of the mR chart is the average of the Moving Ranges and the UCL is 3.27 times the average mR. There is no LCL for the mR chart since the absolute values are used. There are times when one or more data points or Moving Ranges are much larger than others and would skew the average lines unduly. In these cases, it will be more appropriate to use the median of the X values and the median of the mR versus the average (mean) X and average (mean) mR, respectively. When this is done, the statistical scaling factors have to be changed. The value of 2.66 changes to 3.14, and the value of 3.27 changes to 3.87.

Process behavior charts are powerful tools to provide knowledge and help you understand variation in a process. "Points outside the limits are signals – they are opportunities to discover how to improve a process…and ask the right questions" (Wheeler, 2000, p. 59). Wheeler also notes that "if you are not pleased with the amount of variation shown by the Natural Process Limits, you must go to work on the system to change the underlying process, rather than setting arbitrary goals, jawboning the workers, or looking for alternative ways of computing limits" (2000, p. 44). This is accomplished in various ways, including using other CQI tools, such as those presented later in the chapter, e.g., construct a cause-and-effect diagram with a team of people who work in the process to understand the sources of common cause variation.

🔎 PROCESS BEHAVIOR CASE STUDY

In order to illustrate the construction and use of a process behavior chart, in particular an XmR chart, the following hypothetical case study is presented.

University hospital, a large academic teaching hospital, has been undergoing expansion throughout its state. As part of its goal to increase access to quality care in rural areas it has opened a new primary care facility in a rural part of the state. This initiative included transferring well trained, experienced clinical staff as well as hiring/training local staff in administrative roles. Because of her experience in providing quality care and CQI, the new administrator of the rural clinic decided that several measures of quality of care needed to be collected at the initiation of the clinic. Some questions that needed to be answered are as follows (these are provided for readers to consider in their own health care environment):

1. What would be some examples of process measures to collect?
2. How to effectively analyze these measures to understand what the level of quality is?
3. How to decide if and when changes in processes are needed?
4. What specific changes should be made and who decides?
5. How to determine if the changes made were improvements?

These are just a few examples of the kind of questions that should be asked in applying CQI in this setting. We leave it up to readers of this chapter to discuss these questions and to think of others that might be appropriate—especially after completing this chapter; but to illustrate process behavior charts, we will focus on Questions 2 and 3.

To answer any of these questions data collection is required. A useful methodology, especially in this setting when a new center is opening, is to collect daily measures and display them in a process behavior chart. The experienced administrator knows that long waiting times really annoy patients and are symptoms of inefficiency. She also knows that waiting times get increasingly worse throughout the day if the clinic does not get off to a good start. Therefore, she wants the staff to track a simple but important metric that she believes will play an important role in clinic quality and patient satisfaction: Amount of time in minutes to prepare the clinic each morning for the arrival of patients. This metric would not only measure clinic efficiency but could also have a direct impact on several other quality measures, most notably waiting time and patient satisfaction. To answer questions 2 and 3 above the administrator first met with the staff to operationally define how they would measure clinic preparation time, including who would be responsible and when it would be measured each day. She planned to have another meeting with the clinical staff after 2 weeks of data collection and teach them how to display and interpret the data on a process behavior chart. Data were collected each day for the first 2 weeks of operation; the clinic opened on Monday, June 5, 2017, and data were collected until June 18, 2017. Preparation time (in minutes) is shown in **TABLE 4.3A**. The average (mean) amount of time to prepare the clinic each day is approximately 16 minutes (16.3) and fluctuates between 13 and 22 minutes. Some might argue, "We prepared the clinic in 13 minutes on June 7. We should figure out what we did and do it in 13 minutes every day!" This would actually make things worse and unpredictable and would not reflect any understanding of variation. Similarly, asking why June 12 was higher than the prior days would be equally counterproductive.

The optimal way to monitor and assess variation in the clinic preparation process is to use the XmR chart described above. Wheeler (2000) describes reasons for using an XmR chart, which are applicable to this example:

1. It contributes to knowledge about the process because it helps us to understand the right questions to ask; to hear the "voice of the process."
2. It is applicable when the data are collected over time and represent one data element (n = 1) for each time point; in this case the data were continuous (interval scale) data: daily preparation times measured (once a day) in minutes.
3. It allows us to study and learn from the variation in each pair of time points and adds substantial knowledge about the process beyond just knowing the average and range of values.
4. Most important, it provides a methodology for understanding sources of variation and separating "noise vs. signals"; it prevents us from taking unnecessary actions and helps us to know when actions are needed to address special causes of variation.

The initial chart was established using the 14 data points in Table 4.3A and the associated process behavior chart presented in **FIGURE 4.2A**.

Using the data presented in Table 4.3A, the first step in the construction of the XmR chart is to compute the absolute value of the day to day differences in preparation time; for example, the

(continues)

🔎 *PROCESS BEHAVIOR CASE STUDY*   *(continued)*

TABLE 4.3A Clinic Preparation Time in Minutes (June 5–18)

Date	Time
5-Jun	19
6-Jun	15
7-Jun	13
8-Jun	14
9-Jun	15
10-Jun	16
11-Jun	17
12-Jun	19
13-Jun	16
14-Jun	14
15-Jun	14
16-Jun	16
17-Jun	22
18-Jun	18

Average = 16.3 minutes

day 1 (19 minutes) minus day 2 value (15 minutes) leads to an absolute difference of 4 minutes. Each pairwise difference, or moving range (mR), is computed and recorded; the average of the moving ranges in Table 4.3A is 2.23 minutes. As noted above, the average of the individual (X) values and the average of the moving ranges (mR) are needed to compute the upper (UCL) and lower (LCL) control limits of this process behavior chart. (As described above the formula for the control limits are: UCL = average of the individual X values +2.66 times the average of the Moving Ranges; LCL = average of the individual X values −2.66 times the average of the Moving Range). Based on these formulas the LCL is 10.4 and the UCL is 22.2 minutes.

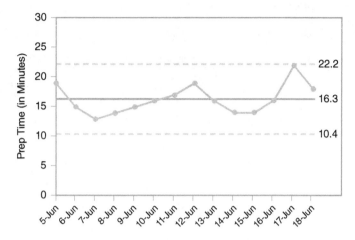

FIGURE 4.2A Process Behavior Chart for Clinic Preparation Time: June 5–18

The chart in Figure 4.2A is the process behavior chart for the data displayed in Table 4.3A; preparation times for the first 2 weeks of clinic operation. This chart reflects the voice of the process. The fact that all of the first 2 weeks of preparation times are within the control limits of 10.4 and 22.2 minutes indicates that the process is stable, and the variability observed is due only to common causes of variation. The process will continue to perform in this range unless a special cause occurs to disrupt the process. If there is a signal of a special cause below the lower limit, the clinic team should investigate and determine if the reason is repeatable or just a fluke. If it is repeatable and could be incorporated into the process daily, then a process change should be planned and implemented since this would represent a shortening of the daily preparation time—an improvement. If there is a special cause signal above the upper limit, the team should also investigate and seek to prevent the special cause from recurring. Lastly, a process that is operating within the control limits does not mean that it should not be improved if it is not meeting the needs of the patient or other downstream processes. It just means that the strategy for improvement will be different. The clinic team would seek to understand the system of common causes and identify what can be changed that would impact every occurrence of the process. This investigation may involve the use of some of the CQI tools that we describe later in this chapter.

After teaching the team how to construct and interpret the initial chart, the administrator explained how to maintain the chart on a daily basis. This simply required the person taking the measurement to extend the limits of the chart into the future, record the date and the daily measurement in the data table, and plot the point. The team should be alerted to investigate immediately if a point exceeds the upper control limit or if runs of data (e.g., a large sequence of times above the mean) are observed. (Please refer to the Run Chart section later in the chapter which defines other rules for detecting patterns or "runs" in the data that may be signals to be investigated further.)

The chart was updated daily and continued to operate within limits until July 4, when preparation time was observed to be 24 minutes, higher than the upper control limit (see **TABLE 4.3B** and **FIGURE 4.2B**). The person taking the measurement immediately polled the team about what was different that day. Obviously, it was a holiday, though that did not explain the special cause. Further discussion with the team indicated that there had been a power outage during the night due to a thunderstorm, and one of the computers used to check in patients failed to reboot automatically. A manual restart was required, and this added to the clinic prep time. No action was taken on the

(continues)

🔍 *PROCESS BEHAVIOR CASE STUDY*   (continued)

TABLE 4.3B Clinic Preparation Time in Minutes (June 5–July 7)

Date	Time	Average	LCL	UCL	Moving Range
5-Jun	19	16.3	10.4	22.2	-
6-Jun	15	16.3	10.4	22.2	4
7-Jun	13	16.3	10.4	22.2	2
8-Jun	14	16.3	10.4	22.2	1
9-Jun	15	16.3	10.4	22.2	1
10-Jun	16	16.3	10.4	22.2	1
11-Jun	17	16.3	10.4	22.2	1
12-Jun	19	16.3	10.4	22.2	2
13-Jun	16	16.3	10.4	22.2	3
14-Jun	14	16.3	10.4	22.2	2
15-Jun	14	16.3	10.4	22.2	0
16-Jun	16	16.3	10.4	22.2	2
17-Jun	22	16.3	10.4	22.2	6
18-Jun	18	16.3	10.4	22.2	4
19-Jun	16	16.3	10.4	22.2	2
20-Jun	15	16.3	10.4	22.2	1
21-Jun	18	16.3	10.4	22.2	3
22-Jun	14	16.3	10.4	22.2	4
23-Jun	17	16.3	10.4	22.2	3

24-Jun	14	16.3	10.4	22.2	3
25-Jun	19	16.3	10.4	22.2	5
26-Jun	14	16.3	10.4	22.2	5
27-Jun	16	16.3	10.4	22.2	2
28-Jun	12	16.3	10.4	22.2	4
29-Jun	13	16.3	10.4	22.2	1
30-Jun	15	16.3	10.4	22.2	2
1-Jul	18	16.3	10.4	22.2	3
2-Jul	16	16.3	10.4	22.2	2
3-Jul	20	16.3	10.4	22.2	4
4-Jul	24	16.3	10.4	22.2	4
5-Jul	21	16.3	10.4	22.2	3
6-Jul	16	16.3	10.4	22.2	5
7-Jul	17	16.3	10.4	22.2	1

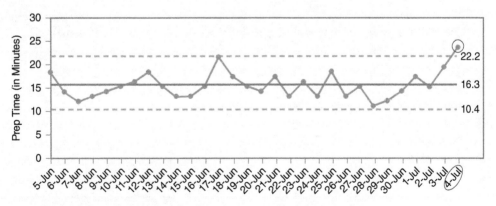

FIGURE 4.2B Process Behavior Chart for Clinic Preparation Time: June 5–July 4

(continues)

🔍 *PROCESS BEHAVIOR CASE STUDY*   *(continued)*

clinic preparation process, and indeed the preparation time the following day fell back within the control limits and continued that way (see **FIGURE 4.2C** and the last three lines of Table 4.3B). The predictability of this stable process allowed the staff to better plan the start of every day and provided opportunities for the staff to establish process behavior charts on other key processes and to systematically select ones to improve. Two important lessons are demonstrated in this case study by the use of the XmR process behavior chart. First, as with any process behavior chart, analysis prevented the team from taking unnecessary actions when a high value was first noted, since it was within the upper control limits. Second, when a value was found that was above the upper control limit a careful analysis was done to gain knowledge about the cause of this high value, and the right questions were asked with input from team members, and in this case the cause was quickly identified. These lessons demonstrate the value of using process behavior charts to monitor and improve processes over time.

Methodological note: In reviewing Figures 4.2A, 4.2B, and 4.2C, it can be noted that Figures 4.2A and 4.2B consist of one time series chart displaying individual preparation time (X) on the vertical axis and date on the horizontal axis; this the traditional display associated with most process behavior charts. The unique and quite important differentiation between these (XmR) charts and other process behavior charts is the use of the average moving range and multiplication factors (2.66) in determining the upper and lower control limits; the use of moving ranges to compute control limits is the most important contribution of the use of XmR charts. In his foundational work on this topic Wheeler (2000) describes the XmR chart as consisting of two charts by adding

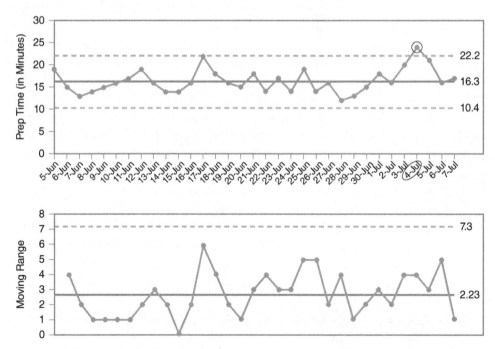

FIGURE 4.2C Process Behavior Chart for Clinic Preparation Time June 5–July 7

a lower control chart display that presents the daily and average moving range and its upper limit. Although useful in many cases as a valuable descriptive tool, it is our experience that this lower (mR) chart is not always necessary to display, as long as the moving ranges have been computed and used to compute control limits for detecting special cause variation. However, it should be also noted that in this case analysis we did compute, but did not display, both charts. Wheeler, in a more recent journal article, presents a good summary of reasons for including the moving range chart when carrying out a process behavior analysis (Wheeler, 2010). Readers should consider these arguments and based on the specific data being analyzed make a decision as to whether both the X and mR charts are needed. For illustrative purposes both the upper chart of individual values of preparation time (X) and lower chart presenting moving ranges (mR) are presented in Figure 4.2C. The average and upper control limit presented in the lower chart are found using the formulas presented above: the average of the mR values $= 2.23$ and the upper control limit of the moving ranges is 7.3 ($= 3.27 \times 2.23$). One other important computational note regarding the XmR charts presented here is that the average of individual values (X) and moving ranges (mR) as well as the upper and lower control limits for all three charts are based only on the first 14 days of data collected. This was done for two reasons: (1) we considered the process to be stable based on the process behavior chart computed for the first 14 days (i.e., it included enough cycles of the process to reflect usual operating conditions); and (2) the first 14 days includes a sufficient amount of data (at least 10 data points). These are two general guidelines that we recommend for computing the initial averages and upper and lower control limits for generating process behavior charts, in general (i.e., not specific to XmR charts). As we continue to monitor this process over a longer period of time the centerline and limits should, of course, be recalculated once it is determined that an actual shift has occurred, hopefully, due to a planned improvement. Further information on the choice of time periods to compute average and control limits in XmR charts is found in Chapter 3 of Wheeler's text, *Understanding Variation* (2000), which has been cited several times in this case study and provides examples that can serve as guidance on the development and interpretation of process behavior charts, in general, and XmR charts specifically. Finally, it should be noted that the analyses and charts presented in this case study were developed using Microsoft Excel™ although other options listed below could also have been used.

Although in this case study, the source of the variation was quickly identified by the team, there are often situations when more complex sources must be investigated. While guesses, "executive decisions" and anecdotal information may seem like an easy way to decide on the action to be taken (e.g., blame one of the new staff), the proper way to proceed is to use input from knowledgeable team members and when necessary use other CQI tools and techniques to gain knowledge about the cause of this change in preparation time. With the knowledge that we have special cause variation, tools and techniques such as those described later in this chapter (e.g., cause-and-effect diagram) or methods that are described by other authors (e.g., root cause analysis; Ross, 2014) might be appropriate. When a process is stable though not performing at the level needed by the customer, strategies for improvement such as applying PDSA cycles to test whether changes that are made lead to true improvement (Langley et al., 2009) and using a team approach (see Chapter 6 for more details on the role of teams in CQI) should be applied. These step wise applications of improvement tools and techniques are always recommended and are especially important to follow when we are analyzing other health care processes that are more complex than the simple example presented here. For instance, please see the patient safety examples in Chapters 9 and 10. The key conclusion of this case study is that the process behavior chart is the most economic method, as originally proven by Shewhart, for gaining knowledge about a process and, more importantly, distinguishing between special and common cause variation. By understanding variation, we will know the appropriate action to take for improvements.

Other Forms of Control/Process Behavior Charts

As noted above there are other forms of control/process behavior charts that can also be used to assess process behavior and may be better known, such as the those that are not based on moving ranges but on means of actual values (X-bar charts) or percentages (P-charts) and are applicable when we have more than one data element per time point. For example, Chapter 5 presents examples of X-bar charts based on samples of patients to track "door to doctor time" in an emergency department.

A good resource for further details and formulae for how to compute control charts for various types of data can be found at: https://www.sqconline.com/about-control-charts.

Another source of software for computing various types of controls charts is the R programming language (R Development Core Team, 2014). However, as with all statistical software, users are urged to study/question findings carefully to understand and gain knowledge from these user-friendly systems before taking actions to change processes.

▶ Quality Improvement Tools

In Chapter 1, the Plan, Do, Study, Act cycle was introduced, with an emphasis on its broad applicability as a framework in which many other CQI processes can be applied. Many organizations, including health care organizations, have adopted the Plan, Do, Study, Act (PDSA) cycle or a tailored version of it as their overall framework for CQI (Langley et al., 2009). Improvement begins with plotting a key quality characteristic of a process over time on a run chart or control chart. Then, depending upon the stability of the process, different tools, techniques, and methods may be used to accomplish the purpose of each phase of the PDSA cycle. (Once again, as noted in Chapter 1, readers are reminded that the PDSA cycle is sometimes described as a PDCA cycle, where "C" stands for check, as in checking your results of the Plan ("P") and Do ("D") phases, which is equivalent to the "S" study phase of a PDSA cycle; i.e., they are two names for the same CQI process.)

There is no one specified point in the CQI process where one needs to use a given method of measurement and analysis. It should be used on a continuous basis. In the context of the PDSA cycle, data and analytical tools may be used throughout the entire cycle. Different tools will be more helpful in different stages of each improvement project, from the initial analysis to monitoring changes that have already been instituted. Reemphasizing the point made earlier in this chapter about using data to learn about improvement, Berwick (1996) notes that it is critical at the studying (S) stage of a PDSA cycle to take the time to reflect and learn about the impact of improvements that have already been made. This should include evaluating whether these changes have actually been improvements and then deciding on what further improvements to make.

There are numerous tools and techniques available to assist managers, clinicians, and organizational teams in improving processes to deliver desired results. These tools include activity network diagrams; affinity diagrams; box-plots, brainstorming; cause-and-effect diagrams; check sheets; concentration diagrams; control charts; failure mode and effects analysis (FMEA); flowcharts (process, deployment, top-down, opportunity); force field analysis; frequency plots; histograms; interrelationship digraphs; matrix diagrams; Pareto charts; prioritization matrices; process capability charts; radar charts; run charts; scatter diagrams; Suppliers, Inputs, Process steps, Outputs, Customers (SIPOC) diagrams; time plots; tree diagrams; and workflow diagrams. These tools are only useful if applied with an understanding of variation described earlier or results may be the opposite of improvement.

While space does not permit detailed description of this entire list of tools, six commonly used tools for CQI efforts in health care are presented here; these are in addition to control charts which were described above and are included by many authors as an important "CQI tool" for understanding variation and knowing when process improvements are needed e.g., *The Improvement Guide*; Langley et al., 2009).

The tools to be described in this chapter in addition to control charts are:

1. Run charts
2. Process flowcharts
3. Checklists
4. Cause-and-effect diagrams
5. Frequency charts
6. Pareto diagrams

This brief list of tools represents a range of types that are useful for preventing errors, describing process flow and for assessing ideas for improvement, which are suitable depending upon the type of variation present in the process. As noted above, one can visualize a life cycle of the improvement team's efforts where these tools (and others not described here) might be applied sequentially at various project stages.

Run Charts

A control chart/process behavior chart has a specific purpose for distinguishing between common and special causes of variation and thereby providing valuable information about process predictability within limits. A run chart is another useful tool with broad applications in health care, to gain knowledge about process performance with minimal mathematical complexity. "Because of its utility and simplicity, the run chart has wide potential application in health care for practitioners and decision-makers. Run charts also provide the foundation for more sophisticated methods of analysis such as Shewhart (control) charts and planned experiments" (Perla, Provost, & Murray, 2011, p. 46). Run charts are graphical time series displays of process measurements along with the median value of that measure; similar to control charts the vertical axis represents actual values of some process measure of interest and the horizontal axis presents a series of time points at which process measures have been collected; however, unlike control charts they do not include upper and lower control limits.

FIGURE 4.3 presents an example of a simple but important run chart, illustrating how (primary) data can be displayed to provide knowledge and information about the effect of making a change in procedures leading to a desired result, consistently fewer medication errors. This illustrates an important concept about how data and tools can provide feedback based on knowledge of systems and processes to not only make improvements but to provide the motivation for improvement (McLaughlin & Kibbe, 2013).

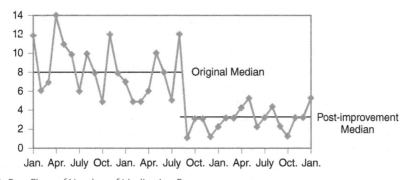

FIGURE 4.3 Run Chart of Number of Medication Errors

Once again, the most powerful tool for distinguishing between common and special causes of variation is the control chart/process behavior chart; but some important uses of the run chart (which it also shares with the control chart) are:

- Displaying data to make process performance visible
- Determining if changes tested result in improvement
- Determining if we are holding the gains made by our improvement
- Allowing for a temporal (analytic) view of data versus a static (enumerative) view (Perla, Provost, & Murray, 2011, p. 47)

As its name implies, one very important use of a run chart analysis is to detect trends defined by runs in the data (i.e., "a consecutive sequence of data points all on the same side of the median"; Balestracci, 2009, p. 147). Balestracci (2009) provides guidance about how many values in a row constitute a run, and in particular, "the guideline" that a run of 8 or more may indicate concern that there are other than common causes of variation in the data. In such cases, an investigation is warranted unless a process change was purposefully made. In the case of a planned change that results in improvement, a shift in the process is expected and a new centerline (median) should be computed starting from the time that the process change was introduced; this is illustrated in the example given in Figure 4.3.

Another useful characteristic of a run chart, which is easily abused if care is not taken, is the ability to identify an "astronomical data point...one that is obviously, even blatantly different from the rest of the points" (Perla, Provost, & Murray, 2011, p. 48). Care should be taken when such points are observed to not assume they are due to special causes or represent signals, which can only be identified using control charts. At most, such points should be discussed by team members to understand possible causes of these values and attention should be paid to note whether

they are repeated over time. A definitive determination of special or common cause can only be made by reanalyzing the process data using a control chart, to determine if the astronomical data points fall outside of control limits.

Further details for how to compute and interpret run charts and, in particular their value in health care CQI, including their strengths and weaknesses are presented by Perla, Provost, & Murray (2011). Most texts on CQI methods in health care/public health describe the construction and interpretation of run charts (Balestracci, 2009; Bialek, Duffy, & Moran, 2009; Langley et al., 2009; Lloyd, 2019; Spath & Kelly, 2017). For an example of how to use run charts, together with control charts and other tools, as part a LEAN management system readers are referred to Chapter 5.

Process Flowcharts

As Langley et al. (2009) point out, CQI projects and teams requires some of the same kinds of tools that are commonly used in project management for describing systems and ensuring that all steps are carried out in the proper sequence. Two tools that fall within this definition are the project checklist and process flowchart. One of the most powerful improvement tools for initiating inquiry into a process improvement project is the flowchart. Flowcharts (also called Flow Diagrams) are pictorial representations of how a process works. Simply put, they trace the steps that the input of a process goes through from start to finish. The input may be a specimen in laboratory tests, a piece of paper in medical records, or a patient in a specialty clinic. Flowcharts are used to describe the sequence of actions that must be carried out in order to complete a particular task or set of tasks. In systems thinking terminology the actions performed on inputs are sometimes described as throughput and the entire process that we are studying/improving can be thought of as a system that can be modeled using three major components: input, throughput, and output

(Grove, 1995). Donabedian (1980) first intro-duced similar systems thinking concepts that were specific to health care when he defined a model of quality of care based on the inter-relationship of structure, process, and out-come. A flowchart is a first step in describing the details (who, what, when) of each of the components in these system models.

To develop a flowchart, one may proceed as follows:

1. Define the basic stages of a process.
2. Further define the process, breaking down each stage into specific steps needed to complete the process.
3. Follow the input through the pro-cess a number of times to verify the process by observation.
4. Discuss the process with the proj-ect team or other employees to clarify the process and include any steps that might be missing.

As the steps of a process are described, they may be documented with simple rectan-gles or, in some cases greater complexity can be described using traditional flowcharting shapes to represent different steps or actions. For example, an activity or action step is rep-resented by a rectangle, a decision step by a diamond, a wait or inventory by a triangle, a document by a symbol that looks like a rectan-gle with a curve at the bottom, a file by a large circle, and the continuation of the flowchart to another sheet of paper by a small circle.

It is very important to note that flow-charts may be as simple or as complex as you wish. It is important to agree on what level of detail is suitable for the purpose. For example, very detailed flowcharts may be used in stan-dard operating procedures (SOPs) for highly technical procedures. A high-level flowchart may be used to describe a general overview of how the process is carried out. FIGURE 4.4 shows a high-level (simple) flowchart of the medication administration process for the inpatient setting; note that this figure also illustrates different shapes that can be used for

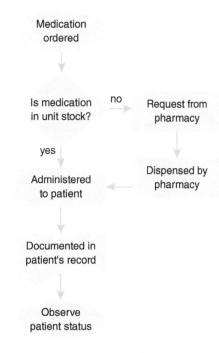

FIGURE 4.4 Simple Flowchart of Medication Administration Process

different activities. Once the general process is described, more detail may be added, depend-ing on the purpose of the analysis.

FIGURE 4.5 shows a more detailed flowchart of a similar process. As more detail has been added, the process has evolved from "medication administration" to "medication management" to include additional process stages involving medication inventory management, pharmacy management, and surveillance for adverse drug events. Each step of this process may in turn be mapped with a finer level of detail.

Members of a work team or improvement project team are likely to find that there is no common understanding of how the current process or system works, especially if multi-ple providers or departments are responsible for carrying out different steps of the process. The development of flowcharts, with input from all team members, allows the team to achieve a common understanding of their work processes and the important customer

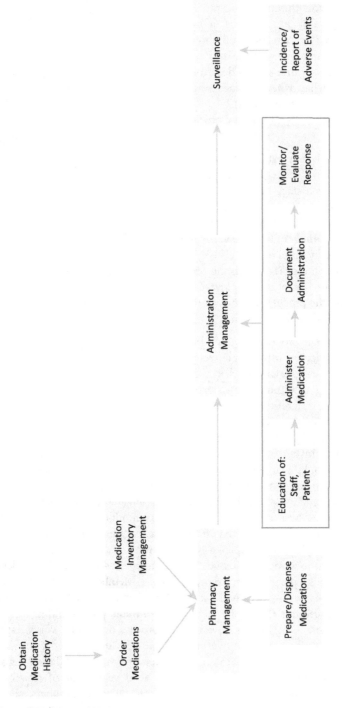

FIGURE 4.5 Flowchart of Medication Management

Modified from VHA and First Consulting Group: VHA 2002 Research Series Publication, *Surveillance for Adverse Drug Events: History Methods and Current Issues* by Killbridge, P. & Classen, D. First Consulting Group

and supplier relationships internal to the processes. These interdependencies are often the key to sustainable process improvement. With an accurate, shared representation of how the process works, the team is then better able to consider how to improve it.

Once agreement is reached on the representation of the current process, the team may begin to ask questions about that process using the flow chart and guided by a control chart of measurements of process outputs, including:

1. How effective is the process in meeting customer requirements?
2. Are there performance gaps or perceived opportunities for improvement?
3. Have the relevant stages of the process been represented? Are "owners" of each stage represented on the team? If not, what needs to be done to gather their feedback and ideas?
4. What are the inputs required for the process, and where do they come from? Are the inputs constraining the process or not? Which ones?
5. Are there equipment or regulatory constraints forcing this approach?
6. Is this the right problem process to be working on? To continue working on?

The potential benefits of flowcharting are considerable. Staff come to know the process much better. A clear understanding of internal customers and suppliers can be gleaned from the overall process flow. The results can be used as a training aid, especially as new staff join the CQI team. People begin to take ownership of the process by participating in this activity, and most importantly, the possibilities and points in the process for improvement become clear almost immediately. And, in the language of project management, the work breakdown structure, timeline, and budget for an improvement initiative can begin to take shape through careful flow chart development (Project Management Institute, 2017).

Other examples of flowcharts are found throughout this text, including a description of their valuable role in Lean Management Systems, in Chapter 5, where flowcharts, also denoted as process maps, are used to describe emergency room patient flow and processes.

Checklists

Although it is neither a statistical tool nor a completely new tool in quality improvement, one that is very basic to both CQI and project management is the checklist. CQI in health care includes as one of its primary goals the prevention of errors (Crosby, 1979), which is an important part of the overall goal of ensuring patient safety, defined as "freedom from accidental or preventable injuries produced by medical care" (AHRQ, 2016). This includes prevention of medical errors, and adverse events (outcomes of medical care); these issues are described in Chapters 8, 9, and 10. (Please note that a checklist is different from another CQI tool with a similar name, the check sheet; see Bialek, Duffy, & Moran, 2009.)

A checklist can take many forms, but in its simplest form it is a list of process activities, usually in a time ordered sequence, that must be carried out by various members of a project or CQI team. As each task is completed, a check mark is made next to the item that was completed; in some cases, greater precision is obtained by indicating the date/time that the task was completed or, if multiple team members are involved in the process, the initials of the team member who completed the task may be entered as a way of ensuring accountability. Checklists should be derived from a process flowchart and apply to performing tasks in a stable process. Checklists have been used for many years in other industries, such as the airline industry, and they have long been an important component of the project manager's tool kit in many different industrial and health care settings. Their role in improving airline safety is well documented and is an important reason that they have now seen an accelerated evolution into medical care, which has had a greater focus on safety issues in the early part of the 21st century (Haynes et al., 2009; Gawande, 2009; Pronovost et al., 2006; Pronovost et al., 2009). Although not without controversy regarding their effectiveness (Bosk et al., 2009), their adoption as part of the medical safety process, to be used in conjunction with other well-established evidence-based practices, continues as we have entered the second decade of this century. Chapter 14 includes a critical review of some of the issues surrounding checklists and other commonly used CQI tools and techniques with a warning that before we assume that a "magic bullet" exists which can be widely applied to guarantee quality we should take time to carefully understand the context in which a CQI tool or procedure has been developed and understand the limits of its generalizability to other settings (Dixon-Woods & Martin, 2016). This advice is particularly important for checklists, whose broad applicability may have been overstated by some, but does not negate their value as a CQI tool if used properly; the same can be said of most tools presented in this and other CQI texts.

In addition to the references cited in the preceding paragraph, Chapters 1, 2, and 8 of this text provide further discussion of the use of checklists in health care. A discussion of how to understand the specific issues surrounding practitioner adoption of checklists through the use of a social marketing approach is presented by Breland (2012) in the form of a case study.

Cause-and-Effect Diagram

Cause-and-effect diagrams, also called Ishikawa or fishbone diagrams, are one of the most widely used tools of CQI. This tool was developed by Kaoru Ishikawa (University of Tokyo) for use at Kawasaki Steel Works in 1943 to sort and interrelate the common causes of process variation (Ishikawa, 1987).

Cause-and-effect diagrams are most useful to begin to identify common causes of variation once the process has been determined to be stable and documented using a process flowchart. However, they are also very useful when special causes have been identified, perhaps via a process behavior chart analysis and the next step is decide what actions need to be taken to prevent the special cause from recurring. Cause-and-effect diagrams are a schematic means of relating causes of variation to the process output and predictability. It is important to note that not all errors are special causes. Errors can be produced by a process with only common causes of variation present. Therefore, it is critical to determine the type of variation that is present before constructing the cause-and-effect diagram, since the strategy for improvement is different. In either case, the first pass at a cause-and-effect diagram may not be enough to understand the cause-and-effect relationships. Therefore, it may be necessary to stratify cause-and-effect diagrams further to achieve finer gradations of error causes. Increasing the level of detail about causes can help with identifying specific action for improvement.

This tool is especially suited for team situations and is quite useful for focusing a discussion and organizing large amounts of information resulting from a brainstorming session. It can be taught easily and quickly, allowing the group to sort ideas into useful categories for further investigation. The diagram is also referred to as a "fishbone" diagram because the shape resembles the skeleton of a fish.

FIGURE 4.6 shows the multilayered process of making a fishbone diagram. Step 1 of the diagram shows the identified performance gap or problem at the right and a big arrow leading to it that represents the overall causation. Step 2 involves drawing spines from that big arrow to represent main classifications or categories of causes, such as labor, materials, and equipment. Step 3 adds the specific causes along each major spine, which also may occur at multiple levels.

Step 1: Draw spine

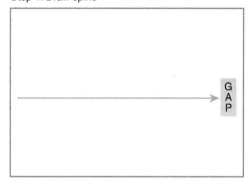

Step 2: Add main causes

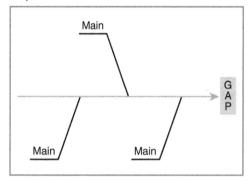

Step 3: Add specific causes

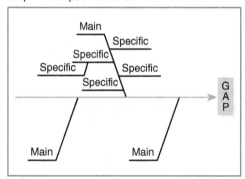

FIGURE 4.6 Multilayered Process of Developing a Fishbone Diagram

Sometimes it is useful to draw the diagram in two stages—one showing the main causes and a separate chart with a spine representing the main cause and its associated levels.

FIGURE 4.7 illustrates a cause-and-effect diagram that may be used to describe common causes of adverse drug events in a hospital setting. The process outcome is "adverse drug events." The main classifications in this example are people, policies, procedures, and plant and equipment, each showing a variety of levels of causes.

Frequency Chart and Pareto Diagram

In some cases, after a cause-and-effect diagram is generated, data are collected to quantify how often the different causes occur. These data must then be presented to the study team and later to others. When measures are based on discrete/attribute data, the simplest display is a frequency chart, a vertical bar chart representing the frequency distribution of a set of data. It is most useful when the measures we are studying are discrete/attribute data but may also be used by collapsing continuous measures in "class-intervals." The bars are arrayed on the *horizontal* (x) axis representing equal or adjacent data intervals or discrete events. The length (height) of the bar against the *vertical* (y) axis shows the number of observations falling on that interval or event classification. The frequency chart displays the nature of the underlying statistical distribution; however, it does not provide any information about process stability and should only be used with a control chart indicating that the process is only producing statistically controlled variation. **FIGURE 4.8** shows a frequency chart of the frequency and causes for the discarding of hospital linens.

A Pareto diagram is a frequency chart with the bars arranged from the longest (most frequent) first on the left and moving successively toward the shortest. The arrangement of the vertical bars gives a visual indication of the relative frequency of the contributing causes of the problem, with each bar representing one cause.

The diagram is named after the 17th-century Italian economist, Vilfredo Pareto.

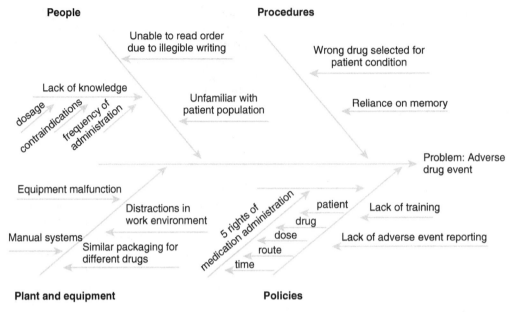

FIGURE 4.7 Cause-and-Effect Diagram of Adverse Drug Events

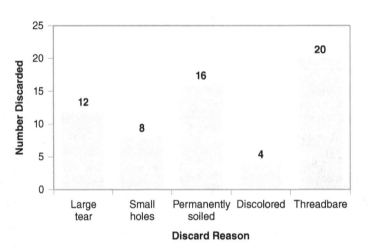

FIGURE 4.8 Frequency Chart of Linen Discard Causes

When he studied the distribution of wealth, he observed that the majority of the wealth had been distributed among a small proportion of the population (Pareto's law). Juran (1988) applied this concept to quality causes, observing that the "vital few" causes account for most of the defects, while others, the "useful many," account for a much smaller proportion of the defects. He noted that these vital few causes are likely to constitute the areas of highest payback to management. Concentrating on the high-volume causes may have the largest potential for reducing process variation once special causes have been eliminated.

On the same Pareto diagram, one also develops a cumulative probability distribution incorporating all the proportions of the observations to the left of and including the bar. It is common to display the frequency scale on the left-hand side of the vertical (*y*) axis and the cumulative percentage scale on the right-hand edge. Segregating the causes that have large frequencies can help identify potential improvements. However, just because a cause is identified as having the greatest frequency does not necessarily mean it should be worked on first. It must also be tractable and not cost more to change than it is worth. It is likely, however, that the first cause to be studied in detail will be among the left-most group. It is important to remember that even though a cause may not be among the most frequent, if it has a devastating result, such as causing a patient death, it must be addressed in the course of the improvement effort.

Once the cause-and-effect diagram, such as the one in Figure 4.7 which identifies possible causes of adverse drug events, has been described data would be collected on the frequency of the specific causes. FIGURE 4.9 illustrates how a Pareto chart can be developed to analyze the frequency of causes identified in the cause-and-effect diagram. For example, Figure 4.9 displays how often the "Five Rights of Medication Administration" contributed to an adverse drug event (ADE). Of 100 ADEs investigated, the Pareto chart shows that "wrong time" occurred most frequently, with "wrong patient" next, and so on.

Through these examples, one can begin to see how the tools fit together to support CQI and patient safety. Since the Institute of Medicine report *To Err Is Human* (IOM, 2000) was published, the topic of medical errors and adverse events has become a priority area for customers and stakeholders of health care organizations. TJC's review process now includes accreditation standards addressing patient safety, medical errors, and adverse events (also see Chapter 12). As illustrated by the preceding examples, various CQI tools, alone and in combination, can be used to address this critical area of concern.

Combinations of tools, such as flowcharts, Pareto charts, run charts, and control charts, may be used together in a lean management process analysis/improvement initiative in an emergency room setting as described in Chapter 5. A good description of the many tools that can be applied in health is found in *The Public Health Quality Improvement Handbook* (Bialek, Duffy, & Moran, 2009). Other examples of applications via case studies illustrating these concepts and tools are found in *Implementing*

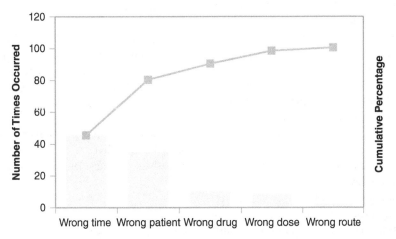

FIGURE 4.9 Pareto Chart: Five Rights of Medication Administration: Cause of Adverse Drug Events

Continuous Quality Improvement in Health Care—A Global Casebook (McLaughlin, Johnson, & Sollecito, 2012).

When faced with the task of developing specific tools there are various types of software, such as those described earlier for developing process behavior charts (e.g., "R"; R Development Core Team, 2014) or Microsoft's Excel™ tool that can be used; there are also websites that provide tutorials and templates to facilitate the understanding, development, and use of the tools discussed in this chapter, and other useful tools and methodologies (e.g., http://asq.org/learn-about-quality/seven-basic-quality-tools/overview/overview.html; also https://www.sqconline.com). As noted earlier, users are urged to study and question findings carefully to understand and gain knowledge from these user-friendly systems before taking actions to change processes.

▶ Sources of Data for CQI

Decisions about process performance and improvements and the application of CQI tools often start by accessing quality data in a step wise "data-to-decision cycle." This cycle begins with data that are transformed into information, which facilitates identification of opportunities for improvement and then leads to the transformation of information into knowledge, about how to redesign processes (e.g., based on best practices). Ultimately these steps result in decisions and actions to make changes and provide feedback on the need for further improvements (e.g., in a classic PDSA cycle; McLaughlin & Kibbe, 2013). Of course, all decisions should be informed by an understanding of variation as previously defined.

In defining sources of data for CQI initiatives, it is important to consider timeliness of the data being collected as well as accessibility. Most critical to this process is the quality of the

data that are the input to this decision-making cycle. As with any good statistical analysis, data collected for CQI must be of the highest quality and every effort must be taken to ensure this. No matter which tool or procedure is used to perform CQI, its findings will only be as good as the data that they are based on. The age-old acronym GIGO (Garbage In, Garbage Out) must always be kept in mind when deciding on data sources for CQI.

Ensuring the highest data quality requires the application of data standards, data management and quality assurance procedures (Loshin, 2011) to ensure that the information used to make CQI decisions is correct. Also important in ensuring data quality is proper training of team members involved in CQI initiatives (McLaughlin & Kibbe, 2013, p. 343):

> Quality improvement teams are temporary systems whose members may or may not be skilled observers and data recorders. Teams may also have to depend on observers who are not team members. Management must make sure that the appropriate team members are trained to observe and record the relevant events and variables. They also should make sure that all those likely to become involved understand the CQI process and the importance of reliable data. This may also be backed up with validation of those data that are most critical in determining which alternative procedure to adopt.

Two major classifications can be used to describe data that are applicable to most CQI initiatives: primary data and secondary data.

Primary Data

For CQI applications primary data can be defined as data that are collected specifically for the purposes of measuring process performance and improvement (i.e., providing information and knowledge about the specific practice setting or other health care environment that allows for improvement decisions to be made).

The data presented in the Case Study earlier in this chapter, which were used to develop an XmR process behavior chart, are a good example of how primary data can be collected to provide knowledge and understanding about the need for process improvements. Another example might be the use of primary data that were specifically collected to provide knowledge about medication errors in a medical practice (e.g., using data collected over a fixed time period and displayed using one of the CQI tools discussed earlier in this chapter—such as the run chart example presented in Figure 4.3).

Sampling Considerations

Primary data analyses can involve collection of all available data for a fixed amount of time, as was done in the case study presented earlier, but quite often, the use of primary data is based on scientific sampling methods. In either case, a clearly defined sampling strategy is a first step.

Any sampling strategy that is used should start with a clear definition of the measures to be selected and the specific sampling methodology that is to be used to select patients or subjects. Two common methodologies in health care are probability (random) sampling and judgement sampling. Also important, especially when process behavior charts involving time-series displays of data are required, is defining how often sample elements will be collected.

Perla, Provost, and Murray present two important concepts, based on the previous work of CQI pioneers, Deming and Shewhart, which provide guidance for sampling in improvement projects:

1. Obtaining just enough data based on past experience to guide our learning in the future.

2. Making full use of subject matter expertise in selecting the most appropriate samples. (2013, p. 37)

Following these guidelines, CQI data are often drawn from judgement or purposive samples. This differs from the types of sampling methods that are used when the goal is to make predictions or derive estimates about large populations, as is the case with probability sampling. Judgement sampling is used in CQI and in health care applications beyond CQI, such as the selection of patients who meet specific entry criteria in clinical trials, by experienced clinical investigators. Judgement sampling is applicable to CQI when collecting data to measure improvement because such data often come from ongoing processes where we rarely have a fixed population of interest, but instead have a population that is changing over time. In process improvement studies, subject matter experts can be relied upon to choose areas, times of the day, or segments of the population to best represent the process being studied for CQI purposes. (Perla, Provost, & Murray, 2013) When random sampling is being used, for example to measure patient satisfaction, the first step is to carefully identify the sampling frame, defined as the source of data for the key elements that are to be analyzed and from which a sample is to be taken in order to make inferences about the larger population of interest, such as the medical care database from the institution whose quality we are assessing. Also critical to successful sampling strategies is careful determination of sample size. Sample size is always important because it plays a role in determining precision of estimates of quality metrics and also directly affects study cost estimates (Levy & Lemeshow, 2008).

Also important in probability sampling is estimating the prevalence of the measures being studied:

Our experience is that the first thing that often happens is that the designers overestimate the prevalence of the phenomenon being studied and hence underestimate the cost of finding enough affected individuals. When the recruitment of participants lags, the perception that the budget is fixed leads to a reduction in those cases surveyed, often jeopardizing what conclusions might be reached. The team must test those prevalence assumptions early on and plan realistically; one of the ways this can be accomplished is through the use of smaller "pilot" studies prior to carrying out the final survey. Interorganizational access to data could make the task of assessing prevalence much easier as well. (McLaughlin & Kibbe, 2013, p. 346)

Whether probability or judgement sampling is used to select primary data an important data quality concern is consideration of "non-sampling" errors (those that cannot be controlled by traditional sample design and statistical analysis adjustments). One very important example of this type of error that is quite prevalent in health care surveys, such as those used to measure patient satisfaction, is non-response (i.e., when the number who respond to a survey is smaller than the number selected to be studies). High levels of non-response can lead to selection bias and under-representation of the patients intended to be surveyed, sometimes also compromising the power of any statistical or process behavior analysis to be carried out based on these data. Quite simply, if a sample of patients is selected, and patients are contacted to provide feedback on patient care they have received, the data derived from such a survey will only be useful if a high response rate is obtained. This fact is true for all types of scientific surveys, but especially health surveys, including those that used to assess and improve quality of care.

An example of this phenomenon in large health care institutions is the use of patient satisfaction surveys, such as those conducted by the Press Ganey organization, which partners with more than 50% of U.S. hospitals to improve health and business outcomes (Press Ganey Associates, Inc., 2017; Wake Forest–Baptist Health, 2016). Measuring patient satisfaction is an important way to ensure a customer focus, a basic tenet of CQI in health care, and such efforts are to be applauded. But two key factors to pay close attention to in these efforts to measure patient satisfaction are adequacy of sample size and consideration/control of non-response. For example, Wake Forest Baptist Hospital in North Carolina, which has earned a "Press Ganey Seal of Integrity" reports that the patient survey results in their organization are based on a random selection of outpatients who receive questionnaires via regular mail or email within a few weeks of their appointments. They also report that the target sample size for computing individual provider ratings is 30, and that the average response rate is 18%, which varies by specialty. Results are posted on-line as part of provider profiles, unless fewer than 30 responses are received, in which case it is the provider's choice as to whether results will be posted. One reason given for this procedure is that it is recognized that smaller sample sizes will lead to high variability in ratings due to extreme values (Wake Forest–Baptist Health, 2016). It may be assumed that this survey process and these numbers are similar for other large hospital systems. A first step to consider when evaluating the knowledge gained from such a survey process, especially for CQI, is to determine whether the response rate is sufficient to make quality of care decisions. While a target of 100% response is a goal, it is not achievable in most cases, so the question remains: What is an acceptable response rate? The answer to this question will vary depending on the decision to be made and should include relevant team members and the use of tools such as those described earlier in this chapter. For example, if survey response rates are considered to be inadequate, then a cause-and-effect analysis may be considered as a way to understand and increase response rates. Also important to consider are other forms of non-response, such as selective responses, which may not be representative of true patient satisfaction—for example, if those who do respond had an extreme experience, whether superb or terrible.

In addition to response rate issues sample size must also be considered before making decisions related to quality of care. For example, when target sample sizes are not achieved, unacceptably high margins of error may invalidate conclusions based on survey data and especially comparisons over time or between departments or providers (Zusman, 2012). Decisions based on patient survey results also require careful consideration of the limits of the data and possible confounding factors that may influence findings; for example, there have been reports of physicians' employment and income being threatened based on poor satisfaction scores and some assertions that patient satisfaction scoring actually leads to poorer quality of care due to some providers altering medical treatment to influence patient satisfaction scores (Zusman, 2012). These examples underline how important it is important to consider both the source of the data being collected in measuring quality and also how the results are used; attention to detail on both extremes—data collection and decision making—is critical.

Despite some criticism of patient satisfaction surveys, their use is increasing, which creates opportunities for continuous improvement. There is a current trend to increase the use of patient satisfaction and spurred by the Patient Protection and Affordable Care Act (ACA) and other legislation attempts to improve and expand such processes are underway. For example, an improved patient satisfaction survey that is being used and is tied to hospital reimbursement is the Hospital Consumer Assessment of Health Care Providers and Systems (HCAHPS; Zusman, 2012).

In summary, the widespread use of patient satisfaction surveys and associated criticisms lead to an important conclusion relative to this chapter and the use of primary survey data in CQI. The key point to be taken from this discussion is not to demean the efforts of measuring patient satisfaction; but in the same way that process improvement actions should only be taken when there is evidence of special cause variation, the same advice applies to only taking action based on surveys of (patients or providers) when data sources are proven to be reliable and high quality and are sufficient to support the level of decisions to which they are being applied. It is important for those who make use of survey data to carefully consider the basic principles of measurement and understanding variation before taking actions and whenever possible use knowledge gained to improve processes, including survey methodology processes.

Secondary Data

Secondary data are data that are collected for purposes other than the specific process performance or improvement initiative that is of interest. Especially with the broad availability of data that can be accessed via the internet and with a proper investment in Health Information Technology (HIT) secondary data have become and will continue to be very useful for carrying out CQI initiatives. Secondary data sources that can support CQI include data registries and claims data. One rich source of claims data represents information available as part of the Medicare program, administered by the Centers for Medicare and Medicaid Services (CMS; McLaughlin & Kibbe, 2013). Although claims data have been frequently criticized for poor quality in the past, more recently, CMS has implemented a number of innovative approaches to drive quality improvement at the national level. These include adopting the use and promoting the development of standard quality measures, public reporting of quality measures, and pay-for-performance efforts to reward physicians for providing better

🔍 *QIO EXAMPLE: CLEMSON NURSING HOME*

An example of how QIOs utilize CMS data to carry out CQI can be seen in the case of Clemson's nursing home. This 95-bed, family-owned nursing home, located in the foothills of North Carolina, was attempting to reduce restraint use in its facility. Clemson received an invitation from the state QIO to participate in a restraint-reduction quality improvement initiative. Using data from all nursing homes in the state (available through the CMS "Minimum Data Set (MDS)" reporting system), the QIO provided Clemson with graphs illustrating that its restraint use was higher than the state and national averages, ranking them as having the fourth highest restraint use rate among nursing homes in the initiative. Working with the QIO, Clemson conducted a root-cause analysis (Ross, 2014) and identified several opportunities for reducing restraints. Testing new processes using PDSA cycles over a period of several weeks, Clemson was able to reduce restraint use from 10% to 6% and ultimately achieved its goal of 3% by the end of the initiative (Schenck, McArdle, & Weiser, 2013, p. 435).

Further details on this example can also be found in a case study (Rokoske, McArdle, & Schenck, 2012) included in our previously published casebook (McLaughlin, Johnson, & Sollecito, 2012).

quality care (McLaughlin & Kibbe, 2013), Quality Improvement Organizations (QIOs), are Medicare's primary agents for carrying out quality improvement initiatives using CMS (secondary) data sources (Schenck, McArdle, & Weiser, 2013). With a presence in every state and most federal territories, QIOs have been called "the nation's main infrastructure for quality improvement" (Hsia, 2003).

Electronic Health Records

An important source of secondary data that is being used more frequently to carry out CQI studies is electronic health records (EHR). Over 90% of hospitals and physician practices now have some form of EHR systems in place. The ubiquity of EHRs is primarily due to the American Recovery and Reinvestment Act of 2009 (ARRA). ARRA established incentive payments to promote the adoption and meaningful use of interoperable HIT and EHRs. Beginning in 2011, the Medicare and Medicaid Electronic Health Record Incentive Programs were established to encourage eligible professionals and eligible hospitals to adopt, implement, upgrade (AIU), and demonstrate meaningful use of certified EHR technology.

Meaningful use is using certified EHR technology to:

- Improve quality, safety, efficiency, and reduce health disparities
- Engage patients and family
- Improve care coordination, and population and public health
- Maintain privacy and security of patient health information

Meaningful Use was implemented in 3 stages.

- Stage 1 (2011–2012) set the foundation for the EHR Incentive Programs by establishing requirements for the electronic capture of clinical data, including providing patients with electronic copies of health information.
- Stage 2 (2014) expanded upon the Stage 1 criteria with a focus on ensuring that the meaningful use of EHRs supported the aims and priorities of the National Quality Strategy. Stage 2 criteria encouraged the use of HIT for CQI at the point of care and the exchange of information in the most structured format possible.
- In October 2015, CMS released a final rule that specifies criteria that eligible

professionals, eligible hospitals and critical access hospitals (CAHs) must meet in order to participate in the EHR Incentive Programs in 2015 through 2017 (Modified Stage 2) and in Stage 3 in 2017 and beyond (CDC, 2017; CMS, 2017a; CMS, 2015a).

CMS has also provided guidance on the choice and use of clinical measures in EHRs through the definition of clinical quality measures (CQMs) that can be used to carry out CQI.

CQMs are tools that help measure and track the quality of health care services provided by eligible professionals, eligible hospitals and critical access hospitals (CAHs) within our health care system. These measures use data associated with providers' ability to deliver high-quality care or relate to long term goals for quality health care. CQMs measure many aspects of patient care including:

- health outcomes
- clinical processes
- patient safety
- efficient use of health care resources
- care coordination
- patient engagements
- population and public health
- adherence to clinical guidelines

(CMS, 2015b; 2017b).

Ultimately, it is hoped that the meaningful use compliance and the use of CQMs will result in better clinical outcomes, improved population health outcomes, increased transparency and efficiency, empowered individuals and more robust research data on health systems.

Most recently, the widespread use of EHRs provides a new source of secondary data that has many useful characteristics for CQI applications, especially in large health systems where direct access to patient data via

primary data collection methods may be costly or infeasible for other reasons.

EHR systems can be very useful especially in large health care systems, because of features such as interoperability, linking patient care across multiple institutions, and the ability to capture details of interactions between providers and patients with linkages to various forms of health indicators (e.g., laboratory results). However, it is most important to recognize that most EHR systems were not designed for the purpose of carrying out detailed analyses required for CQI tools and techniques and although they may include predefined metrics and summaries via "dashboards" these data may not provide the level of specificity needed to meet specific process measurement and improvement requirements. Once again, we advise that wherever CQI studies are not based on primary data collected for the specific purposes of the process evaluation/improvement study of interest, caution must be applied to understand knowledge gained and specifically sources of variation before taking actions.

▶ Conclusions

This chapter described the importance of measurement concepts in CQI. Most important is understanding variation and, in particular, understanding the distinction between special and common causes of variation and how this understanding determines the most appropriate action for improvement. It has been illustrated that the most effective way to understand process variation is to plot data over time, preferably, on a control chart/process behavior chart. Once the appropriate improvement strategy is determined, then the use of CQI tools described here together with other methodologies described in this text (e.g., PDSA, is recommended). A case study designed to facilitate classroom discussion and published data examples have been presented to illustrate the application of these methodologies. This chapter also provided a brief overview of primary and secondary data sources that are a critical input to the "data-to-decision" cycle that is applicable to assessing and improving process performance, with a brief review of the strengths and weaknesses of various data sources, relative to CQI applications.

This chapter has not attempted to exhaustively cover the broad range of topics associated with CQI tools and techniques. In addition to the material presented here, readers are urged to consult other resources referred to throughout this chapter as well as other chapters in this text; for example, Chapter 3, which discusses implementation science and Chapter 5, which addresses LEAN/Six Sigma methodology.

References

Agency for Healthcare Research and Quality (AHRQ). (2016). Patient safety network–glossary. Retrieved October 1, 2017, from http://psnet.ahrq.gov

American Society for Quality. (2017). The 7 basic quality tools for process improvement. Retrieved September 19, 2017, from http://asq.org/

Balestracci, D. (2009). *Data sanity: A quantum leap to unprecedented results.* Englewood, CO: Medical Group Management Association.

Berwick, D. M. (1991). Controlling variation in health care: A consultation from Walter Shewhart. *Medical Care, 29*, 1212–1225.

Berwick, D. M. (1996). A primer on leading the improvement of systems. *British Medical Journal, 312*, 619–622.

Bialek, R., Duffy, G. L., & Moran, J. W. (2009). *The public health quality improvement handbook.* Milwaukee, WI: ASQ Quality Press.

Bodenheimer, T., & Sinsky, C. (2014). From triple to Quadruple Aim: Care of the patient requires care of the provider. *Annals of Family Medicine, 12*(6), 573–576.

Bosk, C. L., Dixon-Woods, M., Goeschel, C. A., & Pronovost, P. J. (2009). The art of medicine—Reality check for checklists. *The Lancet, 374*, 444–445.

Breland, C. E. (2012). Forthright Medical Center: Social marketing and the surgical checklist. In C. P. McLaughlin, J. K. Johnson, & W. A. Sollecito. *Implementing continuous quality improvement in health care: A global casebook.* Sudbury, MA: Jones & Bartlett Learning.

Carey, R. G., & Lloyd, R. C. (2001). *Measuring quality improvement in healthcare: A guide to statistical control applications.* Milwaukee, WI: American Society for Quality Press.

Crosby, P. B. (1979). *Quality is free—The art of making quality certain.* New York, NY: Mentor.

Centers for Disease Control and Prevention (CDC). (2017). Meaningful use. Retrieved September 30, 2017, from https://www.cdc.gov

Centers for Medicare and Medicaid Services (CMS). (2015a). Medicare and Medicaid Programs; Electronic Health Record Incentive Program-Stage 3 and Modifications to Meaningful Use in 2015 through 2017. *Federal Register* 80 FR 62761. Retrieved September 19, 2017, from https://www.federalregister.gov

Centers for Medicare and Medicaid Services (CMS). (2015b). Clinical quality measures basics. Retrieved September 17, 2017, from https://www.cms.gov

Centers for Medicare and Medicaid Services (CMS). (2017a). Electronic health records incentive programs. Retrieved September 17, 2017, from https://www.cms.gov

Centers for Medicare and Medicaid Services (CMS). (2017b). Annual updates to eCQM specifications. Retrieved September 17, 2017, from https://www.cms.gov

Deming, W. E. (1986). *Out of the crisis.* Cambridge, MA: Massachusetts Institute of Technology Center for Advanced Engineering Study.

Deming, W. E. (1993). *The new economics for industry, government, education.* Cambridge, MA: Massachusetts Institute of Technology Center for Advanced Engineering Study.

Dixon-Woods, M., Martin, G. P. (2016). Does quality improvement improve quality? *Future Healthcare Journal, 3*(3), 191–194.

Donabedian, A. (1980). *Explorations in quality assessment and monitoring: Vol. 1—The definition of quality and approaches to its assessment.* Chicago, IL: Health Administration Press.

Gawande, A. (2009). *The checklist manifesto.* New York, NY: Metropolitan Books.

Gold, M. (2004). Geographic variation in Medicare per capita spending: Should policymakers be concerned? Research Synthesis Report No. 6. Princeton, NJ: The Robert Wood Johnson Foundation.

Grove, A. S. 1995. *High Output Management.* New York, NY: Vintage Books.

Haynes, A. B., Weiser, T. G., Berry, W. R., Lipsitz S. R., Breizat A. H., Dellinger E. P., ... Safe Surgery Saves Lives Study Group. (2009). A surgery safety checklist to reduce morbidity and mortality in a global population. *The New England Journal of Medicine, 360*, 491–499.

Hsia, D. C. (2003). Medicare quality improvement: Bad apples or bad systems? *Journal of the American Medical Association, 289*(20), 2648.

Institute of Medicine (IOM). (2000). *To err is human: Building a safer health system.* Washington, D.C.: National Academies Press.

Ishikawa, K. (1987). *Guide to quality control* (trans. Asian Productivity Organization). White Plains, NY: Kraus International Publications.

Juran, J. (1988). *Juran on planning for quality.* New York, NY: Free Press.

Kilbridge, P., & Classen, D. (2002). *Surveillance for adverse drug events: history, methods, and current issues* (pp. 1–35). VHA Research Series. Irving, TX: VHA, Inc.

Langley, G. J., Moen, R. D., Nolan, K. M., Nolan, T. W., Norman, C. L., & Provost, L. P. (2009). *Improvement guide: A practical approach to enhancing organizational performance,* 2nd ed. San Francisco, CA: Jossey-Bass.

Levy, P. S., & Lemeshow, S. (2008). *Sampling of populations—methods and applications,* 4th ed. Hoboken, NJ: Wiley and Sons.

Lighter, D. E., & Fair, D. C. (2004). *Principles and methods of quality management in health care.* Sudbury, MA: Jones and Bartlett Publishers.

Lloyd, R. C. (2019). *Quality health care, a guide to developing and using indicators,* 2nd ed. Burlington, MA: Jones & Bartlett Learning.

Loshin, D. L. (2011). *The practitioners' guide to data quality improvement.* New York, NY: Morgan Kaufman OMG Press.

McLaughlin, C. P. (1996). Why variation reduction is not everything: A new paradigm for service operations. *International Journal of Service Industry Management, 7*(3), 17–30.

McLaughlin, C. P., Johnson, J. K., & Sollecito, W. A. (2012). *Implementing continuous quality improvement in health care: A global casebook.* Sudbury, MA: Jones & Bartlett Learning.

McLaughlin, C. P., & Kaluzny A. D. (Eds.). (2006). *Continuous quality improvement in health care,* 3rd ed. Sudbury, MA: Jones and Bartlett Publishers.

McLaughlin, C. P., & Kibbe, D. C. (2013). The role of health information technology in quality improvement. In W. A. Sollecito and J. K. Johnson (eds.) *Continuous quality improvement in health care,* 4th ed. Sudbury, MA: Jones and Bartlett Publishers.

Nelson, E. C., Splaine, M. E., Batalden, P. B., & Plume SK. (1998). Building measurement and data collection into medical practice. *Annals of Internal Medicine, 128,* 460–466.

Nolan, T. W., & Provost, L. P. (1990). Understanding variation. *Quality Progress, 23*(5), 70–78.

Nolan, T. W., Provost, L. P., & Perla, R. J. (2016). Understanding variation—26 years later. *Quality Progress,* November 2016, 28–37. Retrieved September 17, 2017, from https://healthleadsusa.org

Office of the Inspector General. (2010). Adverse events in hospitals: Methods for identifying events. Washington, DC: Department of Health and Human Services, OEI-06-08-00221. As cited in Landrigan, C. P., Parry, G. J., Bones, C. B., Hackbarth A. D., Goldmann D. A., & Sharek P. J. (2010). *The New England Journal of Medicine, 363*(22), 2124–2134.

Perla, R. J., Provost, L. P., & Murray, S. K. (2011). The run chart: a simple analytical tool for learning from variation in healthcare processes. *BMJ Quality and Safety, 20,* 46–51.

Perla, R. J., Provost, L. P., & Murray, S. K. (2013). Sampling considerations for health care improvement. *Quality Management in Health Care, 22*(1), 36–47.

Press Ganey Associates, Inc. (2017). Outpatient. Retrieved September 30, 2017, from http://www.pressganey.com.

Project Management Institute. (2017). *A guide to the project management body of knowledge, (PMBOK; 6th ed.)* Newtown Square, PA: PMI Publications.

Pronovost, P. J., Goeschel, C. A., Olsen, K. L., Pham, J. C., Miller, M. R., Berenholtz, S. M., ... Clancy, C. M. (2009). Reducing health care hazards: Lessons from the commercial aviation safety team. *Health Affairs, 283,* w479–w489.

Pronovost, P. J., Needham, D., Berenholtz, S., Sinopoli, D., Chu, H., Cosgrove, S., ... Goeschel, C. (2006). An intervention to reduce catheter-related bloodstream infections in the ICU. *The New England Journal of Medicine, 355,* 2725–2732.

Rokoske, F., McArdle, J. A., & Schenck, A. P. (2012). Clemson's nursing home: Working with the state quality improvement organization's restraint reduction initiative. In C. P. McLaughlin, J. K. Johnson, & W. A. Sollecito. *Implementing continuous quality improvement in health care: A global casebook.* Sudbury, MA: Jones & Bartlett Learning.

Ross, T. K. (2014). *Health care quality management—tools and applications.* San Francisco, CA: Jossey-Bass.

R Development Core Team. (2014). *R: A language and environment for statistical computing.* R Foundation for Statistical Computing, Vienna, Austria. Retrieved April 26, 2018, from http://www.R-project.org

Schenck, A. P., McArdle, J., & Weiser, R. (2013). Quality improvement organizations and continuous quality improvement in Medicare. In W. A. Sollecito & J. K. Johnson (Eds.), *Continuous quality improvement in health care,* 4th ed. Sudbury, MA: Jones and Bartlett Publishers.

Shewhart, W. A. (1931). *Economic control of quality of manufactured product.* New York, NY: D. Van Nostrand Company.

Sikka, R., Morath, J. M., & Leape, L. (2015). The Quadruple Aim: care health, cost and meaning in work. *BMJ*

Quality and Safety, 24, 608–610. Retrieved October 6, 2017, from http://qualitysafety.bmj.com

Spath, P. L., & Kelly, D. L. (2017). *Applying quality management in healthcare: A systems approach,* 4th ed. Chicago, IL: Health Administration Press.

Streibel, B. J., Sholtes, P. R., & Joiner, B. L. (2003). *The team handbook,* 3rd ed. Madison, WI: Joiner/Oriel, Inc.

SQC Online. (2017). Online statistical calculators for acceptance sampling and quality control. Retrieved August 17, 2017, from https://www.sqconline.com

Wake Forest–Baptist Health. (2016). About the Press Ganey satisfaction survey. Retrieved July 11, 2017, from http://www.wajkehealth.edu

Wheeler, D. J. (2000). *Understanding variation: The key to managing chaos,* 2nd ed. Knoxville, TN: SPC Press.

Wheeler, D. J. (February 1, 2010). Individual charts done right and wrong. *Quality Digest.* Retrieved October 1, 2017, from https://www.qualitydigest.com

Wheeler, D. J., & Chambers, D. S. (2010). *Understanding statistical process control,* 3rd ed. Knoxville, TN: SPC Press.

Zusman, E. (2012). NCAHPS replaces Press Ganey as quality measure for patient hospital experience. *Neurosurgery, 71*(2), N21–N24. Retrieved August 12, 2017, from www.neurosurger-online.com

CHAPTER 5

Lean and Six Sigma Management: Building a Foundation for Optimal Patient Care Using Patient Flow Physics

Ed Popovich, Hal Wiggin, and Paul Barach

The ultimate arrogance is to change the way people work, without changing the way we manage them.

— **John Toussaint**

High-performing health care organizations differentiate themselves by focusing relentlessly on improving their service and performance and are guided by process-improvement initiatives to advance patient care. Continuous quality improvement offers a powerful way of thinking about how to transform clinical operations and health care teams. Continuous Quality Improvement (CQI), Lean Management Systems (LMS), and Lean Six Sigma (LSS) are philosophies and methods for leadership, management, improvement, and innovation. They offer an approach, a set of tools, and a way of thinking about how to more effectively study, assess, and improve clinical flow, including addressing and reducing variations in processes and operations. LMS and LSS are also broadly generalizable to other health applications such as public health (see Chapter 11) and a broad array of settings, including applying CQI in resource poor countries (see Chapter 13). For illustrative purposes, the primary focus of this chapter will be on traditional health care delivery systems in developed countries.

▶ Lean and Six Sigma Management Defined

Six Sigma, as its name implies (sigma being the Greek symbol used in statistics to measure variation), utilizes statistical methods to identify and reduce variation in processes (Duffy, Farmer, & Moran, 2009). (See Chapter 4 for a detailed description of types and causes of variability.)

In 1986, when Motorola originated and launched the continuous improvement and innovation effort they called *Six Sigma*, it was an evolution of quality methods that originated in in the United States and Japan that then further developed at Motorola. The U.S. and Japanese quality leaders, followed by other companies, learned from each other as they further evolved systems of quality management. Ford Motor Company developed mass production systems that Toyota developed further into the Toyota Production System (TPS) through their emphasis on elimination of waste, which they termed *muda, muri,* and *mura* (Muda, muri, mura—Toyota production system guide, 2013).

Muda: Wasting Resources

Muda is the waste due to nonvalue-added activities, which was translated back by companies in the United States as elimination of waste in the use of seven resources: transportation, inventory, motion during production, waiting time spent during production, over-processing (by doing more than necessary), over-production (by producing more products or items than needed), and defects, such as producing faulty parts or making mistakes in the process. Often, the focus of the Lean Management System (LMS) in health care is reducing *muda*, especially with respect to waiting time experienced by patients, mistakes or "near misses" in patient care, transitions in patient care due to transportation

and/or motion in moving patients between care providers or services, and managing inventory of equipment and supplies. Thus, examples of waste in health care include wasted inventory, rework, excess waiting time—whether by patients or staff members who need results of another provider's inputs to make decisions—lost time, errors, or extra work associated with poor processing of information or outdated procedures, and waste from transporting patients unnecessarily (Spath & Kelly, 2017).

Muri: Overburdening Staff and Equipment

Muri is the waste due to over-burdening the people or equipment in the process, as processes that are balanced are desirable. Less-than-optimal attention paid to *muri* in health care often is evident when physicians and staff feel overwhelmed with the level of effort required for them to provide patient care, document the care provided, address regulatory reporting requirements, attend required meetings, and provide all the support beyond the effort required for patient care. Burnout is experienced by many physicians and health care providers. Improving the balance of processes is an imperative in patient care delivery.

Mura: Uneven Process Workflow

Mura is the waste due to unevenness in the process workflow. *Mura* is the reason for the development of "just-in-time" production systems so that the process flow is more predictable and consistent. In health care, the desire to "get things off your plate" and send it to the next function in the process is common. In other words, rather than providing each person what is needed at the time it is needed, there is a tendency to batch up work and then send it in "one pile" to the next step in the process. Examples include batch reading of radiology exams rather than reading the exam at the time the patient is present and providing the results for each individual patient as they progress their patient care process. Morning blood draws in an acute care setting are another example, as the blood is drawn and sent to pathology in batches to do the analyses.

How Six Sigma Originated

Motorola was very much aware of the quality methodology practiced in Japan, including just-in-time processing, *POKA-YOKE* ("fool-proofing processes"), process simplification, and continuous improvement by all staff (Harry, 1998). They observed that efficient and effective process flow through the elimination or reduction of nonvalued-added processing could not only reduce the number of errors or defects in production, but it also could increase the consistency of performance of the process. Motorola decided to select skilled staff with technical backgrounds and train them in advanced quality, engineering, manufacturing, and statistical methodology, which in turn facilitated their ability to improve or innovate the design of both their products and work processes. Motorola established two improvement goals as part of what they defined as their Total Customer Satisfaction (TCS) strategy:

1. All defects were to be reduced 10-fold every 2 years, which implies a 68% improvement per year. For example, a process yielding a success rate of 90% is expected to perform at 96.8% success rate at the end of Year 1, and 99% at the end of Year 2. Note that in the 2 years, the failure rate would be expected to drop from 10% to 1%, which is a 10-fold improvement.
2. All core processes must reduce their cycle time (lead time) by 50% within 2 years.

To achieve these goals, Motorola recognized that:

- Variation in process performance can lead to greater defect/error rates. Therefore, a reduction in process variation can induce a lower rate of defects, where a defect was defined as the failure of a process to achieve its goals.
- Speeding up processes requires the elimination of unnecessary (e.g., nonvalue-added) tasks or steps since simply doing the same steps faster in order to achieve a 50% reduction in cycle time often will drive more defects while overwhelming workers and which violates the simultaneous goal of a reduction in defect rates.

In 1990, the term "Lean Production" received attention due to the book *The Machine That Changed the World* by James Womack, Daniel Jones, and Daniel Roos. The authors explained that mass production systems emanating from Toyota via Ford and other companies were evolving into a coherent narrative that enabled systems requiring less time for production, less effort from people, lower inventories of supplies, and less capital investment. Remarkably, this new system of work could yield fewer defects, yet it was able to better mass customize by serving smaller and smaller market sizes at lower costs.

In 1996, Womack & Jones published *Lean Thinking*, which distilled the LMS theory into five principles:

1. The customer defines value.
2. Organizations should identify the value stream in every process and seek to eliminate all wasted steps that do not add value.
3. Organizations should make the product (or, in health care, management of the patient's care) flow through the steps of the value-added process continuously.
4. Organizations need subsequent steps in the process that "pull"

products (or patients) from the previous steps rather than push them forward, causing them to batch up waiting for the next step.

5. Organizations should work to continuously improve in order to reduce steps, time, costs, and the information (data) needed to serve the customer (again, the patient in our case; Anthony, Palsuk, Gupta, Mishra, & Barach, 2018).

It was not until the later 1990s that consultants decided to call the time-based techniques "Lean," although these methods had already been incorporated into Motorola's two simultaneous goals of the Six Sigma program. The more technical analyses that incorporated variation and defect reduction were called Six Sigma by many, rather than the more encompassing meaning behind Six Sigma as envisioned by Motorola. Motorola viewed what later became called LMS and Six Sigma as separate management activities that were "two sides of the same coin," which they simply called Six Sigma. For example, having fewer steps to accomplish the same process leads to fewer steps in which to make errors, less variation across the process, and ultimately to better, cheaper, and faster processes.

Michael George is one of the people credited with popularizing the term "Lean Six Sigma." Acknowledging this "two sides of the same coin," he wrote (George, 2002, p. 7):

Lean Six Sigma is a methodology that maximizes shareholder value by achieving the fastest rate of customer satisfaction, cost, quality, process speed, and invested capital. The fusion of LMS and Six Sigma is required because:

- LMS cannot bring a process under statistical control.
- Six Sigma alone cannot dramatically improve process speed or reduce invested capital.

Thomas L. Jackson and Karen R. Jones note that organizations cannot incorporate a LMS overnight. More specifically (Jackson & Jones, 1996, pp. 7–8),

To support lean production, management must build, nurture, and support the logic and machinery that drives lean production. Lean Management is actually a sophisticated practice built around several key conceptual and physical tools. It is about looking at your company in an entirely different way, describing its processes with *a new vocabulary*. The process that delivers lean management has been designed, tested, and refined into what we call the lean management system. This system reflects the principles and methodologies of leading international managers and consultants.

"Lean Six Sigma" (LSS) adoption in health care and public health represents an evolution resulting in part from alliances and interchanges with corporate and government partners, and it promoted the evolution of CQI across several industries (Duffy, Farmer, & Moran, 2009). The combination of LMS and Six Sigma is now being used in a wide range of health care applications, and provides a synergistic methodology for analyzing, and reducing or eliminating waste in health care processes.

The following sections of this chapter will define these methodologies in greater detail by describing their use in health care settings and, in particular, by illustrating patient flow LMS applications.

Patient Flow as an Application of LSS

Organizations that focus on improving value-added activities can develop a strategic and competitive advantage (Byrne, 2013, p. xi).

Improving process "flow" is one of the primary goals of LSS and CQI. A value stream or process with optimum flow would be analogous to a river that cascades over a cliff and rages through a narrow gorge, flowing downhill with no bends, rocks, or other impediments. This is akin to a clinic with high patient flow and demand that has the right number of highly skilled staff working with patients to meet their care needs using well-designed processes that have minimal waste (Sanchez & Barach, 2012). Staff are patient-focused leaders who manage with the "right" data, and they empower staff to continuously improve the workplace as they deliver exceptional care.

With the advent of the 21st century, there have been discernable improvements in the efficiency and effectiveness of care in some settings, including broader applications of what has been called the Triple Aim of Health Care: improving (1) the experience of care and (2) population health while (3) reducing costs (Berwick, Nolan, & Whittington, 2008). However, despite this progress, patients still experience unacceptable harm; processes are not as efficient as they could be; and costs continue to rise at alarming rates, while quality issues remain. The key to ensuring CQI in health care organizations is changing organizational culture, as discussed in Chapter 2. Organizations seeking to be efficient and effective in care delivery need to embed a culture that identifies wasteful effort, seek ways to continually improve existing processes, and design processes for those that do not currently exist in order to increase efficiency and effectiveness in meeting their outcomes with no wasted effort. Womack and Jones correctly observed that "… patients often discover that the time spent on treatment was a tiny fraction of the time you spent going through the "process." Mostly you were sitting and waiting ("patient" is clearly the right word), or moving about to the next step in the diagnosis and treatment…" (2003, p. 50).

If waiting is a nonvalue-adding activity, why do most health care facilities incorporate a formal "waiting" room into their care delivery processes? When flow is attained and information, materials, and activity proceed seamlessly through processes without interruption, then optimal experiences can occur. This is more likely to happen if leaders ensure "rules that require the learning of skills, they set up goals, they provide feedback, and they make control possible. They facilitate concentration and involvement by making the activity as distinct as possible from the so-called paramount reality of everyday existence" (Csikszentmihalyi, 1990, p. 72).

This "ideal state" can be approached and accomplished in real terms by integrating the principals that govern patient flow and variation management—we call it *patient flow physics*, a nod to the universality of the physical rules that govern the universe and LMS. As presented in this chapter, this powerful gestalt can greatly increase the achievement of key process core measures in health care. (Readers are also referred to similar concepts related to time management that are illustrated by control chart analyses of a clinic start up time in Chapter 4.) We begin the discussion with two real-world examples, the first from an emergency department (ED), and the second from an ambulatory screening mammography clinic.

Applying LSS to Patient Flow in Community Hospital Emergency Department

In 2004, one of the authors (EP) was a Vice President for Enterprise Excellence (outside health care, this position is often termed an operational excellence leader) at a non-profit private hospital, where he sought to improve both the patient flow in the ED and the women's mammography service lines. The hospital was located in a wealthy south Florida community that supported the hospital through a large foundation. The board was concerned about reports from some wealthy benefactors that the waiting times to see a physician in the ED were too long. EDs are often called the "front door" to the hospital, in that approximately 65% of patients admitted to the hospital arrive via the ED. Long wait times at various times of the day in the ED lead to patient and family dissatisfaction, frustration by staff and the community, and in turn may lead to reducing charitable donations to a hospital foundation.

One of the authors (EP) was involved in the early days of the evolution of LSS at Motorola and had the opportunity to learn about the use of a concept called Factory Physics™. Although LSS was recognized as a philosophy for process improvement and design, it was in its early days of being utilized by hospital systems. Factory Physics describes the "laws" that govern patient process flow much like physics is a science describing the "laws" that govern the forces on

physical materials in our world. Factory Physics modeling was used to improve the understanding of patient flow through the ED from the time the physician first encountered the patient until a decision was made as to whether to discharge the patient to go home ("treat-to-street" cycle time) or to admit the patient to the hospital ("doctor-to-decision" cycle time). In addition, the time between when a decision was made until the patient left the ED to go home or was moved to an in-patient room was termed the "decision-to-disposition" cycle time. At a high level, patient demand in the ED was addressed by representing the number of patients presenting to the ED at each hour of the day and at each day of the week, as shown in **FIGURE 5.1**.

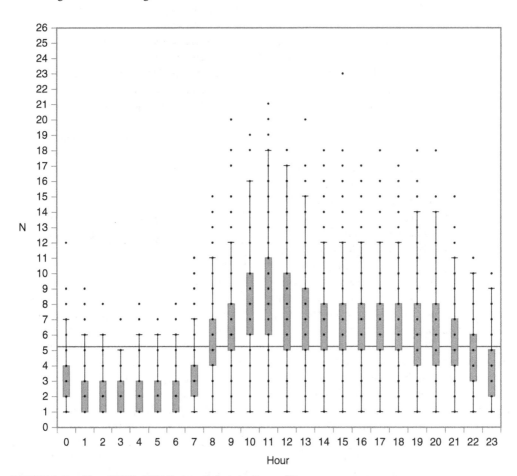

FIGURE 5.1 Box Plot of 2002–2005 Patient Arrivals by Hour of Day

John Tukey introduced the box-and-whiskers plot (aka box plot) as part of his toolkit for exploratory data analysis (Tukey, 1977). The box plot is a compact distributional summary, displaying less detail than a histogram but also taking up less space. Box plots use robust summary statistics and actual data points and they are easy to compute and interpret. They are especially useful for comparing distributions across groups.

Figure 5.1 shows a box plot of patient arrivals to this community hospital by the hour of the day. Each box has a median line in the box that represents the 50th percentile (median) number of arrivals for each hour. The bottom of the box represents the 25th percentile, and the top of the box represents the 75th percentile of patient arrivals each hour. The distant points (outliers) outside the box represent the range of patient arrivals each hour, with those points that are larger than the top of the lines extending from each box representing outliers in the number of patient arrivals that seldom occur but were observed over the period of 2002–2005.

Distinct, daily patterns in patient arrivals were discovered, i.e., days of the week had hourly arrival patterns that were similar from week to week. Knowing the demand patterns helps a health care administrator be better prepared to address the demand. Some of the emerging questions included:

1. How does this demand pattern support decisions and lead to more effective staffing up- and downstream?
2. What are the optimal levels of staffing to meet patient demand?
3. Does the nature of the demand vary over the course of the day?
4. Are there certain "chief complaints" or issues that are seen more often during a certain time of the day or on particular days of the week?
5. Does the type of staff skills needed differ at various times of the day or on certain days of the week?
6. What should the organization do, if anything, to be prepared to handle the variation and demand outliers including during mass casualty or pandemic events?

If the organization is only staffed for the median hourly demand, then 50% of the time, the demand will be greater than expected. This can contribute to increased waiting times and dissatisfaction by patients that choose to stay and wait. Of course, some patients may choose to leave and go elsewhere rather than wait, which may lead to increased patient risk and lowered facility revenue and may undermine the organization's reputation.

Further, the study of time, day, and primary clinical issues of patients that were admitted yielded information about the demand on each floor and unit of the hospital. For example, often hospitals have rules for discharging patients (e.g., all patients going home on a certain day are to be discharged by 2 PM). Unfortunately, the data indicated that the demand for beds within the hospital from patients admitted by the ED did not synchronize with the 2 PM discharge goal. Therefore, some units had patients in beds who were not discharged by 2 PM, although there was a need for these beds to relieve the congestion in the ED. The Patient Flow Physics model predicted the number of beds that were likely to be needed by each unit, stratified by both the day of the week and the time of the day. Knowing the demand requirements for beds in advance allowed each floor to identify the patients most likely to go home each day and determine which patients were likely to be discharged by each hour to meet the bed needs of the ED. Simply put, if the flow out of each unit at least closely approximates the flow into each unit by day of the week and time of day, then there should be less back-up of patients in the ED. In turn, this allows patients to flow smoothly into and out of the ED.

Incorporating process and flow data can facilitate effective handling of patient demand, utilization of resources such as staff skills, and provide input as to where process improvements can be applied to reduce waiting time, poor staff utilization, and other wasteful aspects. Applying the Factory Physics principles to patient flow through the hospital ED led to better-managed patient volume, better provider and staff scheduling, and higher satisfaction among patients and care providers.

Applying LSS to Patient Flow in Community Hospital Mammography Service

The women's mammography service line at the hospital also benefited significantly. At the beginning of the effort, the women who started their diagnostic journey with a self-referral mammography and were diagnosed with cancer would find, on average, that it took 8 weeks to move through the diagnostic journey (e.g., screening, focused mammography views, ultrasound, biopsy, MRI) to treatment, which may include radiation, chemotherapy, and surgery. The journey was reduced to one week or less after detailed assessment of the process and utilization of LSS. The significance of this improvement cannot be understated: The earlier cancer is identified and treatment begun, the greater the chance for improved clinical outcomes, satisfaction, and overall quality of life (Viau & Southern, 2007).

The Patient Flow Physics Framework

The Patient Flow Physics framework provides a performance model that describes how items (patients and information) flow through a patient care process. This framework can help improve the control and predictability of health care operation service lines. This framework recognizes that all processes consist of:

1. Demand
2. Transformation
3. Inventory

Demand is the rate at which patients present to the patient-care organization. *Transformation* is the activity that converts sick patients into healthy ones or, at least, brings wellness from illness or injury. *Inventory* consists of both the supplies used for treating patients and the patients who are waiting for the next stage of their patient care.

Because the health care network consists of interconnected elements, one must be able to characterize and manage patient flows in three different arenas:

1. Flow *into* the patient care process (e.g., ED or out-patient clinic);
2. Flow *through* the patient care process; and
3. Flow *out* of the patient care process.

Whether the flow is smooth or chaotic, fast or slow, restricted or unrestricted, depends on a range of factors internal as well as external to the patient care process. Patient flow *into* the ED is a consequence of patient flows from emergency medical services, nursing homes, transfers from other hospitals, direct patient admits (referrals by outside physicians), and walk-in patients. The patterns and sources of patient arrivals are very important because they critically influence the queuing effects on the input side of the ED or, in general, of any patient-care process.

Understanding the patterns and sources can sometimes allow better management of demand. For example, EDs can choose to divert patients from emergency medical services to other EDs. Also, EDs are often utilized by outside physicians to directly admit patients to a hospital in-patient setting. Why does this happen? Referring physicians recognize that their patients will have tests associated with admission carried out without delay ("stat" orders) in the ED, meaning they are prioritized and completed as soon as possible, versus the expected delays by going to the ambulatory clinic. Therefore, EDs could better work with outside physicians to schedule these direct patient admits for less busy times of the day, thus reducing demand during peak demand times and improving relationships with community providers.

Patients are different in the time and resources required to manage their illnesses. Patient flow through the ED is a function of ED resource utilization and the variability associated with differences between ED providers. Utilization of ED providers is of high concern. These providers include physicians (MDs and DOs), physician assistants (PAs), and nurse practitioners (NPs). Another key resource that often serves as a constraint in EDs are the ED beds. Whenever an ED requires each new patient to be seen in an ED bed, patients may be waiting longer to be seen when beds are filled with patients. Some EDs have recognized that having ED beds as a constraint can be overcome through seeing patients in areas without beds where they can be assessed and treated rapidly (FitzGerald, Jelinek, Scott, & Gerdtz, 2009).

The three-part series published in 2013–2014 called *Cracking the Code: Fixing the Crowded Emergency Department*, written by Dr. Joseph Guarisco, Chair of Emergency Services at Ochsner Health System in New Orleans, captures many of the ideas. The Ochsner Health System uses qTrack for "quick sorting" of patients, which protects ED beds from being over-utilized. Some ED professionals will invoke the rule of thumb that "vertical patients should remain vertical, while horizontal patients should remain horizontal," meaning that those patients who can walk in are vertical and are often able to be treated while standing or sitting. The patients who arrive via emergency medical transport (EMT) are often in a stretcher and should remain lying down on a bed.

Patient flow *out* of the ED is crucial to avoid overly long stays in the ED. The patients who are admitted to the hospital yet are "blocked" from being transported to in-patient units will remain in the ED until an in-patient unit can accept the patient. These patients are referred to as "ED boarded" patients. The reason ED boarding arises may be due to a lack of transport personnel, unavailability of consulting physicians (consults), and insufficient beds (either in the hospital or perhaps destinations outside of the hospital). Patient flow out of the ED is an issue during winter seasons when demand is greatest; for example, during the winter in Florida, there is often a significant increase in part-time residents and visitors, which may lead to an increase in in-patient census.

Cycle times through a care process can depend upon flow through and out of a care process. This, of course, can be influenced by the design of the care process. For example, whether processes are arranged in series or in parallel, and whether process steps serve a useful function or exist merely because of tradition and organizational legacy.

Patient Flow and the VUT Equation

Patient flow through and out of a patient care process is often the focus of clinical operations. The flow *into* patient care processes is impacted by the demand that operations try to manage. The flow *through* patient care processes is impacted by the utilization of key resources (e.g., staffing levels, providers available, and room availability) to keep patients flowing smoothly through the care processes. The flow *out* of patient care processes is impacted by both internal resources and readiness of resources outside of the current patient care process. For example, it is more difficult to discharge some older patients if there are not enough skilled nursing facilities (SNF) in the community. Likewise, limited behavioral health program options impact the release of patients needing those services.

In their book *Factory Physics: Foundations of Manufacturing Management*, Hopp & Spearman (2008), provide the "laws that govern process flow" in manufacturing systems. Interestingly, just as the laws of physics are those

---

BOX 5.1 VUT Equation

Average Patient Flow Care Time = Variation (V) × Utilization (U) × Process Time (T)

---

that define and describe motion, the principles of process flow can also describe flow in health care processes. One of the concepts discussed in the book is the VUT Equation (BOX 5.1).

It is sufficient for our discussion to understand that anything that increases the variation (V), increases resource utilization (U), or operates in processes that are designed to take a long time (T) leads to increases in average patient flow care time. In other words, to reduce the overall cycle time in the care of patients requires efforts to reduce the variation in the clinical processes, reduce utilization of key resources (e.g., having extra capacity in terms of resources), and optimize the inherent process design to eliminate wasted time.

The following paragraphs describe V, U, and T and provide examples as they relate to patient care and flow.

Variation

Knowledge of process variation is one of the four parts of W. Edwards Deming's System of Profound Knowledge (Deming, 1993, pp. 98–99):

> Variation there will always be, between people, in output, in service, and in product. What is the variation trying to tell us about a process, and about the people who work in it? .... A process may be in statistical control or it may not be. In the state of statistical control, the variation to expect in the future is predictable. Costs, performance, quality, and quantity are predictable. [Walter] Shewhart called this the stable state. If the process is not stable, then it is unstable. Its performance is not predictable.

Variation is either common or special. *Common cause variation* can be the routine patient census number increases and decreases across hours, days, and seasons. *Special cause variation* is not random, and it can be assigned to special events or circumstances such as with extremely high patient count in an ED due to a major, mass casualty event. It could also be attributed to an increase in medical errors due to new equipment failures.

Causes of variation in data can be detected with control charts, which are run charts (or time series graphs) that incorporate upper and lower control (sigma) lines (see Chapter 4 and examples later in the chapter). There are eight universally accepted decision rules that are applied to detect extreme points from the mean, trends, and the unusual patterns that are low probability events. Wheeler (2000) prefers the name *process behavior charts* because it better describes the variation as the "voice of the process." These charts can help distinguish between routine, always occurring "noise" vs. "signals" that are hopefully less frequent indications of some special cause variation. Finally, data and variation can only be understood in the context in which they were collected (Hesselink et al., 2013). More specifically, the analysis must be applied to a specific process; individual or group; period of time; or the use of specific material or equipment. This latter point is critical and often misunderstood.

Control charts must use rational sampling and rational subgrouping to produce valid results (Wheeler, 1995). Selection of the time and data must be consistent and based on logic. When data collection is properly conducted, the three sigma limits *and* within-group variation will help identify legitimate process "signals." The goal of rational subgrouping is to identify differences between short- and longer-term process variation at single points in time. The variables that effect variation are random if there were no deliberate changes to the process. Purposeful modifications could include staffing changes, new devices or equipment, such as more bronchoscopes or surgical microscopes, or the introduction of new treatment protocols, etc. If data are regularly collected and analyzed, staff will more likely know "what is different."

Jensen and Mayer (2015) propose the terms natural and artificial variation. Natural variation is commonly occurring and due to chance, bias, or an artifact in data collection. Variation is natural and it is going to happen. It cannot be eliminated but it can be managed. On the other hand, artificial variation "is neither necessary nor random. It is driven by largely unknown, ignored, or unchallenged priorities." It is like the self-inflicted wound of scheduling elective surgeries during busy, prime hours.

Variation can be attributed to:

■ Demand for patient flow into the processes
■ Differences in patient needs (e.g., ambulatory vs. handicapped, older vs. younger)
■ Differences in how care is delivered by clinical staff
■ Reliability of patient care and handoffs to avoid errors, and rework
■ Availability of resources outside current patient care processes (e.g., rehabilitation, assisted living or skilled nursing facilities, family support, and in-patient care units)

Hospital management seeks to find ways to understand variation in demand, patient care processing, and readiness of rate limiting resources to which patients are flowing out of the patient care process. We have found the following observations about managing variation to be helpful.

Learn the patterns of demand. Although demand of clinical processes can vary significantly from day to day or within a day, there are tools, including run charts, control charts, and box plots, that can lead to a better understanding of demand variation in terms of when it may occur and how much variation it can cause. For example, grocery stores use forecasts to manage inventory along with staffing matched to demand. Some stores will provide extra capacity by having enough check-out lanes for each hour in a day for each day of the week. They also call "all baggers" to the front when lines start forming. And just as grocery stores know the customer demand by day of week and hour of day, in EDs, Mondays will look like other Mondays, Tuesdays like other Tuesdays, and so forth. Dave Eitel, an emergency medicine physician who co-created the Emergency Services Index Triage protocols, would often say that he knew the typical patient that was coming to the ED, but just did not know their name (AHRQ, 2012). Eitel recommended that EDs adopt grocery store practices for forecasting peaks and valleys in demand and adjust capacity accordingly.

Standardize care for typical patients. Clinical practice variation can be addressed through some form of standardization as discussed later in this chapter in LMS practices. Health care systems often use standard order sets to address the 80/20 rule, where 80% of the patients presenting with known conditions can be handled with a basic order set. For example, although patients that visit an ED may be unique, experienced providers will recognize that most of these patients present a similar patient pattern, and standard order sets can be used effectively. The care for these "typical" patients will therefore be more consistent and standardized. The patients presenting with unusual conditions or an unusual manifestation of these conditions can then be addressed with extra attention or with different procedures.

Standardization of activities is also an effective way to reduce variation by ensuring that staff perform the same duties in the same preferred ways. Only best practices are standardized so this also increases quality. According to Imai (2012, pp. 54–55), "standards represent the best, easiest, and safest way to do a job." They also preserve organizational knowledge and expertise and facilitate valid measurement of organizational performance. Standards can also help clarify cause and effect relationships and expedite maintenance and improvement.

Put population data to work. Population health analytics allows tailoring the management approach for various patient demographics and conditions thus reducing the practice variation and lessening the time needed to address each patient's needs. This knowledge can be readily applied to disease management.

Learn from other organizations dealing with high variability. High-reliability organizations (HROs) have characteristics that parallel many features of the health care environments (i.e., EDs, operating rooms, intensive care units, etc.), including the use of complex technologies, a fast-paced tempo of operations, and a high level of risk, yet they manifest spectacularly low error rates (Sanchez & Barach, 2012). HROs are required to respond to a wide variety of situations under changing environmental conditions in a reliable and consistent way. Examples of HROs include aircraft carriers, nuclear power plants, and firefighting teams. Weick and Sutcliffe (2001) have studied these industries and found that they share an extraordinary capacity to discover and manage unexpected events resulting in exceptional safety and consistent levels of performance despite a fast-changing external environment. HRO methodologies and practices can offer clinical care with greater patient safety, less process rework, improved patient outcomes, and greater patient satisfaction (Oster & Braaten, 2016; Tamuz & Harrison, 2006).

Create buffers. Buffer management is an effective approach for reducing and mitigating the negative aspects of excessive and/or uncontrolled variation. Buffers are like shock absorbers on cars. Instead of reducing bumps in the road for a car, buffers reduce or dampen the effect of variability when trying to synchronize demand to transformation (Pound, Bell, & Spearman, 2014, p. 51). There are time, capacity, and inventory buffers. Time buffers include waiting times and extra available time that can be used. Capacity buffers are the numbers of staff, beds, and equipment that can be used to treat patients. Inventory buffers can be supplies or patients' waiting for the next step in a process. Buffers must be properly managed, and they cannot be too large. Patients do not like to wait and unused capacity and inventory costs money. The creative use of buffers can greatly reduce patient length of stay. A family practitioner liked to spend extra time with certain patients to socialize. Unfortunately, this usually altered the carefully constructed patient schedule. He did not want to give up this "special" time so it was suggested that he see those patients just before his lunch break or at the end of the day. It proved an effective compromise.

Utilization

Utilization refers to the use of resources. Utilization without any waste or nonvalue-added activities is an "efficient" process (see the previous *Muri* discussion). These resources are more technically referred to as "capacity." Utilization is impacted by:

- Available staffing capacity each hour to handle variation in demand
- Availability of resources such as computer systems, beds/treatment rooms, equipment in imaging/labs, and transportation
- Sufficient availability of inventory such as blood, medications, medical devices including stents/splints, transport equipment, or patients ready for the next procedure

- Financial resources to access services
- The time to complete clinical and administrative activities
- Resources for training and other staff development

This "capacity" must be available across the basic value stream (**FIGURE 5.2**) and at each step of the microlevel processes.

When the population does not have adequate and effective prevention services, they can develop serious health conditions that require secondary or tertiary treatment. Families without health insurance tend to use more expensive ED services because they cannot access ambulatory and out-patient care. A lack of in-patient beds contributes to ED boarding, as does limited availabilty of SNFs. Inadequate staffing levels adds to length of stay and decreases the quality of patient care. Both under and over-utilization of resources can be problematic.

Capacity issues, poor process design, and/or unsatisfactory staff performance contribute to process bottlenecks which are the slowest activity steps. One way to address capacity is to build in "slack" as "a cushion of actual or potential resources which allows an organization to adapt successfully to internal pressures for adjustment or to external pressures for change in policy as well as to initiate changes in strategy…" (Lawson, 2001, pp. 125–131). Slack is uncommitted staff, space, and equipment. It is the antidote for the "myth of 100% efficiency." First, if people are always busy with regular work duties, they have no flexibility or time for reflecting, thinking, planning, training, or quality improvement (DeMarco, 2001). CQI projects require staff time and resources. Busy staff resent these projects being dumped

on their already "full plates" (Barach & Kleinman, 2018).

Experienced hospital executives know that ED boarding tends to increase when in-patient bed usage exceeds 80%. The Toyota Production System (TPS) has been the very effective model for many LMS turnaround initiatives in hospitals systems like Virginia Mason (Kenney, 2010). TPS frees up time for quality by empowering workers to "fix" errors when they occur, even if it slows down or stops "the line." They have lower manager- and supervisor-to-staff ratios, which aids in problem solving and coaching. They also take more time to plan new products and services to "get it right," thus saving significant resources before production and delivery commences.

There are many ways to keep utilization of key resources low:

1. Keeping key resources such as providers and beds in an ED utilized less than 80% of the time allows for better management of demand and enables the system to address more effectively variation in patient flow (see *Muri* discussed previously);

2. Understanding variation in demand and patients will allow for better scheduling of people resources (see *Mura* discussed previously); and

3. Applying box plots of variation as explained earlier in this chapter allows for determining the 75th percentile of demand and process variation so that adjusting scheduling to meet the demands of the 75th percentile will lessen the impact of overall process demand and minimize flow variation.

FIGURE 5.2 Generic High-Level Health Care Value Stream

Time

Slow and inefficient health care processes negatively impact patient satisfaction. Management dictates that "time is money." More importantly, slow treatment can contribute to poor health outcomes. Time includes the activities or tasks within each step and the space between steps. Delays can occur during handoffs and transitions; departmental or functional group boundaries can also contribute to these "white space" management challenges (Rummler & Brache, 1995).

The cancer screening mammography example discussed earlier in the chapter illustrates the impact that the passing time has on the effectiveness of the process. Each step in the diagnostic journey for cancer screening (e.g., initial screening, additional digital imaging, ultrasound, MRI, biopsy, surgical treatment, oncological treatment) may be well-defined and managed. However, the time between steps may be increased due to the unplanned or poorly managed transitions between each step. If an initial screening mammography is completed and no "suspicious" areas of the breast are observed, then the process may stop. If a suspicious area in the mammography is observed, then the provider may either ask the patient to stay longer for additional imaging or, for those providers who do not read the initial imaging in real time while the patient is there, the patient's primary care physician may receive a report later indicating more work-up is needed. The patient is contacted and requested to make an appointment for a follow-up visit with either the primary care physician or the mammography center, or both. Therefore, the transition from initial screening imaging and follow-up imaging may have wait times built in that can increase patient anxiety. Furthermore, delay may allow time for ongoing growth of a cancerous tumor.

In 1915, Gilbreth used time motion studies to show convincingly that the actual time needed to complete a process, such as imaging, reading the results, and determining the next clinical steps, may be short relative to the time spent between steps (Gilbreth & Gilbreth, 2002). Reducing transition time between steps (i.e., eliminating wait time) is often worthwhile in reducing patient anxiety, determining clinical concerns earlier, perhaps reducing the effort needed for treatment if caught earlier, and honoring the patient's personal time. It is not unusual for transition times to be increased for the convenience of the providers, other staff, the facilities in which patients are seen, and to complete documentation consistent with regulatory or compliance requirements. Putting the patient first (beyond paying lip service) takes significant effort and may be a challenge to the "way things are done here."

Time is also defined by the process:

- The design of a patient care process can determine the minimal amount of time a patient will spend, flow through, and out of a process if there were no impediments or variation in the process.
- Addition of nonvalue-added steps in the process that only adds time, potentially increases variation, and increased opportunity for errors. For example, in an empty ED, are all patients required to go through a separate step called "triage," or can they immediately proceed directly to being seen by a provider?

We have learned by managing dozens of clinical projects that finding ways to reduce the length of time spent in the patient flow care process may require staff to:

1. Eliminate or reduce nonvalue-added process tasks or steps such as unnecessary waiting times. The longer the process, the more things can go wrong for patients and the more costs for the system.
2. Implement LMS (see discussion that follows) to draw attention to time spent on identifying and reducing nonvalue-added process steps.

3. Create value-stream managers that control all the resources needed for their service lines (i.e., ICU patients, hip repairs, etc.). This reduces boundary or interface issues.

It is not coincidental that the philosophies and practices of CQI as espoused by Six Sigma, LMS, and LSS, all lead to reducing variation in processes and overutilization of resources as well as streamlining patient flow care processes, leading to reduced time to care. In the next part of this chapter, we provide an overview of the principles of LMS.

▶ Lean Management System (LMS)

The VUT equation described is a relatively simple model to understand, but it is more challenging to implement. LMS models provide for an effective system to optimize process management as suggested by the VUT equation. The active joining of these two models will be discussed later. Specifically, managers and their staff need to direct and set examples about required behaviors to reduce or manage variation, maximize human and equipment utilization, and decrease process cycle times.

First, a comparison is in order. If a Lean organization is like an automobile, then the engine is similar to the organization's capacity to provide services and the transmission is anologous to a LMS. The transmission sends power to the wheel axel to move the vehicle forward. It also changes gears to better match power and resource demands. An automatic transmission smooths these shifts and helps reduce variation. An organization's LMS coordinates resources and directs them to efficiently satisfy customer work orders (demands). When managers apply the "right" tools, this stimulus and response situation can be virtually seamless.

Management in Lean organizations has "two major functions: maintaining or controlling the existing processes, and improving existing processes" (Charron, Harrington, Voehl, & Wiggin, 2015, p. 1). Performance management occurs through continuous improvement, and emphasizes staff development, socio-technical (belief) systems, and change management. High performing companies are paying increasingly more attention to organizational culture that focuses on reliability and safety (Weick & Roberts, 1993).

Organizational goal success can seem entirely random without effective management. On some days, the production might be successful, and on others it will produce near misses and process failures. Management and front line staff will not know when or why either will occur. This is akin to employees starting each day with the important question, "Do I feel lucky?" This mode of operation is very stressful and costly, and one never feels in control of their processes or environment because so much of the output is ruled by chance.

LMS approaches have been successfully applied in hundreds of organizations and two prominent examples in health care are at Virginia Mason and Baylor, Scott & White (BS&W). A recent book, *The Power of Ideas to Transform Healthcare: Engaging Staff by Building Daily Lean Management Systems* by Steve Hoeft and Robert W. Pryor (2016), thoroughly documents the BS&W Lean journey. The authors credit the successful LMS implementation to the continuous implementation of staff-generated ideas. Lean management is the vehicle for this staff engagement and the continuous infusion of suggestions successfully implemented in both the clinics and administrative activities. The basic principles apply across the board in both health care services and manufacturing (Hoeft & Pryor, 2016). A more in-depth treatment can be found in Mann (2015) where he shows how it can become even more powerful when attention is devoted to organizational culture.

The LMS model shown in **FIGURE 5.3** is adapted from Mann (2015) and is represented as a Venn diagram because there are

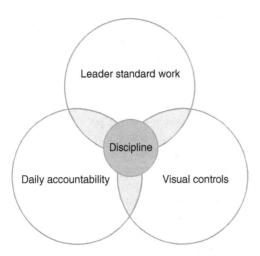

FIGURE 5.3 Lean Management System Model

interconnections and overlaps between the three components. Everything begins with the Leader Standard Work, because that is where supervision through executive activities and the standardization of the processes of the other elements are spelled out. For example, how do leaders select and maintain the data in Visual Controls (see the following sections), how is their Daily Accountability (see the following sections) implemented, and how are staff held to account on a regular basis.

The three interconnected variables of leader standard work, visual controls, and daily accountability are influenced by the important factor of discipline. Discipline and stable leadership are needed to ensure that long term success and flow are maximized at the juncture where important parts of the model align.

The Toyota Production System argues that organizational culture can change through the inculcation of principles delineated in the *Four P Model* (Liker & Ross, 2017, p. 48) and include:

1. **P**roblem solving for continuous organizational learning and alignment to objectives and plans
2. **P**eople are respected, challenged, engaged and developed

3. **P**rocesses are improved and stabilized based on customer defined "value"
4. **P**hilosophy of long-term focus

Staff must be allowed to devote time to completely understand and reflect on their work activities in order to identify waste and standardize best practices. To understand variation in one's work flow, one must carefully review multiple data points. Ideally, at least 20 data points are needed for a significant "minimum" trend, but a minimum of seven data points should be used when tracking seasonal changes that are so crucial for health care planning (Balestracci, 2015). When more data is available, it is easier to differentiate between common- and special-cause variation.

Lean management is a very hands-on activity requiring supervisors and line managers to actively apply these principles on the work floor or "*gemba*." They cannot manage this from their offices while reviewing data or reports and answering emails. This begins with Leader Standard Work.

Leader Standard Work

LMS does not assume that employees, including managers and leaders, know what they are supposed to do. Best practices or standards are clearly spelled out in detail and often posted in activity areas. Common examples include hand washing directions in rest rooms or graphical safety directions for using dangerous equipment. These best practices are updated as new standards and improvements are made.

A lack of standardized work increases variation and can produce very strange data distributions. Variation is a key element in the VUT equation. Different types of patients or invoices require specialized "handling" and will require multiple methods and change-overs, etc. This tends to reduce cycle time. On the other hand, a generalized approach can restrict flow and slow down processes. The following LMS tables (see **TABLE 5.1**, **TABLE 5.2**, and **TABLE 5.3**) have been adapted from *Creating a*

Lean Culture (Mann, 2015, pp. 58–59). The three tables are divided to show the frequency of application and levels within the organization. Note that the supervisors or team leaders repeat tasks more frequently than managers or directors. They also do not have the same responsibilities and there is no universal application of this approach across the organization.

Supervisors and managers "go to the *gemba*" or where the work is done on the shop floor—or in the clinical context, the operating room, the intensive care unit, or the ED, many times every day (Imai, 2012). They observe, listen and question. Staff are encouraged and rewarded to speak up and find simple solutions (*kaizens*) to improve the value work stream. Staff are coached and developed in an apprentice model. Working with staff, managers assist in removing barriers, search for ways to improve flow capacity, and reduce process variation, capacity restraints, and cycle time.

This direct contact between management and frontline workers builds trust, and provides opportunities for much learning, data collection, and problem identification before it is filtered by middle management. Managers can directly observe how buffers are managed to ensure that patients, transactions and information are being effectively used. They can directly observe staff (and machines) working at a manageable pace or breakneck speed? Is there any "slack" that can be used in positive ways? Finally, standard work is monitored and modified on the production line (floor) as

TABLE 5.1 Leader Standard Work for Activities Completed Many Times Each Day				
Frequency	**Supervisors/ Team Leaders**	**Managers**	**Directors**	**Hospital Administrators**
Many times every day	Go to the *gemba* (work floor) to:	Go to the *gemba* (rounds) to:	Communicate with key stakeholders and customers	Communicate with key stakeholders and customers
	Coach employees	Coach employees	Coach employees	Encourage and praise staff
	Remove barriers and help solve problems	Remove barriers and help solve problems	Remove barriers and help solve problems	Remove barriers and help solve problems
	Monitor standard work	Encourage and praise staff	Encourage and praise staff	
	Encourage and praise staff			
	Monitor time and capacity buffers			
	Prevent accidents			

Modified from Creating a Lean Culture (Mann, D., 2015, pp. 58–59).

TABLE 5.2 Leader Standard Work for Activities Completed At Least Once Daily

Frequency	Supervisors/Team Leaders	Managers	Directors	Hospital Administrators
Once daily, every day	Check call-ins Coordinate shift changes Administrative tasks	Monitor and adjust staffing plans Administrative tasks	Administrative tasks	Administrative tasks
	Review performance data from previous day	Review performance data from previous day all supervisors	Review performance data from previous day for area	Review highest level hospital metrics
	AM review of patient schedule	AM review of patient schedule by type of patient	Review end of day patient totals	Review patient census trends for whole hospital
	AM review of supply inventory		Go to the *gemba* (rounds)	Go to the *gemba* (rounds)
	AM review of repair needs			
	Prepare data for huddle boards	Prepare data for huddle boards		
	Huddle with staff for about 10 minutes to: ▪ Review performance data ▪ Discuss data variation, obstacles, and capacity issues	Huddle with supervisors for about 10 minutes to: ▪ Review performance data ▪ Discuss common variation, flow, and capacity issues	Huddle with managers for about 10 minutes to: ▪ Review performance ▪ Discuss common variation, flow, and capacity issues	Huddle with executive staff for about 10 minutes
	Monitor standard work	Monitor standard work		
	End of shift review of work			
	Follow up on urgent assignments	Follow up on urgent assignments		

Modified from *Creating a Lean Culture* (Mann, D., 2015, pp. 58–59).

Frequency	Supervisors/ Team Leaders	Managers	Directors	Hospital Administrators
TABLE 5.3 Leader Standard Work for Activities Completed Weekly or Less Frequently				
Weekly or less frequently	Hold weekly staff meeting for supervisors	Hold weekly staff meeting for supervisors	Hold weekly staff meeting for managers	Hold weekly staff meeting for executive staff and directors
	Participate in improvement projects when assigned.	Participate in improvement projects when assigned.	Champion improvement projects	Champion improvement projects
				Review progress on strategic plan

Modified from Creating a Lean Culture (Mann, D., 2015, pp. 58–59).

different work methods can be a leading cause of process variation.

Many more activities such as huddles occur daily. These short staff meetings at the beginning of each shift employ a very data driven approach to planning and problem solving. Key management data are displayed on a wall that is convenient for staff to view during the daily huddles. Huddles will be addressed more completely in the Daily Accountability Section (later in the chapter).

Staffing levels, equipment and inventory are checked because that also impacts capacity. Supervisors and managers should also briefly review the day's work before going home and especially consider visiting the hospital on weekends where they can help focus on work that can prevent excessive harm on weekends (Shulkin, 2008). Directors and hospital administrators should also go to the *gemba* or "rounds" at least once a day in one of their many areas or locations (Saposnik, 2007). This helps managers understand the value streams and their regular presence motivates staff to stay focused and continuously improve (Bendavid et al., 2007).

These activities are less frequent but no less important. Note the importance of regular champion meetings to address ongoing improvement needs. These weekly or biweekly staff meetings are longer, sit-down events that communicate important organizational changes, deal with near miss or process failures, etc. Discussions can also be more in-depth, but this is not time for microlevel problem solving. That can be assigned to people to handle outside the meeting and report back. Finally, senior leaders need to regularly review strategic plan implementation.

Visual Controls

Visual controls in Lean management should always begin with some type of "as is" value stream or process map. This provides an important context and a reference point for any discussion of related metrics or issues. FIGURE 5.4 illustrates an ED process map.

A process map or flowchart is a visual representation of the care process that is created with information provided by team members. The process mapping exercise can

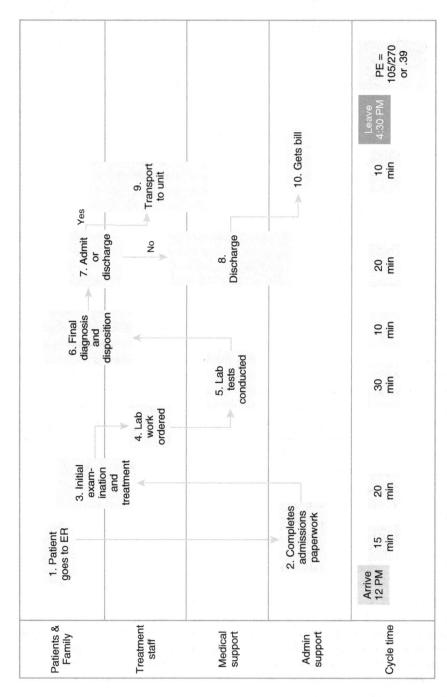

FIGURE 5.4 Emergency Department Process Map Example

help clinicians clarify through visualization what they know about their environment and determine what they want to improve about it (Barach & Johnson, 2006). The process maps use common flowchart symbols and can describe the current state or baseline, the improved state in transition, and the optimal state. The exercise helps clinicians make assumptions and expectations explicit and can provide insights into reflections on their current state and, importantly, into how to improve the process of care or to overcome barriers they perceive to its improvement (Johnson et al., 2012). The numbered steps facilitate an honest discussion and the process efficiency times are a useful ratio for assessing what is value-added time versus nonvalue-added timed activities (Hollingsworth et al., 1998).

An important part of a LMS is "learning to see" what is happening in the value stream or process. The visual display of the right data facilitates this awareness and is crucial because measurement influences behavior. In this approach, the "right" data focuses attention on variation, utilization/capacity, and time (VUT). Clinical microsystems should monitor and analyze no more than four to five key performance indicators (KPIs) because staff focus can easily be distracted and overwhelmed (Mohr, Bataden, Barach, 2004). Ideal health care metrics might include the cycle time, patient wait times, medical errors, scheduling errors, patient volumes, provider volumes, and takt times.

Takt is the German word for the baton that an orchestra conductor uses to regulate the tempo of the music. In Lean, *takt* time is the rate at which a finished product needs to be completed in order to meet customer demand, and patient satisfaction, etc. (Rother, 2010). The data collection should include important variables such as types of patients, providers, and errors.

Every metric selected should include a numerical target and these need to be "stretch goals" to help motivate improvements. You may also collect data for the important parts of the clinical process such as times

for door-to-doctor; doctor-to-decision; and decision-to-disposition. This enables stratification or the necessary "drilling down" into the datasets to find specific answers to the many important management questions.

It is important that an appropriate sampling plan be developed, as described in Chapter 4 and throughout the CQI evolution, including the earliest work of Deming. There are various approaches that can be used to select primary data for CQI processes (Perla, Provost, & Murray, 2013). For many organizations, the management metrics used to understand and manage work processes are often based on averages rather than understanding actual variation in processes (Kim, Spahlinger, Kin, & Billi, 2006). For example, the length of stay (LOS) is often reported as an average length of stay (ALOS) and resource utilization is also reported in averages, etc. This would be adequate if the data did not fluctuate much around the average. As previously stated, patient demand tends to vary hour to hour, day to day, and seasonally, while patient conditions can also markedly differ. How do we better manage and ultimately improve our health care processes?

Ideally, the data would be automatically collected by the electronic health record (EHR) or another database aligned throughout the organization. This produces a synergistic effect of added value. "Like magnetism, alignment is a force. It coalesces and focuses an organization and moves it forward" (Labowski & Rosansky, 1997, p. 6).

The data points need to be collected for every patient or transaction for any desired time period. The data needs to be easily exported into a standard data format that facilitates data analysis. Unfortunately, this is not the current reality in most organizations, as process data (e.g., waiting time, variation in test and treatment order sets among physicians, real-time utilization of key resources, errors or near-miss causes, etc.) are often not tracked or readily available in the IT applications used in clinical processes. Instead, the data tracked in the IT systems are related to activity transactions per patient such as orders made and fulfilled, tests or procedures applied, and medications administered, etc.

The huddle board design template (**FIGURE 5.5**) was successfully implemented at a large health care revenue cycle management organization. Some data examples will follow later. Each team constructed their own board and creative differences were encouraged. It was important to display the current process map for quick reference and context. Finally, each team posted a list of what their successful outcomes would contribute to the next downstream group in the value stream. For example, chart recovery staff had time and accuracy goals to expedite coding. This helped employees understand how they contributed to the "big picture." Suneja and Suneja (2010) use the term "Glass Wall" for the same concept.

The top row contains trends for the macro level KPIs that are aligned to the highest level of the organization. Where appropriate, the metrics should include mandated core measures such as patient satisfaction or median length of stay. The run chart shown in **FIGURE 5.6** is an example of a displayed metric on the huddle board.

A quick glance at the trend reveals nonrandom patterns, including what some authors define as "astronomical" data points (i.e., the two unusually large values at 10:00 AM and 12:00 AM) (Perla, Provost, & Murray, 2011). Unfortunately, explanations are not apparent. These warrant further analysis using other CQI tools; the analysis methodology and these CQI tools are presented below and described further in Chapter 4. This leads to the second row on the huddle board, where "drilldowns" or stratification charts can be displayed.

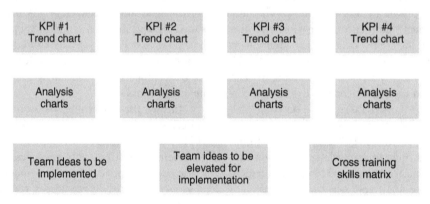

FIGURE 5.5 Huddle Board Template

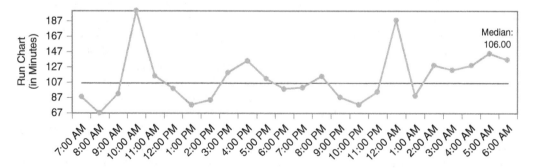

FIGURE 5.6 Average ED Process Cycle Times for Sampled Patients on November 15, 2016

These charts can be tacked under each high-level chart from the first row and can be presented in a chronological "pile" that can be easily explored. Appropriate charts include Pareto charts for medical errors/harm and controls charts for both trended errors and process times (Johnson & Barach, 2017). A typical control chart can be seen in **FIGURE 5.7**.

The XbarR charts in Figure 5.7 displays the means (Xbar) of each sub-group (solid lines). The dashed lines represent different standard deviation levels. In these control charts, four patients were tracked at the beginning of each hour in the initial door-to-doctor phase of an ED redesign process. This is in-between group variation, and there are some obvious special cause outliers and other patterns (see Chapter 4 for further description of special cause variation). The accompanying range (R) chart in Figure 5.7 shows the corresponding within group variation.

Box plots (**FIGURE 5.8**) are great graphical tools for comparing distributions of variable data such as time passed and costs of care. This graph looks at how much time ED physicians take from when then they first talk to their patients to the time when they make their clinical decisions. Box plots provide an interesting perspective on managing variation in care.

A quick glance at Figure 5.8 shows that the physicians labeled #12214, 11288, and 12215 are spending relatively more time with their patients than physicians labeled #139, 309, 378, 11215, 11082, 12214, and 13179. The physicians labeled #13159, 13259, and 13179 had a wider range of times to come to their decisions. This time data is important because it impacts both utilization (capacity) and process time. It would be important to drill down and compare physician times across common patient type variables such as chief complaints or diagnostic related groups (DRG).

How can the information in a box plot be used to understand variation (V in the VUT equation)? When comparing attending ED physicians, patient LOS in the ED can be measured before they are ultimately admitted to an in-patient room at a hospital. If we only

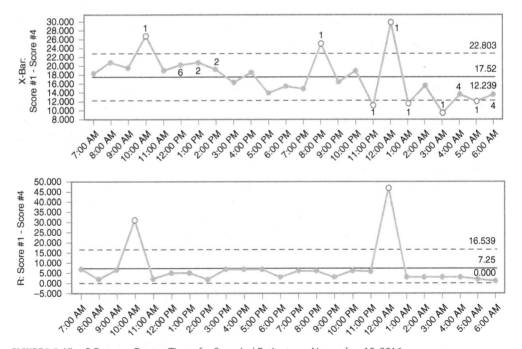

FIGURE 5.7 XbarR Door-to-Doctor Times for Sampled Patients on November 15, 2016

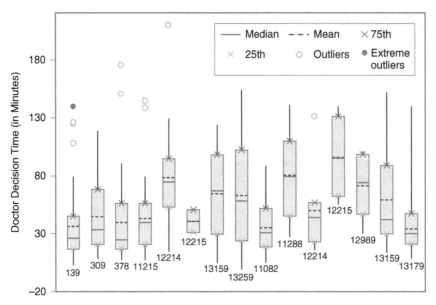

FIGURE 5.8 Box Plot for Physicians to Assess Their Decision Times

compare patients who are admitted with respiratory distress related issues (e.g., flu, pneumonia) then it is expected that although there may be outliers in LOS, in general the middle 50% of the patients admitted for respiratory reasons by different physicians should be similar. Rather than looking at the exceptions as represented by outliers outside the boxes, compare the size of the boxes representing the amount of variation in the middle 50% of the LOS data. It is reasonable to expect similar results between physicians for the middle 50%. If the variation in the LOS for these physicians is quite different, then the natural question is what might be causing the variation in outcomes. The reasons may include physicians ordering more tests and treatments than their colleagues which may result in longer LOS for their patients. Some physicians may either use standard order sets or have a very well-defined process for handling respiratory challenged patients, hence they are more consistent in their LOS results.

Rather than challenging staff to explain to others the reason for differences in variation, it is better to provide staff with the information in a graphical format and let them discuss it among themselves. Having variation data

displayed with box plots is useful as it is easy to understand if applied on a regular basis and often sparks dialogue among providers to understand why variation is occurring.

A Pareto chart (first introduced in Chapter 4) is a powerful tool to help graphically illustrate variation, as illustrated in **FIGURE 5.9**.

It is obvious in Figure 5.9 that some providers need to sign their charts before the charts can be coded and billed. Missing signatures accounted for 71% of the sampled errors. A second level Pareto analysis can drill down to show which providers are the primary offenders. Knowing the "real" times to complete documentation or see patients provides essential information for improving the process.

If "production" is one of the first row KPIs, then pitch charts (**FIGURE 5.10**) can be used to track work output during specific periods of time against goals. Examples of production might include numbers of tests completed in the lab, images read by radiologists, or charts coded during revenue cycle management (RCM).

The chart can also be modified to add an individual worker column. These charts can

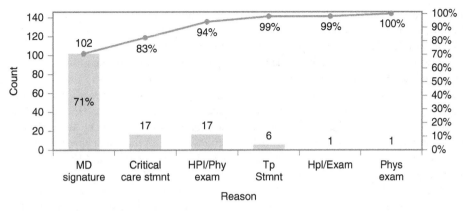

FIGURE 5.9 Missing Chart Elements From a Coding QA Review

Pitch times	Goal pitch/ Cumulative	Actual pitch/ Cumulative	Variation pitch/ Cumulative	Reason for misses
8–10 AM	20/20	18/18	–2/–2	10 minutes start up meeting. Went over 2 minutes—safety issue
10–12	30/50	30/48	0/–2	
1–3 PM	20/70	15/63	–5/–7	Computers down for 20 minutes
3–5 PM	30/100	27/90	–3/–10	Rework needed
Overtime 5–6 PM	10/100	10/100	0/0	2 staff worked
Totals	100/100			

FIGURE 5.10 Pitch Chart for RCM Chart Reviews

facilitate demand and capacity planning. This is an example from revenue cycle management (RCM) but it could be used in any repetitive work environment. Color can be added to highlight good, fair, or bad performance. A simple review of the numerator/denominator differences show that adjustments need to be made after a quick review. The traffic light colors make it even easier to understand, and "red" really stands out. The colors would be selected based on some standard, agreed-upon levels of performance. Another application for traffic light colors could be for the Centers for Medicare and Medicaid Services (CMS) Five Star Quality Rating System. The 4s and 5s would be green; yellow would be used for 3s, 2s, and 1s would be red. Lighter and darker color shading could also be used for the reds and greens.

The third row of the huddle board is a great place to show capacity and other data such as a training matrix (**FIGURE 5.11**). This is a simple way to show the most "strategic" skills and which staff members have mastered them. Dates of attainment could be used instead of the Xs.

Another helpful capacity tool is an overlay run chart (**FIGURE 5.12**). An overlay run chart can be used to calculate the demand and

	Mary	John	James	Susan	William
Skill 1	X		X		
Skill 2	X	X	X		X
Skill 3	X		X	X	X
Skill 4	X	X		X	X
Skill 5	X			X	

FIGURE 5.11 Staff Skills and Cross-Training Matrix

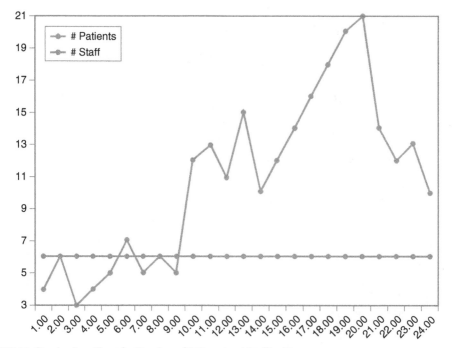

FIGURE 5.12 Overlay Run Chart for Number of Patients and Staff by Times

Date	Item	Who suggested	Who to implement	Start date	Due date	Status
1/2/15	Idea 1	Bob	Bob	1/2/15	1/3/15	Successfully completed
1/2/15	Idea 2	Arif	Arif	1/2/15	1/6/15	In process on schedule
1/3/15	Idea 3	Sue	Sue	1/3/15	1/4/15	Successfully completed
1/3/15	Idea 4	Linda	Linda	1/3/15	1/5/15	Successfully completed
1/4/15	Idea 5	James	James	1/4/15	1/10/15	In process on schedule
1/5/15	Idea 6	Willie	Willie	1/5/15	1/10/15	In process late

FIGURE 5.13 Staff Suggestions and Their Implementation

capacity, both important aspects of the VUT equation. Managers must successfully juggle patient volume (demand) with staff availability. These two trend lines can easily show what capacity existed during that reporting time period given the varying patient demands. Was there adequate coverage later in the day? What happened to the patient length of stay after 10:00?

Staff suggestions are an important part of continuous quality improvement and they should be tracked and posted on the board (**FIGURE 5.13**). The similar companion chart for supervisors can also be maintained and displayed because the staff deserve responses and tracking increases action.

Traffic light colors make it "easier to see" (unless someone is color blind!). Line graphs could also be used to display this data over time (**FIGURE 5.14**).

Daily Accountability

Daily accountability is the most interactive part of the LMS model. Management actively engages with staff when they "go to the *gemba*" and during huddles (Ben-Tovim et al., 2007). This can also include regular follow-up discussions on clinical improvement projects. *Gemba* walks are at the core of Lean practice. Going to "where the work occurs" is the best place to collect real time data. This happens when supervisors and managers observe, listen, challenge and question each other. We want the staff to think and derive the growth and satisfaction that comes from their own problem solving efforts. We want them to actively "see" what is happening and actively engage their colleagues to look for waste. The simple tool shown in **TABLE 5.4** can help this exploration.

This list of waste types enables managers to remember what to look for and reminds them to record brief observations and improvement ideas (Fine, Golden, Hannam, & Morra, 2009). Managers should ask the same four questions during *gemba* walks:

1. What are your team's targets or goals today?
2. How well are you meeting these targets (facts)?
3. What is your plan or planned actions to close the performance gap?
4. How can I help you implement your ideas?

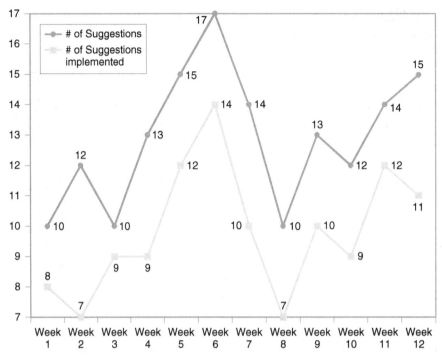

FIGURE 5.14 Trend Chart for Suggestions Made and Implemented by Staff

TABLE 5.4 Waste Walk Tool		
Waste	**What do you see?**	**How to Improve**
Defects/errors		
Overproduction		
Under-utilizing people		
Motion/transportation		
Transitions		
Over-processing		
Inventory		

The Huddle Board examples shown in FIGURE 5.15 and FIGURE 5.16 are the focus of brief, 10- to 15-minute, stand-up meetings that might involve different staff at different levels. They address more than just the exchange of important shift change information or communication "from above." This is an opportunity to briefly review the highlights of KPI data and to focus on both positive and negative variation. Why did that data point increase (or decrease)? What explains the trend? Write comments on the charts, involve staff in these discussions, and have them all take turns leading the huddles. Encourage staff to come back and think about the data. Assignments can be given for later report backs and good facilitation is imperative.

Coaching is another important piece of daily accountability because it is the preferred way to development staff and improve accountability (Sherrard, Trypuc, & Hudson, 2009). Managers must respect their workers to be effective coaches. This is accomplished by asking staff how something should be done as opposed to just telling them the correct way to complete a task. Coaches model appropriate behaviors and use shaping and modeling to help staff perfect new skills. Shaping involves reinforcing each successive approximation until mastery is achieved. Incorrect behaviors are corrected but that can be initiated by asking the worker if the task was completed correctly. If they acknowledge the error, then the follow-up question can be "How would you improve it?"

Continuing to engage staff and attentively listening to the staff suggestions are the most important output of daily accountability meetings. This "sense-making" is a huge part of engendering trust, accountability and organizational loyalty (Barach & Phelps, 2013). Empowering staff jump starts creative problem solving. Observing and questioning also facilitates critical thinking. This on-going generation of staff ideas is important that the number of suggestions made and implemented should be recorded and tracked on the huddle board. Management responses and follow-up should also be posted.

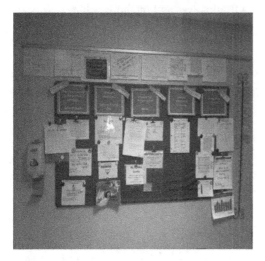

FIGURE 5.15 Huddle Board Example 1

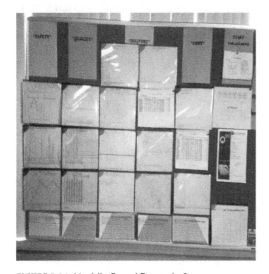

FIGURE 5.16 Huddle Board Example 2

▶ Conclusions

Lean Management Systems (LMS) and Lean Six Sigma (LSS) offer an approach, a set of tools, and a way of thinking about how to more effectively assess and study clinical flow, including addressing variation in process and operations.

These methodologies are widely applicable in studying and improving quality and efficiency of health processes spanning health care, public health and other settings. A particular LSS example illustrated in this chapter is an application to the Patient Flow Physics Framework. It illustrates that improvement requires an understanding of the patient care process flows (e.g., process maps or flow charts), the factors that drive variation in the process, resource utilization impacts on the process, and the relationships of patient care flow cycle times are impacted by poor or inefficient process design.

Improving clinical teamwork is an important factor in improving patient outcomes. In fact, it is a requirement for effective use of the tools described in this chapter. Indeed, quality improvement efforts are not about which tools are used but about how these tools can produce insight, engage the team members, and track patient progress. Their purpose is to help people function as a team, as well as to improve patient outcomes. The importance of teamwork in LMS and LSS as well as other CQI initiatives and methods will be discussed further in Chapter 6.

References

Agency for Healthcare Research and Quality (AHRQ). (2012). Emergency Severity Index (ESI): A Triage Tool for Emergency Department (AHRQ publication no. 05-0046). Retrieved April 27, 2018, from www.ahrq.gov

Antony, J., Palsuk, P., Gupta, S., Mishra, D., & Barach, P. (2018). Six Sigma in healthcare: A systematic review of the literature. *International Journal of Quality & Reliability Management, 35*(5), 1075–1092.

Balestracci, D. (2015). *Data sanity: A quantum leap to unprecedented results*, 2nd ed. Washington, D.C.: Medical Group Management Association.

Barach, P., & Johnson J. (2006). Understanding the complexity of redesigning care around the clinical microsystem. *Quality & Safety in Health Care, 15*(Suppl 1), i10–i16.

Barach, P., & Kleinman, L. (2018). Measuring and improving comprehensive pediatric cardiac care: learning from continuous quality improvement methods and tools. *Progress in Pediatric Cardiology, 48*, 82–92.

Barach, P., & Phelps G. (2013). Clinical sense-making: a systematic approach to reduce the impact of normalised deviance in the medical profession. *Journal of the Royal Society of Medicine, 106*(10), 387–390.

Bendavid E., Kaganova Y., Needleman J., Gruenberg L., & Weissman J. S. Complication rates on weekends and weekdays in US hospitals. *American Journal of Medicine, 120*, 422–428.

Berwick, D. M., Nolan, T. W., & Whittington, J. (2008). The triple aim: Care, health and cost. *Health Affairs, 27*(3), 759–769.

Ben-Tovim, D. I., Bassham, J. E., Bolch, D., et al. (2007). Lean thinking across a hospital: redesigning care at the Flinders Medical Centre. *Australian Health Review, 31*(1), 10–15.

Byrne, A. (2013). *The lean turnaround*. New York, NY: McGraw Hill.

Charron, R., Harrington, H. J., Voehl, F., & Wiggin, H. (2015). *The lean management systems handbook*, Boca Raton, FL: CRC Press.

Csikszentmihalyi, M. (1990). *Flow: The psychology of optimal experience*. New York, NY: Harper Perennial Modern Classics.

DeMarco, T. (2001). *Slack: Getting past burnout, busywork, and the myth of total efficiency*. New York, NY: Broadway Books.

Deming, W. E. (1993). *The new economics for industry, government, education*. Cambridge, MA: Massachusetts Institute of Technology Center for Advanced Engineering Study.

Duffy, G. L., Farmer E., & Moran, J. W. (2009). Applying lean six sigma in public health. In R. Bialek, G. L. Duffy, & J. W. Moran (Eds.), *The public health quality improvement handbook*. Milwaukee, WI: ASQ Quality Press.

Fine, B., Golden, B., Hannam, R., & Morra, D. (2009). Leading Lean: A Canadian healthcare leader's guide. *Healthcare Quarterly, 12*(3), 32–41.

FitzGerald, G., Jelinek, G. A., Scott, D., & Gerdtz, M. F. (2009). Emergency department triage revisited. *Emergency Medicine Journal, 27*, 86–92.

George, M. L. (2002). *Lean Six Sigma: Combining Six Sigma quality with Lean speed*. New York, NY: McGraw Hill.

Gilbreth, F., Jr, & Gilbreth, C. E. (2002). *Cheaper by the dozen*. New York, NY: Harper Perennial Modern Classics.

Guarisco, J. (2013). Cracking the code: fixing the crowded emergency department. *AAEM News*, CommonSense, September/October, 18–20; November/December, p. 24.

Harry, M. (1988). The nature of Six Sigma quality. [Online]: Motorola University Press.

Hesselink, G., Vernooij-Dassen, M., Pijnenborg, L., Barach P., Gademan, P., Dudzik-Urbaniak, E., ... European HANDOVER Research Collaborative. (2013). Organizational culture: an important context for addressing and improving hospital to community patient discharge. *Medical Care, 51*(1), 90–98.

Hollingsworth, J. C., Chisholm, C. D., Giles, B. K., Cordell, W. H., & Nelson, D. R. (1998). How Do physicians and nurses spend their time in the emergency department?" *Annals of Emergency Medicine, 31*(1), 87–91.

Hoeft, S., & Pryor, R.W. (2016). *The power of ideas to transform healthcare: Engaging staff by building lean management systems.* Boca Raton, FL: CRC Press.

Hopp, W. J., & Spearman, M. L. (2008). *Factory physics: Foundations of manufacturing management,* 3rd ed. New York, NY: McGraw-Hill.

Imai, M. (2012). *Gemba kaizen,* 2nd ed. New York, NY: McGraw-Hill.

Jackson, T. L., & Jones, K. R. (1996). *Implementing a lean management system.* Portland, OR: Productivity Press.

Jensen, K., & Mayer, T. (2015). *The patient flow advantage.* Pensacola, FL: Fire Starter Publishing.

Johnson, J., & Barach, P. (2017). Tools and strategies for continuous quality improvement and patient safety. In J. Sanchez, P. Barach, H. Johnson, & J. Jacobs (Eds.), *Perioperative patient safety and quality: principles and practice.* New York, NY: Springer.

Johnson, J., Farnan, J., Barach, P., Hesselink, G., Wollersheim, H., Pijnenborg, L. ... HANDOVER Research Collaborative. (2012). Searching for the missing pieces between the hospital and primary care: mapping the patient process during care transitions. *BMJ Quality & Safety, 21,* i97–i105.

Kenney, C. (2010). *Transforming healthcare: Virginia Mason Medical Center's pursuit of the perfect patient experience.* Boca Raton, FL: CRC Press.

Kim, C. S., Spahlinger, D. A., Kin, J. M., & Billi, J. E. (2006). Lean health care: What can hospitals learn from a world-class automaker?" *Journal of Hospital Medicine, 1*(3), 191–199.

Labowski, G., & Rosansky, V. (1997). *The power of alignment.* New York, NY: John Wiley & Sons.

Lawson, M. B. (2001). In praise of slack: Time is of the essence. *Academy of Management Perspectives, 15*(3), 125–135.

Liker, J. & Ross, K. (2017). *The toyota way to service excellence: Lean transformation in service organizations.* New York, NY: McGraw-Hill Education.

Mann, D. (2015). *Creating a lean culture: Tools to sustain lean conversions,* 3rd ed. Boca Raton, FL: CRC Press.

Mohr, J., Batalden, P., & Barach, P. (2004). Integrating patient safety into the clinical microsystem. *Quality and Safety in Healthcare, 13,* 34–38.

[No Author]. (2013 May 31). Muda, muri, mura—Toyota production system guide. The Official Blog of Toyota GB. Retrieved from http://blog.toyota.co.uk/muda-muri-mura-toyota-production-system

Oster, C. A., & Braaten, J. S. (2016). *High reliability organizations: A healthcare handbook for patient safety & quality.* Indianapolis, IN: Sigma Theta Tau International.

Perla, R. J., Provost, L. P., & Murray, S. K. (2011). The run chart: a simple analytical tool for learning from variation in healthcare processes. *BMJ Quality and Safety, 20,* 46–51.

Perla, R. J., Provost, L. P., & Murray, S. K. (2013). Sampling considerations for health care improvement. *Quality Management in Health Care, 22*(1), 36–47.

Pound, E. S., Bell, J. H., & Spearman, M. L. (2014). *Factory physics for managers: How leaders improve performance in a post-Lean Six Sigma world.* New York, NY: McGraw-Hill Education.

Rother, M. (2010). Toyota kata: Managing people for improvement, adaptiveness, and superior results. Ann Arbor, MI: Rother & Company LLC.

Rummler, G. A., & Brache, A. P. (1995). *Improving performance: How to manage the white space on the organizational chart,* 2nd ed. San Francisco, CA: Jossey-Bass.

Sanchez, J., & Barach, P. (2012). High reliability organizations and surgical microsystems: Re-engineering surgical care. *Surgical Clinics of North America, 92*(1), 114.

Saposnik, G., Baibergenova, A., Bayer, N., & Hachinski, V. (2007). Weekends: a dangerous time for having a stroke? *Stroke 38,* 1211–1215.

Sherrard, H., Trypuc, J., & Hudson, A. (2009). The use of coaching to improve peri-operative efficiencies: The Ontario experience. *Healthcare Quarterly 12*(1), 48–75.

Shulkin, D. (2008). Like night and day—shedding light on off-hours care. *The New England Journal of Medicine, 358,* 2092–2093.

Spath, P. L., & Kelly, D. L. (2017). *Applying quality management in healthcare: A systems approach,* 4th ed. Chicago, IL: Health Administration Press.

Suneja, A., & Suneja, C. (2010). *Lean doctors.* Milwaukee, WI: ASQ Quality Press.

Tamuz, M., & Harrison, M. I. (2006). Improving patient safety in hospitals: contributions of high-reliability theory and normal accident theory. *Health Services Research, 41*(4 Pt 2), 1654–1676.

Tukey, J. W. (1977). *Exploratory data analysis.* Boston, MA: Addison-Wesley.

Viau, M., & Southern, B. (2007). Six sigma and lean concepts, a case study: patient centered care model for a mammography center, *Journal of Radiology Management*, 29(5), 19–28.

Wheeler, D. J. (1995). Advanced topics in statistical process control. Knoxville, TN: SPC Press.

Wheeler, D. J. (2000). *Understanding variation: The key to managing chaos*, 2nd ed. Knoxville, TN: SPC Press.

Weick, K. E., & Roberts, K. H. (1993). Collective mind in organizations: heedful interrelating on flight decks. *Administrative Science Quarterly, 38*, 357–381.

Weick, K. E., & Sutcliffe, K. M. (2001). *Managing the unexpected: assuring high performance in an age of complexity*. New York, NY: John Wiley and Sons, Inc.

Womack, J. P., & Jones, D. T. (2003). *Lean thinking: Banish waste and create wealth in your corporation*. New York, NY: Free Press.

Womack, J. P., Jones, D. T., & Roos, D. (1990). *The machine that changed the world*. New York, NY: Free Press.

CHAPTER 6

Understanding and Improving Team Effectiveness in Quality Improvement

Bruce Fried

There is no substitute for teamwork and good leaders of teams to bring consistency of effort along with knowledge.

— **W. Edwards Deming**

Teams play a major part in all aspects of health care. In quality improvement, the team is the primary vehicle through which problems are analyzed, solutions are generated, and changes evaluated. Effective teamwork is a key factor influencing the diffusion and successful implementation of quality improvement (QI) in health care.

In this chapter, brief case studies are used to illustrate the potential of teams for fostering improvement in organizations and the problems encountered when teams are poorly organized. **CASE STUDY 6.1** illustrates both the positive and negative potential of teams.

State University Hospital (SUH) sought to assemble an integrated, multidepartmental team to address a complex problem involving many organizational components that rarely interacted in a concerted, coordinated manner. Each department had developed systems addressing end-of-life records and documentation for its own processes. However, because these were not integrated with other departments' systems, all departments experienced problems that were badly compounded by an unpredicted environmental change brought to light by State Donor Services (SDS). In its initial attempt to address the organ donation problem, the team was given inadequate time to get organized, leading to a production schedule that was unrealistic. The tight time frame did not provide adequate time to determine the composition of the team. Several members lacked

🔍 CASE STUDY 6.1: STATE UNIVERSITY HOSPITAL AND STATE DONOR SERVICES

State Donor Services (SDS) centrally manages the state's organ procurement and donation process. There had been a trend of declining organ availability for transplant, despite efforts to increase awareness and success in registering donors through the Division of Motor Vehicles. To help solve the problem, SDS approached State University Hospital (SUH), one of the biggest sources of and utilizers of donated organs through its renowned organ transplant programs. Initial exploration of the problem quickly indicated a consistent demand for organs, but organ donations at SUH were down, matching the pattern seen by SDS.

Chris Carter, the new administrator for SUH's emergency department, was asked to build a team to solve this problem for SUH. The hospital's Chief Operating Officer (COO) told Chris that this was a top priority because of the high visibility of the transplant programs, the revenues it brought to the institution, and the fact that the Chairman of Surgery had just threatened to leave the institution if SUH "didn't fix this problem it had obviously created." The COO gave Chris 2 weeks to get a team together and develop a solution, which Chris would present at SUH's monthly Executive Committee meeting. Chris asked the COO for advice regarding whom to have on the team, and the COO referred him to the Chief Nursing Officer (CNO).

Chris went immediately to the CNO, but the first available meeting time she had was in 3 days. In the meantime, Chris gathered as much information as possible. On the third day, the CNO's secretary called to cancel the meeting but suggested that he talk with the Nursing Division Director for Medicine. She met with Chris that afternoon, and together, they formulated a list of people they thought would be able to address the issue. SUH was a functionally structured organization, so they built a team with nursing directors from each of the transplant services and the emergency department, the Director of Patient Care Services, a clerk, a physician from the emergency room, and the State Medical Examiner—whose office was located at SUH and who was responsible for autopsies—as well as a clerk from his office.

The earliest possible meeting time for this group was in 3 weeks— well beyond the COO's deadline. Nonetheless, Chris set up a meeting with as many team members as possible and met with the others individually. The team would be able to meet only once or perhaps twice given the aggressive deadline and members' schedules.

Fearing the approaching deadline and wanting to waste no time, Chris got right to business when the group met. He told the group his goals and invited an open discussion of each team member's experiences with organ procurement. It quickly became evident that several members of the team were too new or too junior to be helpful, with some of Chris's invitees having asked more junior colleagues to be a part of the team in their stead. The Medical Examiner immediately called into question the validity of the group and the authority by which he had been called to this meeting. When Chris told him this was a high-priority project for the COO and CNO—stating only their names and not their titles—the Medical Examiner indignantly replied that he had never heard of these people and that this was a waste of his time. When Chris clarified their titles, the Medical Examiner became less vocal, but remained indignant. He had been focused on solving a problem of declining autopsies, which placed SUH at risk of violating a state regulation. He was angry to have been diverted from this pressing problem and felt that Chris's group would draw organizational focus and energies away from his own needs. His resentment spread to others in the group, which, coupled with their inexperience and a lack of appropriate representation, rendered the meeting—and the group—effectively useless.

In an effort to avoid a public display of this disaster, Chris reported his lack of success to the COO prior to the Executive Committee meeting. The COO realized the impossibility of the goals he had set for Chris. He extended the deadline 3 months and also utilized his own authority by agreeing to attend the next team meeting. These two key factors allowed Chris to rebuild a more knowledgeable, representative, and experienced team.

Ultimately, the organ donation problem was traced to a series of new federal regulations and SUH's fragmented approach to processing end-of-life paperwork. In summary, each operational unit had established its own processes for responding to the regulatory requirements, none of which were integrated with the other operational units, thus creating hours of work for the clinical staff, most of whom gave up trying to secure organ donations. Interestingly, the Medical Examiner's problem of a declining autopsy rate was also a result of this same disjointed method of paperwork processing.

experience, and while they were supportive of the team's goals, they could not contribute in a significant way to the team's work. Senior management provided inadequate support to the team, neglecting to extend the authority of organization leaders to the team and its chair. This led some key team members to dismiss the team as inconsequential and to an overall lack of commitment.

The events at SUH illustrate multiple violations of building a successful, high-performing team. The situation was improved, however, as senior management became more involved, setting an appropriate timeline, changing membership, and conveying the importance of the team to the organization. As team composition and size were restructured to include the appropriate participants, senior management also granted the team visible and legitimate authority to undertake its tasks, and an environment of psychological safety was created where open communication was encouraged and individual team members could contribute with no risk of rebuke by others.

Teams are pervasive in health care and used for virtually every activity carried out in health care organizations, including clinical and management-focused activities. While our knowledge of evidence-based practices continues to grow, implementation of these practices has been uneven and fragmented. The recent development of the field of implementation science, introduced in Chapter 3, has sought to address the challenges of putting evidence into practice (Nilsen, 2015). While there is an array of obstacles to implementation, the application of medical knowledge to clinical service delivery is limited by the effectiveness and efficiency of teams charged with putting that knowledge into practice. Similarly, as new management techniques and technologies are developed, including QI methods, successful use of these approaches is dependent upon appropriately staffed, well-functioning teams. Clearly, we have moved well beyond the era of the autonomous heroic clinician (or manager, for that matter). It is not a stretch to state that behind every successful clinician or manager is a high-functioning team (or teams). And given what we know about the effectiveness of teams in most organizations, it can safely be said that the performance of virtually all clinicians and managers could be markedly improved by improvements in team effectiveness.

Teams also play a critical role in improving the performance of health care systems, whether a medical group practice, a hospital inpatient unit, a long-term care facility, or local public health departments. While effective patient care certainly requires that physicians and others possess current clinical knowledge, patient outcomes often depend upon how well patient-care teams work—whether team members understand and agree on patient-care goals, how members communicate with each other, and the effectiveness of team leadership. In sum, teams are the building blocks of health care organizations and are absolutely essential to implementing plans, caring for populations and individual patients, and identifying and successfully solving quality problems. Teams are not an option but a necessity. As such, it makes great sense to examine these building blocks and see how they can be strengthened.

In this chapter, the concept of *team* is applied very broadly, and shares characteristics with the concept of *microsystems* (Nelson et al., 2002), which are also discussed in greater detail, with specific application to patient safety, in Chapter 9. A microsystem is one of several subsystems of a larger system that is integral to system performance. This perspective, drawn from systems theory, is not a new concept but clearly helps us understand how the human body, an automobile, or an organization, operates. When examining the performance of any system, it is essential to examine (among other factors) the effectiveness of each component subsystem (e.g., the respiratory system), how these subsystems work together (e.g., the nature and adequacy of coordination between a hospital pharmacy and an inpatient unit), and the adequacy of information about system and subsystem performance (e.g., the extent to which the driver of an automobile is provided with information about the automobile's performance).

According to this view, a health system is composed of many subsystems. In patient care, these may be referred to as *clinical microsystems* or *frontline systems*, referring to teams charged with meeting the needs of the patient population. It is these smaller microsystems that actually provide those services that result in positive patient outcomes, provider and patient safety, system efficiency, and patient satisfaction. And as is true with any large system, the effectiveness of any large health care system can be no better than the microsystems of which it is composed (Nelson et al., 2002).

Using the terminology of the microsystem, it is apparent how a microsystem is in fact one type of team, as defined by Nelson et al. (2002):

A clinical microsystem is a small group of people who work together on a regular basis to provide care to discrete subpopulations of patients. It has clinical and business aims, linked processes, and a shared information environment, and it produces performance outcomes. Microsystems evolve over time and are often embedded in larger organizations. They are complex adaptive systems, and as such they must do the primary work associated with core aims, meet the needs of internal staff, and maintain themselves over time as clinical units. (p. 474)

This definition may be slightly altered to apply to all other types of teams in health care. The key concepts in relation to teams are as follows:

- People work together toward specific goals.
- They use multiple interconnected processes.
- They produce performance outcomes.
- They have access to information about the team's performance.

In addition, teams must adapt to changing circumstances, ensure the satisfaction of team members, and maintain and improve their performance over time.

In this chapter, we bring together several traditions of research on teams. We demonstrate how our knowledge of teams informs our understanding of team performance and the important role of teams in QI efforts.

Most of the research on team effectiveness has been carried out in relatively permanent teams with stable membership and opportunities for face-to-face interactions. However, many teams in health care and other sectors exist for only a short period of time, perhaps as short as a nursing shift. Because QI teams typically draw from multiple parts of an organization, these teams may exist for a limited period of time. These types of teams must organize themselves rapidly, and may not have the luxury of going through extended stages of team development. In this chapter, attention is given to traditional as well as temporary teams. Simply put, today's teams do not always fit into traditional team structures and processes, and we need to account for these variations when discussing health care teams.

▶ Teams in Health Care

As medical knowledge grows increasingly complex and medical specialties continue to develop around specific focus areas of that knowledge, there is a risk that health care organizations will lose their patient-centered orientation. There is a paradox in relation to the adoption of new medical technologies and procedures. On the one hand, increasingly specific diagnostic and treatment procedures imply a narrowing of focus. This is desirable because we all support the discovery and implementation of procedures to improve the sensitivity and specificity of diagnoses and the development of pharmaceuticals, technology, and procedures that treat a disease in a manner that is most specific to the individual and the disease state. However, to diagnose, treat, and provide continuing care to a patient requires information from multiple sources and, very often, the involvement of multiple individuals. For example, psychopharmacology has become increasingly specific and sophisticated. However, better utilization of new pharmaceuticals for the benefit of the patient requires that psychiatrists have an understanding of a patient's social environment, which may require the knowledge base of social workers and others. That is, a team of individuals (e.g., social worker, psychiatric nurse) is likely required to ensure that patients are compliant and that home support and respite services are available to caregivers. Thus, the need for patient-centered multispecialty teams becomes ever more important as health care providers and organizations specialize and strive to deliver the best and most appropriate care possible.

Health care system complexity extends beyond the clinical care arena and into administrative areas. Teams fill an organizational need of helping to identify and respond to changes brought about by legal and regulatory changes, more complex payer contracts, and increasing accountability and pressure for value.

At the most basic level, clinical health care teams are comprised of health care providers including nonclinical personnel from multiple disciplines, focusing on a patient or patient population with similar health care needs. This patient-centeredness has extended upward and outward to all aspects of many health care organizations. Indeed, the industry has seen a trend away from organizational structures based on functional areas of technical expertise (e.g., nursing, environmental services, registration, medicine, surgery) and toward functionally integrated organizational structures with clinical care teams based on patient needs (e.g., children's services, women's services, cancer care services). Individual clinical specialists serving on these teams report not only to their disciplinary head (e.g., chief of nursing, chair of medicine), but also to team leaders associated with specific patient-centered service areas. This "dual reporting" format is described in organizational management literature as a matrix structure (Grove, 1995; Burns, Bradley, & Weiner, 2011). As discussed later in this chapter, dual reporting requirements pose challenges for managing multidisciplinary teams.

While the multidisciplinary team model has been adopted to improve patient-centered health, these teams and supporting organizational structures do not spontaneously form, nor are they easily managed. In fact, reward systems often work against the formation and effectiveness of teams. Reward systems are typically designed around performance of one's particular discipline or function, rather than on an individual's role on teams. Where teams do exist, performance is, more often than not, suboptimal. A substantial body of research demonstrates that key elements are necessary for teams to perform to their maximum potential (Hackman, 2002). If these elements are not attended to, dysfunctional teams can result in team member and patient dissatisfaction, disjointed care provision, and inefficient and ineffective operations nested in a cumbersome bureaucracy.

▶ High-Performance Teams and Quality Improvement

The focus of this chapter is on the critical role of high-performing teams in QI efforts, and on strategies to improve team effectiveness. The value of teams was established in the earliest applications of QI as a way to ensure the multidisciplinary sharing of knowledge (Deming, 1986). In modern health care, teams are critical to success in QI for a number of reasons.

1. Quality problems are often not visible to managers at middle or senior management levels, but the impact of problems can be experienced by the entire organization, as shown in the organ donation case (Case Study 6-1). Hospital staff nurses, for example, may see repeated examples of poor communications between shifts that result in a myriad of problems for patients and families, physicians, and other hospital staff. Each occurrence of a problem may be dealt with and resolved in a satisfactory manner; however, in aggregate, these communication problems may become costly in terms of wasted time, reduced quality and patient safety, and lack of continuity of care. Individuals on the front lines are quite frequently aware of systemic problems requiring methodical analysis.

One can easily make the case that the farther one is from the front lines of care, the more removed one is from seeing and solving day-to-day problems. Thus, if we wish to identify quality problems and optimal solutions, we need individuals on our teams who are close to the problem and can help uncover root causes.

2. Health care organizations accomplish their work through a myriad of processes, which may be flawed, confusing, or inefficient. In some instances, a process itself may be ineffective, while in other cases, a well-designed process may be poorly implemented. That is, what appears theoretically on paper as an effective process flowchart may be entirely inaccurate when compared to how the process actually operates. Regardless, much of QI involves process analysis and improvement. Individuals working in dysfunctional processes are often most knowledgeable about process impacts and causes. Therefore, to understand a process, it is essential to have participation from individuals who have the most accurate and detailed understanding of the process.

3. Individuals at the front lines often have unique knowledge and insight into organizational problems and are thus in a position to offer effective and feasible suggestions for improvement. It has long been known that individuals at relatively low levels of the organization often acquire considerable knowledge about the organization and are positioned to reduce uncertainty in the organization, and, in some cases, may use this knowledge to acquire

power (Crozier, 1964). For example, a receptionist who has worked in a pediatric group practice over several years may have a very clear understanding of why waiting times are unacceptably long at certain times of the day. As a result of that experience, he or she may have a well-reasoned understanding of how the practice operates and may have valuable suggestions about how scheduling and staffing may be altered to help ameliorate the waiting time problem. Note as well that because the receptionist is a "nonprofessional," this person may never have been asked to provide input. If we are interested in solving such a problem, it is important to have individuals on a team who understand the problem and can suggest changes that are both effective and feasible.

4. Addressing quality problems requires the support of all affected individuals, not simply those at middle or senior management levels. Identifying and proposing solutions to quality problems is central to QI efforts, but unless those involved in solution implementation understand fully the rationale for the effort, implementation is likely to fall short. Those involved in implementing the solution must be involved so that they understand the QI strategy and can identify possible obstacles to effective implementation.

5. High-functioning teams empower people by providing opportunities for meaningful participation in problem identification and problem solving. Participants feel they are contributing in a positive way to the larger success of the organization,

and not simply through their particular discipline. Among the consequences of empowerment is that people feel greater commitment to the organization and have a stronger sense of ownership. Empowerment also has a direct impact on increasing team members' motivation, a critical element in successful QI initiatives (Daft, 2015). Together, these consequences promote in people a greater willingness to participate in developing and implementing solutions.

As seen in the introductory organ donation example, the well-intentioned manager tasked with solving an institution-wide problem was unable to constitute a team with appropriate members. As a result, the team was frustrated in its inability to achieve its goals. However, one cannot place the blame entirely on the manager. An unrealistic timeline and the absence of initial support by senior management both played a role in the team's failure. Given a second chance, and provided with a more appropriate timeline and sufficient authority, the manager built a team comprised of individuals with appropriate experience and organizational diversity; this team was able to develop, perform, and reach its goals. Such well-designed and managed teams can maximize communication, collaboration, patient and staff satisfaction, and effective and efficient clinical care provision in an organization that is continually able to adapt and improve in the changing environment.

How do we develop and sustain high-performing QI teams? There is much that we know about successful teams, and while there is no guarantee that using all of the concepts and recommendations in this chapter will bring success, the chapter provides a framework to increase the likelihood of team success and avoid many of the pitfalls faced by teams. Understanding key aspects of team dynamics can help to guide improvement efforts.

▶ Understanding and Improving the Performance of Quality Improvement Teams

In this section, we present evidence about teams and team management, relate this information to QI teams, and apply case examples to illustrate selective concepts and principles.

Team Tasks and Goals

As a point of departure, all teams have goals and specific tasks. Understanding the fundamental purposes of a team guides other aspects of team development and management, including team composition, decision-making processes, and the types of interdependencies the team has with other entities in the organization. In general, we can state that QI teams are, by definition, focused on identifying and analyzing quality and patient safety problems, designing interventions to address these problems, and evaluating the impact of changes. In one form or another, teams complete tasks aligned with the Planning, Doing, Checking, Acting (PDCA) cycle, which was first introduced in Chapter 1 and is discussed with various applications throughout this text. The clarity of the task as well as the authority/empowerment of the team to carry out improvement efforts is very important in engaging team members. Essentially, team members should have a shared understanding of the goals of the team.

Although some teams have clear and self-evident goals, QI teams may face ambiguity. The nature of QI itself is a process of discovery; as root causes of problems are uncovered, teams may find that the task of the team changes. For example, a team working in a clinic in a low-income country may be

investigating the problem of drug stock-outs. The team may find that a key root cause of the problem is an inconsistent supply chain, and supply chain problems in turn are due to poor communication between clinic staff and a central supply depot. Further, communication problems may be due to frequent gaps in electricity in the clinic as well as in the supply depot. An intervention to reduce stock-outs may therefore require team members with expertise in addressing problems of power outages and connectivity. In this case, the initial composition of the team may be inadequate to address the root cause of the problem. The team may wish to add a team member from the supply depot to help suggest changes in how and when the clinic communicates with the supply depot. The point here is that as fundamental underlying problems are identified, a team's tasks may change. In the preceding example, a new task emerged: addressing power outages.

A common problem in teams is related to a lack of clarity about the team's authority to implement change. The question arises as to whether a team has the authority to make decisions and implement changes, or simply to make recommendations. There is no single answer to this question; many highly variable factors ranging from organizational politics to intra-organizational dynamics to environmental changes may influence a team's authority. What is most important is that teams have a clear understanding of the limits of their authority. It is disheartening and demotivating for team members to believe the team has the authority to implement a change only to face the reality that the team is limited to providing suggestions or recommendations.

As illustrated in the Greenwood Family Medicine example (**CASE STUDY 6.2**), goal definition presents a problem. The initial goal in the case study's situation was to improve the provision of preventive services. However, little analytic effort was spent trying to understand the important causes of the problem. The team adopted a premature solution, and the goal

☌ *CASE STUDY 6.2: PREVENTIVE SERVICES AT GREENWOOD FAMILY MEDICINE*

Greenwood Family Medicine is a five-clinician family medicine practice serving a largely middle-class suburban population. In addition to the medical staff, the practice employs four nurses, one receptionist, and three medical records and insurance technicians.

The practice recently identified two priority areas: attention to family concerns and greater emphasis on ensuring the provision of timely preventive services. The latter effort was prompted by one of the physicians, who had recently attended a continuing medical education program on preventive services. Upon her return, she decided to assess the practice's provision of preventive services.

With a nurse and one of the medical records technicians, she reviewed a sample of children's patient charts. She and the other physicians were surprised when she distributed the results:

- Half of the children were behind schedule in at least one immunization.
- No patient charts noted that children had had vision screening.
- Fifty percent of children had not had anemia screening.
- Seventy-five percent of children had not had their blood pressure recorded in the chart.
- Eighty-five percent had not had tuberculosis screening.
- Eighty-seven percent of children had not been screened for lead exposure.

The medical staff was surprised by these findings, but medical records personnel and nursing staff found this information consistent with their impressions. The review indicated that even children who were seen for an annual physical were often not updated on preventive services—or if they were, this information was not recorded in the patient chart. It was felt that high patient volume made it impossible to ensure that appropriate preventive services were provided to all children. In addition, the practice saw many drop-in patients. The nurses felt that while these drop-ins caused added tension from the increased workload, they also presented an opportunity to check on patients' needs for preventive services.

The findings were discussed at the monthly meeting for all staff, and it was decided to form a team to address the problem. A medical records technician was asked to schedule a meeting. It was decided that two nurses and four physicians would participate on this team.

The first meeting was scheduled over the noon hour (12:00 PM to 1:00 PM). One physician arrived at 12:20, while another had to leave early, at 12:45. Virtually the entire meeting was spent attempting to find an appropriate date and time for follow-up meetings.

At the next meeting, the physicians stated that during an acute visit, physicians simply do not have time to go through the chart to determine if a patient needs updating on preventive services. It was decided, therefore, that the nurses would review each chart for the day's patients and fasten a form listing all preventive services. Services needing updating would be circled. The medical records staff was asked to design this form.

When the physicians saw the resulting form, they felt it was poorly designed. Some services were not included, and immunization schedule information was not included. The physicians asked the medical records technician to redesign the form. The technician and a nurse added the immunization schedule and other information. When presented to the physicians, they discovered disagreements in several areas. Immunization schedules differed, and practices varied on lead and TB screening. They decided that the form should include separate columns for each physician, each column specifying a physician's preventive services preferences. A form was created reflecting each physician's preventive service preferences.

(continues)

🔍 CASE STUDY 6.2: PREVENTIVE SERVICES AT GREENWOOD FAMILY MEDICINE *(continued)*

After the new preventive services chart was developed, the nurses expressed concern about the lack of time available to record preventive services needs but agreed reluctantly to start reviewing charts and entering preventive service information on each chart. After 6 weeks of working with this system, the following events unfolded:

- Nurses complained that medical records staff were not making charts available in time to do the preventive services review.
- Physicians complained among themselves that preventive service information was incomplete or inaccurate in more than 50% of the cases.
- Nurses were spending an additional 1 to 2 hours in the office preparing the next day's files and complained that the charts were very hard to decipher. The nurses requested, and were denied, overtime pay. One nurse left the practice.
- Confusion was rampant when charts were prepared for one physician but another physician actually saw the patient. This caused increased patient waiting time. An even more difficult problem was caused by drop-ins for whom the record review was not prepared. Nurses spent up to 30 minutes reviewing drop-in charts and recording relevant information. Backlogs resulted, and nurses neglected their other roles.
- The system was eliminated, and physicians decided to independently deal with preventive services.

The Case Studies are reprinted with permission from a chapter by these authors in S. M. Shortell and A. D. Kaluzny, *Health Care Management: Organization Design and Behavior*, 5th ed. Albany, NY: Thomson Delmar Learning, 2006.

drifted away from improving preventive service rates to constructing and implementing a preventive services chart. While such a chart may have been useful as part of the solution to the performance gap in preventive services, the team became fixated on this as the solution, at the expense of generating other more impactful alternatives. Implementing a solution became the goal, and the team lost its initial focus on the problem of low preventive services rates. Team member time was spent constructing a tool instead of trying to understand the fundamental causes of the problem. Basically, a "solution" presented itself, and the solution became the goal in itself. A key problem faced as a result of this is that the team did not work on what seemed to be a very major problem facing the practice, namely, the variation in protocols for preventive services. The team also did not sufficiently examine the problem of record keeping and never came to an understanding of whether their rates were really low or whether the problem was an artifact of poor record keeping. The use of a cause-and-effect diagram, first introduced and explained in Chapter 4, may have helped, and most important, effective leadership may have kept the team on task and focused on its primary goal.

Team Characteristics

Team characteristics refer to basic physical and social psychological aspects of a team and include team composition and size, relationships between team members, status differences, level of psychological safety, team norms, and the team's stage of team development. All of these characteristics potentially affect the team effectiveness.

Team Composition and Size

What is the optimal composition and size of a team? This answer obviously depends upon the nature of the team, its goals, and tasks. In some cases, team size and composition are mandated, such as sports teams and accreditation teams. Teams must be sufficiently large to have the requisite expertise to get the work done, but not so large that they are cumbersome and difficult to manage. In the Greenwood Family Medicine example (Case Study 6-2), the team faced multiple problems because of its unwieldy size and difficulty scheduling meetings, keeping order during meetings, establishing a protocol for discussion, and decision making.

Interestingly, although the team was too large, it did not in fact contain all of the expertise required to address the preventive services problem. The Institute for Health Improvement suggest that successful QI teams require four general types of expertise. A *clinical leader* is an individual who has authority in the organization to test and implement changes and to overcome implementation problems. A team member with *technical expertise* has a thorough understanding of the systems and processes of care. A third key area of expertise is a team member who is a *subject matter expert* and is in a position to drive the project on a day-to-day basis—a project manager of sorts. Finally, teams need a *project sponsor* who has the executive authority to serve as a link with senior management; this individual may or may not be a member of the team on a day-to-day basis (IHI, 2017), but is essential for success.

In the Greenwood Family Medicine example, the medical records staff, who foresaw the difficulties with the new system, were not included on the team—even to selectively provide input or react to proposed solutions. When deciding upon team composition, one needs to consider the tasks facing the team. For example, if information is required about information technology, it would naturally be helpful to have someone knowledgeable in this area. In the Greenwood Family Medicine case, abstracting information from medical records was a key aspect of the intervention. Medical records staff familiar with the structure of the medical record could have contributed substantially to the design of this intervention.

Team size therefore goes hand-in-hand with team composition. The team must have adequate diversity and expertise to inform all aspects of the team's tasks and goals. Yet the team must not be so large that reaching consensus or following an appropriate timeline is impossible. In Greenwood Family Medicine, it would have been advisable to cut the team size by 50% and ask team members to consult and obtain input from their constituencies about the team's work.

In today's work world, team size and composition may vary significantly over short periods of time. An individual may join a team for a short period of time to address a specific technical problem. In addition, it is common for members in team meetings to rotate attendance. For example, if the nursing perspective is required to address a problem, it would not be uncommon for different nurses to attend team meetings over time. This type of arrangement is often necessary because of the realities of organizational life; people have multiple commitments and time pressures that may require flexibility in team membership. Furthermore, teams also vary in terms of their permanence and longevity. We traditionally think of teams as relatively permanent and stable groups of people. However, there are instances where a team must quickly form and work together over a short period of time. In health care organizations, teams may form and disband over a period of a shift. Edmondson (2012) coined the term "teaming" to refer to an organization capable of collaborating and coordinating without the necessary team structures, such as stable team membership. She refers to this capability as "team on the fly." As described by Edmondson, individuals working in hospital emergency departments must work as a team, although each shift may bring different team members who may not have previously worked together. Valentine and Edmondson (2015) used the term "scaffolding" to describe a number of ways in which organizations can support the development and effective operation of temporary teams on a continuous basis.

Team Relationships and Status

Because we often learn about quality problems from individuals situated at different levels and units of an organization, a central tenet of QI is participation of a broad array of team members. These include individuals at relatively low levels in the organization without formal authority but with considerable tacit knowledge. In fact, it is often those on the front lines who bring unique perspectives and insights into a situation.

Involving an appropriate range of people is only the first step, however. In any team, people bring with them their roles and status from regular organizational life. Physicians working on a team with nurses bring with them their higher professional status and authority. The physician–nurse relationship, however that is characterized in a particular organization, is thus "imported" into the team. These pre-formed relationships and status systems may influence the participation of team members and affect the effectiveness of a team. Individuals from a lower status group are less likely to contribute than those of higher status. They may feel condescended to or intimidated, or they may simply feel that their input is not valued. For QI teams, such status differences are dysfunctional. To engage all team members and ensure that the team can utilize each member's knowledge, QI team leaders need to find a way to diminish the impact of status differences.

The important role of nurses as equals on QI teams should not be underestimated. For example, this recognition has contributed to the important leadership role of nurses in the development and implementation of a number of quality initiatives, such as surgical safety checklists (Gawande, 2009).

Team members bring to the team previously formed relationships. We may find two individuals with a history of interpersonal problems serving on the same team. Unfortunately, relationship problems and dysfunctional status differences can dramatically affect the work of a team. It is truly the remarkable team that can dispose of status differences and interpersonal animosities in the interest of team goals. At the very least, team leaders need to be aware of status differences and the impact of those differences on communication and team effectiveness. One way to avoid the problems of status difference and interpersonal conflict is to have a team leader with sufficient authority and respect act as moderator, encouraging lower status members to participate, keeping higher status members in check, and defusing tension driven by team member conflict. A key characteristic of effective team leaders that is often absent in science and health care activities is the ability to resolve conflicts (Sapienza, 2004); this is a characteristic which can increase motivation and help to ensure a team's success.

People who work on QI teams typically have "regular" jobs in the organization, and their participation in improvement efforts requires time away from their normal work. It is therefore important to reduce the amount of time lost to process issues, or issues that are not part of the actual task of the team. These include dealing with logistical issues such as scheduling meetings, as well as managing conflict. Teams may come together amidst great enthusiasm about tackling a difficult problem. However, the work of a group may create frictions and bring to the surface latent conflicts or reignite old disputes. Interprofessional rivalries, which may have been part of the organizational culture for many years, may surface, and leaders should devise strategies to manage and minimize these conflicts. Otherwise, a substantial amount of work time may be lost managing these conflicts. QI teams, like other teams, are also prone to personality clashes that may be very destructive to the work of a team. Health care is particularly prone to difficulties posed by status differences because of the traditional professional hierarchy common in most organizations.

In Greenwood Family Medicine, status differences were destructive to the work of the group. First, medical records staff were not included, likely because they were considered nonprofessional staff and their perspectives and opinions were discounted. Status differences, with likely elements of intimidation, also prevented both nurses and medical records staff from voicing their reservations about the use of the preventive services chart. There was also tension and status differences between the two "high-volume" physicians and others in the practice. These differences were not beneficial to the work of the team.

Psychological Safety

Team psychological safety is defined as a shared belief that the team is safe for interpersonal risk taking (Edmondson, 1999). A central tenet of QI is the belief that people must be forthcoming and honest about quality problems, even where they themselves were responsible for, or shared responsibility for, a quality or patient safety incident. Individuals involved in improvement efforts must feel that their suggestions will be heard without fear of intimidation, condescension, or castigation (Deming, 1986). Where people feel safe, there is a greater likelihood of their participating effectively in QI efforts. Furthermore, psychological safety is an important prerequisite for implementing organizational change. People need to feel psychologically safe if they are to feel secure and capable of changing (Schein & Bennis, 1965).

Status differences certainly affect psychological safety. Where status differences have an oppressive presence, it is very unlikely that team participants will feel the willingness to participate in discussions of quality. In the Greenwood Family Medicine case, the medical records staff had a clear sense that the

preventive services chart plan was doomed to failure, but felt uninvited. Although they voiced reservations about the plan privately, they did not feel comfortable voicing their concerns. They had a fear, likely justifiable, that they would have been criticized by others in the practice for being negative, resistant to change, or perhaps lazy. This is similar to the Donor Services case (Case Study 6-1), where many of the lower-status team members were reluctant to participate actively or positively given the negative and highly vocal nature of the Medical Examiner, a higher-status individual with whom many of the team members had to work on a daily basis. They felt that if they didn't follow his lead in the team meetings, they would incur repercussions later.

Team leaders need to consider questions of psychological safety: Do participants feel safe in making recommendations, participating in discussions, and perhaps of greatest importance, expressing skepticism and disagreement? Leaders must examine their own behavior and assess the extent to which their leadership style and manner of interaction invites participation and promotes safety. It is only by creating such a climate that team members will not become "yes-men" and "yes-women," also described by Grove (1995) as "peer group syndrome," a situation that results when group members fear stating an opinion that goes against the group.

Team Norms

A norm is a standard of behavior that is shared by team members. Norms set expectations and establish standards of behavior and performance. Norms have a strong impact on individuals in organizations, essentially establishing the "rules" under which people function. Behavioral norms consist of rules that govern individual behavior and attitudes. In a team context, behavioral norms define how people are expected to behave on a team. These may include expectations about attendance, preparation for team meetings, and the manner in which members communicate with each other during and between team meetings. Norms are different in every team. In the Greenwood Family Medicine case study, we see the interaction between status differences and norms. Although there was likely a superficial belief in the desirability of a democratic and participative climate, it was clear that behavioral norms emphasized a high regard for hierarchy. For example, nurses were directed to produce a form (and then several versions), and physicians declared the termination of the QI initiative. Norms about attendance at meetings were very loose—at least for the medical staff. One meeting, in which arguments ensued about whether the preventive services issue was office wide or specific to the physicians, ended with no conclusion, summary, or future plans. Evidently, norms were never established for how meetings would be conducted or expectations for attendance. Norms were nonexistent or dysfunctional. Participation was inhibited, full discussion of issues was repressed, and meetings were inefficient and ineffective.

In contrast to behavioral norms, performance norms govern the amount and quality of work expected of team members. In the Greenwood Family Medicine case, performance norms were broken, leading to difficulties for the practice. While there were expectations about working hours for nurses, the new preventive services chart system required that they work up to 3 hours after regular working hours—a break from normal working hours. This change in work demand was not anticipated, and breaking this performance norm caused morale problems and the departure of at least one nurse.

Stages of Team Development

Teams go through various life cycle stages, and different tasks and levels of productivity characterize each stage. We can conveniently think of teams going through four stages: forming, storming, norming, and performing. These stages, first described by Tuckman (1965), are best viewed as guides, and not rigid expectations. The speed with which teams proceed through these stages varies greatly and some teams never move to the final stage of performing. A team begins in the forming stage when goals and tasks are established. It is characterized by generally polite behavior among team members, which may mask underlying conflicts. Individuals often do not feel psychologically safe at this time and may be reluctant to contribute and unlikely to disagree. Team members, still unclear about the norms of the team, may stand back until they get a sense of norms and "rules" of the team.

When team members begin to feel more comfortable, there may be a period of "storming," which may be mild or severe. Team members may compete for roles, may argue about team goals and processes, or may simply attempt to stake their ground. This type of conflict is normal, and if managed well by the team leader, can result in a resolution of important issues.

If the team resolves its storming stage (which does not always happen), a norming stage emerges in which there is agreement on team norms and expectations. Team member roles are clarified, although these may change during the life of a team.

Following the norming stage is a performing stage in which the team is in the best position to accomplish its goals. Conflicts have mainly been resolved, roles are clear, norms are established, and team time can be spent on the substantive work of the team rather than on process issues.

Teams can function at all stages of their development. However, at earlier stages, much energy is lost to "process loss"—that is, focusing the team's energies and time on team maintenance functions rather than on the substantive work of the team. Teams are most effective when they have matured, meaning they have successfully progressed through the first three stages and are able to focus on team goals and tasks.

What stage of development did the Greenwood Family Medicine team reach? The team that was assembled for the preventive services improvement project included virtually all members of the practice. This team did not show evidence of maturity. Norms of behavior were unclear (for example, attendance at meetings), decision making and rules for discussion were not well developed, and perhaps most importantly, role relationships among participants still reflected their roles in the practice. Physicians assumed a rather superior role in the practice, which may or may not have been appropriate. On the improvement team, however, such a role was clearly inappropriate and blocked the team from accessing information needed to address the preventive services problem. It is likely that the events that transpired in this case could have been predicted from observing the team's inability to move through stages of development.

▶ Resources and Support

As open systems, teams require resources in order to survive and flourish. Resources come in a number of forms, including financial resources; intellectual resources; information; people with the necessary knowledge, skills, and abilities; equipment; communication systems; and moral support and credibility. Furthermore, individual team members require support, including recognition for their work on the team and rewards for their performance. At the most fundamental level, a team functions best when ensconced within an organization that supports the concept of teamwork and, more specifically, respects the work done by the team. We begin our discussion of resources and support at this level, with a brief review of the definition and concepts related to organizational culture.

Organizational Culture

Many definitions have been suggested for organizational culture. Broadly speaking,

organizational culture refers to the fabric of values, beliefs, assumptions, myths, norms, goals, and visions that are widely shared in the organization (French, 1998). An organization can have a single culture, although there are often subcultures within the organization. Among health care organizations, for example, we would expect to see cultural differences between a large teaching hospital and a small, rural medical practice. Within an organization, teams themselves can develop their own culture; as with ethnic cultures, these organizational cultures may include rituals, a specific language, particular modes of communication, and unique systems of rewards and sanctions.

Organizational culture has a number of implications for teams. First, effective teams are usually characterized by a culture that is respectful and supportive of team members, with appropriate levels of empowerment. In a QI team, for example, we would hope to see a culture characterized by interdisciplinary respect, open communication, and a collective spirit. It would be very difficult to imagine a successful QI team that does not share these and other cultural characteristics.

Consider an organization characterized by intense and dysfunctional competition, low staff participation in decision making, and interprofessional rivalries and antagonism. We can consider this type of organization as having a *dissonant culture* (Fleeger, 1993). Notwithstanding the skills of an effective team leader, can we really expect team members drawn from such an environment to perform effectively on a multidisciplinary team? It's more likely that team member attitudes would mirror their attitudes and behaviors outside the team. Team members would probably exhibit distrust, a "them vs. us" norm, and skepticism about their role in decision making.

Consider the behavior and attitudes of team members drawn from a positive or *consonant culture*. We would expect team members to bring with them the very supportive cultural attributes of the larger organization; this would contribute to team growth and performance. We can see how the larger organizational culture can be viewed as a resource: The larger culture can be highly supportive, unsupportive, or destructive to the work of the team.

Although challenging, a team can develop a strong and appropriate culture while enmeshed in an organization with a contrary culture. This is not ideal and requires leadership that can help to build a team culture that does in fact serve the interests of team effectiveness.

Changing Culture

Cultures are very difficult to change, so team leaders and participants must understand the impact of the culture of the larger organization on the work and culture of the team. Team members' negative or dysfunctional attitudes may simply reflect how they are treated in the larger organization. Team leaders should acknowledge the difficulty of leading a

participative improvement team within a larger organizational culture that is nonparticipative and autocratic. Staff who work in a rigid, overbearing culture are likely to become skeptical when suddenly asked to participate in decision making, wondering whether their opinions will be valued, and so forth. QI efforts in health care often confront this contradictory culture issue, experiencing the difficulties of attempting to introduce a culture that is inconsistent with the dominant organizational culture.

In the state regulatory agency case (CASE STUDY 6.3), there was a culture that stressed the importance of customer relations. Value was placed on the need to provide accurate and timely information. The team that was formed to analyze and make recommendations about the problem of providing inaccurate information was motivated by the same belief in the importance of its service mission. Multiple teams were formed, each adopting this organizational culture, leading to improved communication and overall influence on policy; and ultimately more accurate information to customers.

🔍 CASE STUDY 6.3: ERRONEOUS INFORMATION AT A STATE REGULATORY AGENCY

The Department of Health and Emergency Services is a state regulatory agency dealing with a variety of health care professional issues. Its roles include credentialing emergency medical service (EMS) personnel, providers, and educational institutions; developing and enforcing administrative code; and serving as a primary collection point for statewide EMS data. Among its most important roles is responding to requests for information about credentialing requirements for health and EMS personnel. These requests come from physicians, hospitals, EMS providers, city and county governments, and other organizations.

The agency has one main office and three regional offices. The main office has 30 staff members; each regional office is staffed by 5 to 7 people. Each regional office has a regional manager reporting to the Operations Section Chief. Since each regional office serves approximately one-third of the state, the volume of requests can be overwhelming. Each staff member is responsible for serving as primary contact for 8 to 14 counties.

The agency recently learned that a significant amount of inaccurate information has been distributed by regional staff. The agency learned about this problem from complaints that inaccurate and contradictory information had been given out. For example, a hospital requested information about how nurses could challenge the EMS exam. The hospital was informed that nurses could challenge the EMS exam when in fact agency policy prohibits any health care provider from challenging a credentialing exam.

In response to this problem, the agency director formed an education/credentialing team with one liaison in each regional office and the team leader in the main office. The team's goals included improving consistency among the three regional offices, ensuring accurate information distribution, and educating regional staff on agency policy. In addition to the team leader and regional office liaisons, the team also included members representing each specialty within the agency. These specialists would provide technical information about their particular specialty and serve as the primary contact for regional offices in their area of expertise.

The team met monthly for 12 months to discuss issues and develop policy. One of its first tasks was to determine the underlying reason(s) for its information dissemination problem. The team obtained information from its membership and through discussions with other staff in the state and regional offices, EMS providers, physicians, and educational institutions. Information was obtained through formal and informal discussions, surveys, and a Web-based forum.

Among the team's discoveries was that staff did not have clear channels of communication with senior management and were not informed about changes in regulatory requirements. The team also learned that regional office staff were trying to be "experts" in too many different fields.

The team suggested a number of changes, including the following:

- Each regional staff member will be assigned an area of specialization; thus, each member will serve the entire region instead of 8 to 14 counties. For example, one provider specialist would be the primary point of contact for all provider issues for the entire regional office.
- Each of these specialists will serve as the regional office representative on all statewide and intra-agency committees that focus on that area of specialization.
- Each regional manager will serve on a committee with senior management that will meet monthly to ensure that up-to-date information is distributed to each regional office.

These changes were implemented at the state and regional offices. Mandatory committee attendance was difficult because of statewide travel restrictions and budget shortfalls. These obstacles were overcome by using advanced computer technology and telecommunications. Other obstacles included changes in job descriptions that were resisted by several "old timers." Their fears were eased by giving them an opportunity to assist with writing their job description.

Six months after these changes were put in place, the distribution of incorrect credentialing information dramatically decreased. Specialists in the regional offices actively consulted other specialists to learn about current policy in their area. An informal telephone survey found consistent information dissemination from each regional office. Among the most successful strategies was formation of teams. This promoted consistency in information exchange and developed interagency communication between all regional offices and the main office. It was also felt that success was attributed in large part to the manner in which team members were selected and how the teams functioned.

The team concept has continued to grow within the agency, and currently every staff member within the agency serves on at least one team. Some members serve on several teams and have taken on additional work responsibilities because the team approach has provided them the opportunity to have a strong voice within the agency. Senior leadership was careful not to push the team approach too fast and did not force anyone to join a team right away. Since the education team was formed first, management emphasized the work that team performed and allowed the education team to provide monthly updates to staff. This helped show that voice is important within the agency and that if staff members work together as a team, the team will have a significant influence on agency policy as well as administrative code.

Material and Nonmaterial Support and Recognition

Regardless of their function, effective teams require material resources. As noted previously, material resources take a number of forms and vary depending on the goals and needs of the team. Provision of necessary material and nonmaterial support to a team is a reflection of the moral support and encouragement given a team by the larger organization and, in particular, senior management or other authority. Consider a team that is given appropriate space and time to meet, where senior managers on occasion voluntarily drop in on team meetings to provide information and support, or simply to reinforce the importance of a team's task, and where support staff are assigned to the team to assist in its work. Furthermore, while the team is given a specific mandate and set of goals, team members collectively decide on the manner in which it carries out most of its work. Finally, upon presenting a preliminary report, detailed feedback and questions are provided the team by all relevant stakeholders. In all likelihood, team members will feel as if their work is valued and that the team's work is indeed making a contribution to the larger organization. Consistent with the motivational and satisfying qualities of jobs defined in the *Job Characteristics Model*, such a team provides members with autonomy, feedback, a sense of meaningfulness, and a belief that their work is having a broad impact (Hackman & Oldham, 1980). In sum, giving teams appropriate support can be highly motivating. Where this support is absent or ambiguous, teams will be starved for support and will be unlikely to produce at an optimal level.

The state regulatory agency case (Case Study 6-3) provides a good example of how a team was provided with adequate support. Perhaps the most important resource provided was the time and energy of various individuals internal and external to the agency. Time was provided for team meetings, and team members felt that the work they were doing was worthwhile and valued by others in the larger organization. Where travel restrictions posed obstacles to team members' ability to meet in person, computer technology—telecommunications and teleconferencing—was used. This again reinforced the importance not only of the team's work but also of each team member's contributions.

Rewards and Motivation

Related to support and recognition is the need for team and individual rewards. From the perspective of the team, rewards typically come in the form of recognition and commendation for the team's work. In QI, team rewards usually consist of the intrinsic satisfaction of overcoming some quality challenge, that is, achieving results. Rewards may also consist of the positive feelings created by a successful team effort. Factors that contribute to team members' intrinsic motivation are of critical importance in QI efforts (Deming, 1994).

In addition to team rewards, individuals on teams need to be rewarded. Participation on teams is sometimes ambiguously defined as something between the person's job and a voluntary effort, that is, it may not be perceived as part of a staff member's "real job." Job descriptions themselves may indicate little about team participation. Performance appraisals may not include team participation criteria, and compensation and promotion decisions may not take into consideration a staff member's contribution to the work of a team. A team-oriented organization will be more likely to recognize individual contributions on teams by including teamwork in job descriptions, performance appraisal systems, and incentive compensation programs. Team-oriented organizations may also provide training in teamwork. Rewards are therefore important from the perspective of both the team and its individual members. Like individuals, teams are motivated by appropriate recognition and rewards. Individuals working on teams should receive the message that their participation on teams is important, necessary, and a key part of their jobs. As with team recognition these concepts represent intrinsic individual rewards that have a strong impact on motivating team members to achieve quality outcomes (Deming, 1994). A key step in this process of ensuring intrinsic motivation is empowerment of team members in order to achieve their highest levels of performance (Daft, 2015).

Members of the state regulatory agency team from Case Study 6-3 were able to see the consequences of their work, namely, a substantial decrease in the amount of erroneous information provided and better relations with their customers. Team members also saw their recommendations put into action, which communicated to team members the value of the team's work. This set the stage for a more team-focused agency and the likelihood that future team efforts would meet with success.

▶ Team Processes

Team processes refer to those aspects of the team dealing with leadership, communication, decision making, and member and team learning. Each of these factors can have an important impact on the effectiveness of a team.

Team Leadership

Ideally, the leader of a QI team should have thorough knowledge of the organization and the problem being addressed, as well as the authority to implement changes and overcome barriers to implementation. The leader should also have an appreciation of the implications of suggested changes on other units in the organization, as well as authority over all areas affected by proposed changes. Finally, the leader should be authorized to allocate space, time, and human resources to the team (HRSA, n.d.). As noted, these are ideal conditions, but there are times when the team leader is appointed or emerges from group

deliberations. Individuals assuming team leader roles may lack some of these characteristics. Absent these qualities, successful teams require support from key people outside of the team who are in actual positions of authority. These are discussed later in the chapter in a section devoted to external support. Discussion on leadership below applies to team leaders who have the formal authority as described above, as well as leaders who lack many of these qualities.

Leadership has taken on many meanings through the last century, with early writing on leadership emphasizing plans, details, roles, budgets, processes, and schedules. These perspectives were based in an era when technology was simple and predictable, products and customers were uniform, and scientific principles could be applied to work to maximize productivity. The legacy of this era is still with us, evidenced by management attitudes toward workers and the use of fear as a means of controlling workers. We are, of course, in a very different era in which uncertainty and unpredictability are normal, and where the ability of an organization or team to be successful requires it to put itself in a position to learn.

Where a team task is clear and unambiguous, a top-down leadership style may be justified, although even in such settings, input from team members may be valuable. In essence, the traditional role of a leader in low-uncertainty settings is to see that the job is done and that team members communicate and coordinate their work. In the QI area, however, leadership must take on a different look. Quality improvement is based on learning and discovery; while the team leader should be very knowledgeable about the issues under examination, no one person has all of the information to solve or even identify the sources of quality challenges. QI is by definition ambiguous and is largely a problem-solving process. Team members participate on a QI team because they have expertise relevant to the problem. Team members do not need to be told what to do, but rather encouraged to participate actively in identifying problems, analyzing causation, developing interventions, evaluating the impact of change, and so forth. Team members are brought onto a QI team because no single person has the expertise to solve a particular problem. Team member passivity is most definitely not an appropriate strategy.

In an era where uncertainty is the norm, leadership styles are required that emphasize eliciting information from others, sharing of information, and using that information to collaboratively design change initiatives. In sum, the need for a participative style of leadership is unavoidable if we hope our teams be effective. Learning how to use a participative leadership style is not easy, and it is much easier to exercise an autocratic style, although it is doubtful that this style will result in positive outcomes. A participative leader does not simply listen to others but encourages and seeks out information from team members and

individuals outside of the team (Daft, 2015). A participative leader must recognize that teams have both formal and informal leaders. A sports team, for example, may have a coach or manager, but there clearly can be informal leaders, usually not specifically appointed as such, but nevertheless assuming a leadership function. A multidisciplinary health care team may have a nominal team leader, but typically power and authority flow to nonleaders who have specialized knowledge or expertise; this is the root of the concept of empowerment (Daft, 2015). A leader must be able to recognize informal leaders, ascertain how to best use their expertise and authority, and empower team members to apply their expertise and authority for the good of the team. Consider the case of Jones Hospital (CASE STUDY 6.4), which has many different, unique programs and program leaders with specific clinical expertise. These providers sometimes work independently, but more often than not work in concert to

🔍 CASE STUDY 6.4: FORMATION OF A MEDICAL CENTER SERVICE LINE TO ADDRESS NEEDS FOR COMMUNICATION AND QUALITY IMPROVEMENT

Jones Hospital is an academic medical center with 850 beds and an operating budget of more than $1 billion. In 1998, the hospital decided to develop service lines in an effort to better coordinate administrative, clinical, and business development needs of the institution. The objectives of this initiative were to integrate hospital and physician practice operations and bring together support services in an effort to develop more efficient and effective operational planning, market development, and patient-care QI. To accomplish this, the hospital divided all functional areas into 13 service lines, one of which was the Oncology Clinical Service Unit (CSU). This CSU encompassed, among others, inpatient medical oncology units, radiation oncology, and the adult bone marrow transplant program.

A few of the organization's goals were realized in the first 4 years after the creation of the CSU structure: communication among functional areas was enhanced, identification of strategic opportunities was improved, and day-to-day management was stronger. However, expectations were not met regarding strategic plan development, collaborative business plan development, resource allocation, and revenue management. It was noted that the challenges of meeting organizational goals were in part due to the continuing decentralized management of several critical areas. Even with the creation of the CSU, other oncology areas remained independent of the service line: The Jones Oncology Network, the NCI-designated Comprehensive Cancer Center, the Tumor Registry, the Cancer Protocol Coordination Team, the medical school clinical departments, and the faculty practice plan's outpatient clinics. These, along with various support functions such as Management Engineering and Medical Center Finance, were critical to success with oncology strategy and operations. Yet there was no structure that pulled the various constituencies together to work toward improving cancer patient care.

To address this problem, the medical center conducted a review of all oncology service areas and related support functions, including an assessment of specific challenges attributable to the current infrastructure. The review and assessment revealed operational fragmentation due to a lack of coordination and communication, independent priority-setting among areas, few change-implementation efforts, and a misalignment of incentives regarding both compensation and patient flow. Furthermore, the review pointed to the near impossibility of developing strategic and business plans for growing patient populations since there was not an agreed-upon process for developing and approving such plans among the many stakeholders.

In response, the CSU developed an internal program model to enhance efficiency and effectiveness by taking a patient-centered, QI approach. Based on the major cancer patient populations, specific programs were created inside the CSU, including the Adult Bone Marrow Transplant Program, the Breast Oncology Program, the GI Oncology Program, and the GYN Oncology Program, among others. Each program operated using a matrix model centered on the cancer patient experience (Grove, 1995). This structure allowed the CSU and others to focus on the needs of specific patient populations regardless of location or type of service. It reduced the organizational unit to a more manageable size in which problems could be more easily identified, analyzed, and solved by the people who were (1) the most familiar with the specific needs of each type of patient and (2) the most capable of developing a solution.

Two groups provided the leadership for this new structure: The Strategic Governance Council and the Program Meeting. These groups comprised representatives from all areas of oncology. The Strategic Governance Council addressed issues of strategic direction and included the most senior physician from each of the major areas of oncology in addition to the senior administrator from the service line, physician practice plan, oncology clinics, and oncology outreach program. This council set the strategic direction and approved all plans in a well-defined planning process. The Program Meeting led the operational implementation of the strategies and plans created by the Strategic Governance Council and further served as the central forum for communication of strategic priorities and progress reports on major projects and issues for all oncology operations throughout the hospital system.

Critical factors contributing to the successful creation of this new structure included agreement on planning processes and sufficient resourcing by centralized services such as informatics, finance, clinical laboratories, pharmacy, and radiology. The creation of the new model resulted in significant improvements in communication, planning, and resource management; cooperation among the many stakeholders; shared decision making regarding strategic and operational plans; expedited operational problem resolution; and a dramatic financial improvement in the service line overall.

collaboratively provide multidisciplinary care for a heterogeneous oncology patient population. While these individuals guide their individual programs' operations on a daily basis, these program leaders are unified under the constructs of the Strategic Governance Council and the Program Meeting, where the roles and influence of each are formalized, and they are each able to communicate in a fairly respectful and egalitarian environment. These forums provide information to the Oncology Leadership Group, which distills the information of the larger forums into guiding principles and strategies for oncology services as a whole. While the Leadership Group has a physician head who holds authority within the group, it is not possible to say that this position holds unilaterally directive authority over all the programs. The position and indeed the group serve to integrate the perspectives and needs of the multidisciplinary programs and as such provide continuity and uniformity of vision, strategy, and upward and outward communication for oncology services as they seek to continuously improve clinical care and the health care experience for the oncology patient population.

We can see that the style of leadership most appropriate in QI is one that emphasizes participation and that builds trust among team members. It is a style that encourages members to express their views and to take risks, and that develops the team and helps it to become mature and more effective. All of these characteristics can be seen in the Jones Hospital oncology service line. Leadership must also focus on keeping people engaged, motivated, and stimulated to create and innovate. Quality improvement teams are, if not voluntary, dependent upon the goodwill of participants for their success. Some successful teams encourage shared leadership by allowing specific individuals on a team to take on leadership roles for particular phases of the QI process. The overall leader therefore also assumes a training role, helping to develop team members' skills in team leadership and project management.

In sum, a participative leadership style is required not because it is humane and fosters a happy workforce (although it is likely to do so), but because team members' active participation is absolutely essential to success. Because QI teams often do not exist within the formal hierarchical structure of the organization, team leaders must be conscious of the impact of formal and informal lines of authority, on team member motivation and commitment.

Communication Networks and Interaction Patterns

A key maintenance task in any team is the exchange of information. Methods of communication are essential and central in any team activity, whether it is an operating room team, a string quartet, a sports team, or a QI team. Communication is necessary not only within the team but also between the team and the larger external environment, including other teams.

Communication is critical and cannot be left to chance. Consider the consequences, for example, of there being no formal means of communication between attending physicians and nursing staff in a hospital—or if there were no forum for communication among the 30 or more oncology programs at Jones Hospital. This is actually what drove Jones Hospital to completely restructure its organization to a service-line format. Communication and coordination deficiencies were identified as the underpinning factors contributing to less-than-optimal performance, declining patient care coordination and patient satisfaction, and a perception of reduced quality of care.

In any team, information must be conveyed, and a key question is, how? And how effectively and accurately is the information that is being exchanged? A key concept to help with understanding how to achieve the highest levels of communication is that information exchange requires responsibilities of both the sender and receiver of information. This is especially true in teams where exchanges between team members and team leaders do not rely solely on the hierarchy implied by a team structure, but also on the expertise of each team member. One way to ensure optimal exchange between senders and receivers of information is to make use of the important concept of *active listening*. Active listening requires drawing out of opinions of fellow team members, through open and deliberative stances that are nonjudgmental, and may require asking clarifying questions and other skills to reduce distortions that prevent mutual understanding. This idea relates not only to team members listening carefully to each other, but also to external stakeholders (Sapienza, 2004).

To ensure that communication is carried out in the most effective manner, teams—and especially QI teams—require a communication structure. Interestingly, a substantial proportion of health care quality problems reside in communication structure problems in the organization. Communication networks come in several varieties, and each situation demands a different type of communication structure (Longest & Young, 2006). Where the team task is simple, it may be most efficient to use a centralized structure in which information passes from the team leader to other team members. Alternatively, information can be passed from the team leader to another team member who, in a hierarchical manner, passes it down to the next individual. Neither of these models allows for or encourages upward communication. In other teams, one individual assumes the role of network hub and communicates with other members. Information from team members must pass through the hub in order to reach other team members. An all-channel communication structure is dense; communication lines are open and encouraged between all members of the team (Longest & Young, 2006). Such a structure is most useful for complex situations where the work of each team member is interdependent with others' work. In such situations, formal lines of authority are blurred or meaningless. In teams focused on patient care, QI, research, or management, it is important for team members to have ready access to other team members, as is seen in the service line of Jones Hospital, which provides such access through formalized communication forums. Information is passed not only from the team leader but also among team members, making centralized models inappropriate. Similarly, going through an intermediary is inefficient and may use up valuable time.

Quality improvement activities require a rich and dense communication structure. The work of QI teams is complex, and communication lines must be open between all members. For example, an intervention aimed at decreasing waiting time in a clinic requires interaction between clinicians on the team, support staff within the clinic, those involved in data collection, and so forth. The leader of such a team would assume the important role of ensuring that communication networks are in fact open and that team members are able to communicate with each other.

Communication between a team and its external environment is also important. As an open system, teams are often dependent upon other individuals and other teams inside or outside the organization. Leaders here assume boundary-spanning roles, in which they ensure that relationships with critical outside groups are workable (Longest & Young, 2006). This is particularly important in a hospital setting, where a particular work unit's operations are highly dependent upon interactions with other units (for example, patient-care units are highly dependent upon the pharmacy, dietary department, and so forth). The Oncology Leadership Group fills this role within the oncology service line at Jones Hospital. The Leadership Group is the broker between the oncology department and the medical center's senior administration for such needs as major redeployments of resources to support oncology's strategic priorities, redesign and reallocation of clinical space, or needs for changes in the operational interface with independent departments such as Pharmacy Services, which, to fit strategic and political needs, maintains an independent departmental structure in the organization. A QI team likely relies on information and resources from outside the immediate team and just as communication networks among team members are critical, so are strong and reliable networks between the team and other units and teams. An isolated team that neglects its external relations is likely to perform poorly because key relationships will not be well managed.

Decision Making

Decision making is a task of all teams, and the manner in which decisions are made is critical to team success. Ideally, a formal systematic approach starting with free discussion and ending with full support of the entire team is a goal to be strived for in making team decisions (Grove, 1995). There are various ways to achieve this ideal, but in some cases, full consensus cannot always be achieved or needed to make correct decisions. Teams may reach decisions by consensus or voting, or team members may simply advise the team leader, leaving the final decision to the leader. There is no single, best way for a team to make decisions, and the mode of decision making often depends upon the circumstances and goals of the team. The president of a hospital, for example, may charge a team with the task of analyzing an acquisition possibility. The team may return with recommendations and options, but the final decision and accountability for consequences remains with the president. In a multidisciplinary mental health treatment team, it is likely that decisions will be based on team consensus, although the team leader (who may be the psychiatrist) may reserve the right to override the team's recommendations. In still other teams, particularly those where there is no single person in a position of formal authority, the team as a whole may make decisions. In such situations, team members should discuss how decisions are to be made—by voting, by working toward consensus and compromise, or perhaps by deferring to the individual most knowledgeable about a particular issue to be decided.

In the Jones Hospital example (Case Study 6.4), the decision-making process and the people who make the decisions are highly dependent on the decisions themselves. Depending on the nature and criticality of the issue at hand, there are decisions made by formal vote in the Strategic Governance Council, by informal consensus in the Program Meeting, and by mandate in the Leadership Group. The success of such decision making is dependent upon open communication among the members of these groups; all information is shared, and a record of decisions made is kept through meeting minutes of all bodies. When an individual has a problem with a decision made by the Leadership Group, for example, the forum for discussion of such concerns is formally built in to the service line structure via the other two groups.

Regardless of the mode of decision making, it is critical that team members understand their role in decision making. Assuming an advising rather than decision-making role is acceptable to team members as long as they do not expect to be in the position of making decisions. The decisional authority of the team and that of team members needs to be specific and clear.

Teams often strive for cohesion, and in general cohesion is a positive force. Efforts should be made to develop a team such that members understand each other, are at ease communicating with each other, and feel a unified sense of purpose and solidarity. Taken to an extreme, however, cohesion can develop into conformity and "groupthink," where team members become so cohesive that they lose their independence as free thinkers and may fear expressing views opposed to what they consider to be the prevailing team consensus (Daft, 2015).

Member and Team Learning

Peter Senge popularized the idea of the learning organization in his book *The Fifth Discipline* (1990). Briefly, a learning organization is one that proactively creates, acquires, and transfers knowledge and changes its behavior on the basis of new knowledge and insights (Garvin, 1993). The implication of this definition for teams is clear. First, effective teams continuously look for new information to improve their performance, whether new technology, new organizational processes, or new concepts. They are open to new ideas and seek them out. They do this by seeking diversity among team members, including people on teams with new expertise and alternative perspectives, and by ensuring that team members are engaged in continuous training and learning. Effective teams then attempt to use new information, ensuring that new knowledge is transferred to the team. This new knowledge is then used to change the team's behavior in pursuit of higher levels of achievement. Teams may enhance their ability to learn and apply new knowledge through the use of a number of facilitating factors, including scanning the environment for new information; identifying performance gaps within the team; adopting an "experimental mindset," such that team members are open to new approaches; and having leadership supportive of change. (See Moingeon & Edmondson [1996] for a more in-depth discussion of facilitating factors.)

Team and organizational learning are key aspects of QI, and it is no surprise that the capacity to learn is a hallmark of effective QI teams (Upshaw, Steffen, & McLaughlin, 2013). A QI team is faced not only with solving problems, but also with the responsibility for helping the larger organization transition into a learning organization. Effective QI teams review their own performance and the satisfaction of members and seek to develop strategies and new team management techniques that will enhance their performance. Some teams "debrief" after each meeting to review the progress of their work and the manner in which they worked and seek to learn from this and improve their capabilities. Learning from experience and learning from the broader external environment are trademarks of effective organizations and teams.

▶ Conclusions

In this chapter, we have reviewed the importance of teams and effective teamwork in health care and most importantly in regard to the successful implementation of QI efforts. Steps in team development and team processes were reviewed; these include development of balanced team relationships and equal status to ensure participation of all team members, and open communication and feedback, which will ensure efficient team performance through empowerment and high levels of motivation. Critical to the success of any team effort is the role of team leaders, who can come from within the team or from traditional leadership positions; also critical to success is developing a team's culture. Finally, ongoing team learning was described as one of the most important aspects of teamwork in CQI; it provides a means for sharing knowledge and improving performance of a team as well as the larger organization in which the team exists.

References

Burns, L., Bradley, E., & Weiner, B. (2011). *Health care management—Organization design and behavior*, 6th ed. Clifton Park, NY: Delmar Cengage Learning.

Crozier, M. (1964). *The bureaucratic phenomenon.* London: Tavistock.

Daft, R. L. (2015). *The leadership experience*, 6th ed. Stamford, CT: Cengage Learning.

Deming, W. E. (1986). *Out of the crisis.* Cambridge, MA: Massachusetts Institute of Technology Center for Advanced Engineering Study.

Deming, W. E. (1994). *The new economics: For industry, government and education,* 2nd ed. Cambridge, MA: Massachusetts Institute of Technology Center for Advanced Engineering Study.

Edmondson, A. (1999). Psychological safety and learning behavior in work teams. *Administrative Science Quarterly, 44*(4), 350–383.

Edmondson, A. C. (2012). *Teaming: How organizations learn, innovate, and compete in the knowledge economy.* San Francisco, CA: Wiley.

Fleeger, M. E. (1993). Assessing organizational culture: A planning strategy. *Nursing Management, 24*(2), 40.

French, W. L. (1998). *Human resources management*, 4th ed. Boston: Houghton Mifflin.

Garvin, D. A. (1993). Building a learning organization. *Harvard Business Review, 71*(4), 78–91.

Gawande, A. (2009). *The checklist manifesto.* New York, NY: Metropolitan Books.

Grove, A. S. (1995). *High output management.* New York, NY: Vintage Books.

Hackman, J. R. (2002). *Leading teams: Setting the stage for great performances.* Boston, MA: Harvard Business School Press.

Hackman, J. R., & Oldham, G. R. (1980). *Work redesign.* Reading, MA: Addison-Wesley.

Health Resources & Services Administration. (n.d.). Improvement teams. Retrieved from https://www.hrsa.gov/sites/default/files/quality/toolbox/508pdfs/improvementteams.pdf

Institute for Health Improvement. (2017). *Science of improvement: Forming the team.* Retrieved from http://www.ihi.org

Longest, B. B., & Young, G. T. (2006). Coordination and communication. In S. M. Shortell & A. D. Kaluzny (Eds.), *Health care management — organization design and behavior*, 5th ed. Clifton Park, NY: Thompson Delmar Learning.

Moingeon, B., & Edmondson, A. (1996). *Organizational learning and competitive advantage*. Thousand Oaks, CA: Sage.

Nelson, E. C., Batalden, P. B., Huber, T. P., Mohr, J. J., Godfrey, M. M., Headrick, L. A., & Wasson, J. H. (2002). Microsystems in health care: Part 1. Learning from high-performing front-line clinical units. *The Joint Commission Journal of Quality Improvement*, *28*(9), 472–493.

Nilsen, P. (2015). Making sense of implementation theories, models and frameworks. *Implementation Science 10*, 53.

Schein, E. H., & Bennis, W. (1965). *Personal and organizational change via group methods*. New York, NY: Wiley.

Sapienza, A. M. (2004). *Managing scientists — Leadership strategies in scientific research*, 2nd ed. Hoboken, NJ: Wiley-Liss Inc.

Senge, P. M. (1990). *The fifth discipline: The art and practice of the learning organization*. New York, NY: Doubleday.

Tuckman, B. W. (1965). Developmental sequence in small groups. *Psychological Bulletin, 63*(6), 384–399.

Upshaw, V. M., Steffen, D. P., & McLaughlin, C. P. (2013). CQI, transformation and the "learning" organization, in W. A. Sollecito & J. K. Johnson (Eds.), *McLaughlin and Kaluzny's continuous quality improvement in health care*, 4th ed. Sudbury, MA: Jones and Bartlett Publishers.

Valentine, M., & Edmondson, A. C. (2015). Team scaffolds: how mesolevel structures enable role-based coordination in temporary groups. *Organization Science, 26*(2), 405–422.

CHAPTER 7

The Role of the Patient in Continuous Quality Improvement

Joanne F. Travaglia and Hamish Robertson

It is much more important to know what sort of a patient has a disease than what sort of disease a patient has.

— **William Osler**
(Canadian physician, 1849–1919)

Health systems and services around the world have one primary function: to care for the health and well-being of individuals and populations in the most effective way possible. This is true whether the people are working in a laboratory, managing a hospital, triaging at an accident or disaster site, performing cardiac surgery, or counseling a patient with schizophrenia. Whatever the setting or service, the measures of quality for the professional, staff member, team, ward, and/or service are clear. Such measures are established by a range of mechanisms, including legislation, regulatory practice, professional registration, peer and management review, government and organizational policies, guidelines, and research, and evidence-based practice.

Despite all best efforts over the last 15 years, the role of the patient (and the patient's family and carers) in maintaining and improving the quality of health care remains poorly understood (Peat et al., 2010; Schwappach, 2010). This lack of clarity arises from three sources. First, at least in part, the lack of clarity is a result of the historical, political, organizational, and managerial agendas that converge on this issue, making it difficult to define and compare the different logics, types and levels of approaches across services, systems and countries (Tritter, 2009). Second, while there exist a wide variety of policies (including, in some cases, no policy at all) and mechanisms, methods, and tools aimed at increasing patient involvement in health care, there is very limited evidence addressing their role specifically in quality improvement. As Groene and Sunol (2015) argue, patient engagement "... takes multiple forms in health care and there is not a single strategy or method that can be considered to reflect best practice" (p. 563).

Third, it remains difficult to connect patient involvement in health care services and the quality of outcomes either for particular individuals or for patients in general.

While this lack of clarity can make the involvement of consumers in quality improvement difficult, it does not negate the importance of their involvement in continuous quality improvement (CQI). One of the markers of CQI, compared to other quality systems, is that CQI acknowledges customer input as a vital source of evidence at every step of the improvement process. At an institutional level, health care services have sought information from customers through surveys, market research, advertising, and outreach efforts. From the health customer perspective, feedback is often measured via word of mouth referrals, complaints, service reputation, service demand, and litigation.

The value of these sources of information is unquestionable. Patient or consumer "involvement" in health care, however, is about more than the collection of patient satisfaction surveys. There is an increasing recognition that efforts to increase the safety and improve the quality of care have mainly focused at the technical, managerial, or professional levels. These approaches tended to leave both the patient and the wider community outside of the improvement processes. A meta-analysis of eight public inquiries into large-scale breaches of patient safety around the world showed that there were common features in the breakdown of care. Despite the diversity of country of origin, health care system, type of error(s), and clinicians involved, several key themes were identified across the inquiries. These themes included a lack of patient and family involvement; poor communication and teamwork; and inadequate quality monitoring processes (Hindle et al., 2006). This confluence of factors points clearly to the importance of the integral involvement of patients in the CQI process. The question remains, however: How do we

best gain and maximize the benefit from the active involvement of patients in the quality improvement process?

In this chapter, we begin by reviewing the rationale, models, mechanisms, and current evidence base for patient involvement in quality improvement. We then present a model of patients' involvement in health care that defines three dimensions (active to passive involvement, proactive to reactive responses, and micro to macro levels). Lastly, we consider the barriers to involvement in CQI of patients—especially vulnerable patients—and the ways in which health care services can address this issue.

▶ Patient Involvement in Health Care Improvement: A Brief Overview

The call for active patient involvement in CQI activities is in line with changes to the "traditional" patient–clinician relationship that have occurred over several decades. This space for engagement emerged as a consequence of broader social changes. We briefly consider five such changes that impacted the way in which not only patients but health care as a whole was perceived. These changes included shifts in social structures, which in turn have had an effect on the patient–clinician relationship.

From the late 1960s onward, individuals and groups became more critical of institutions of power, including medicine and health care (Illich, 1974). A greater questioning of the relationship between medical practitioners and their patients as well as other clinicians has led to a decline (albeit a slow one) in medical and provider dominance (Dent, 2006; Wade & Halligan, 2004). The increasing diversity of the health professions has also meant that the disciplinary scope of the health sciences has expanded, along with types and numbers of services available (Borthwick et al., 2010).

Several unforeseen global developments also contributed to a shift in the perceived location of health expertise. The emergence of HIV/AIDS in the 1980s produced profound social and clinical changes. Because of the rate of this condition's progression, the patients themselves knew more about the illness than the clinicians and researchers, introducing the concept of the lay (or patient) expert (Epstein, 1995). The slow response to the scale and severity of AIDS saw some significant shifts in political policy generally and health policy in particular. Not only did communities become directly engaged in providing education about and treatment of the disease, but the attitudes and responses of health services and governments to patient involvement also changed as powerful community lobby groups emerged (Shilts, 2007).

Similar trends developed in the United States in the 1990s relative to information services that became available to cancer patients and other seriously ill patients. These services continue to be rich sources of patient information, leading to greater patient empowerment. For example, the U.S. National Cancer Institute sponsors a "Cancer Information Service" that allows patients direct access to the latest information by cancer site and type, providing access to both physician- and patient-level information, including information on treatment options, treatment centers, and the latest news about clinical trials. These services can be accessed utilizing multiple modes: telephone (1-800-4-Cancer), the Internet, and more recently, social media platforms, including Twitter and Facebook. These services provide patients with the knowledge to help choose and even direct the level of care they are receiving, ensuring the highest level of quality and thereby playing a direct role in quality improvement.

The politicization of various social groups and their efforts to reestablish and legitimize their medical traditions as part of their disenfranchised cultures and epistemologies have contributed to the growth in calls for direct

patient involvement in the governance of health care. These have combined with a growing recognition of the impact produced by differences in these groups access to and quality of care (Betancourt & King, 2003). The concept of cultural safety in health care was developed by the Irihapeti Ramsden in New Zealand and has now spread internationally as a way of conceptualizing the importance of indigenous perspectives, ideas, and values in health care systems. Ramsden's argument was that health care systems were already political and that for disenfranchised peoples to have their perspectives acknowledged by these systems was, in actuality, a political act of both self-definition and resistance (Ramsden, 1993, 2000a, 2000b).

The growth in "alternative" or complementary medicine since the 1980s has been associated with both globalization and the dissatisfaction felt by many people with mainstream medical care. It has, in effect, produced a secondary health care system, one more directly controlled by the consumer and their preferences (Mak & Faux, 2010; Senel, 2010). The emergence of invigorated cultural health traditions means that mainstream systems need to address demands for the improved recognition and inclusion of, for example, traditional healers, medicines, and conceptual health schemata in treatment regimens (Gottlieb, Sylvester, & Eby, 2008). Where medical systems have resisted these shifts, they have often been forced by political pressure and policy shifts to make some accommodations of these more patient-centered and patient-driven approaches.

Lastly, the arrival of the Internet has changed patients' access to information in quite profound ways. Patients now have readily accessible information about their conditions from an expanding range of sources (Bylund et al., 2010). They can also gain information about the treatments, services, or clinicians available locally, nationally, and internationally. The media, both public and private, now produce or host regular information programs, websites, and columns addressing health care concerns, treatments, and services. In addition to breaking news stories, there is now a constant stream of health-related programs ranging from documentaries to "reality" television programs on hospitals and clinicians, all the way to the cult of the celebrity clinician (e.g., Crouch et al., 2016; Jeong & Lee, 2017). Medicine has gone from the rarefied and private to the increasingly commonplace and public.

It is not only patients and the media who make use of these technologies. Health departments and services exhibit growing use of websites and social networking sites to distribute information. Prominent clinicians also use the technology; for example, Atul Gawande, a leading patient safety researcher, has a regular column in *The New Yorker*. Other researchers and practitioners use iTunes to disseminate their messages to clinicians and patients alike. The Institute for Healthcare Improvement (IHI) offers an online interprofessional educational community for clinicians and students wanting to learn more about quality and safety.

For patients, the Internet has produced another profound effect. It has become a platform through which support and discussion groups have emerged. Even individuals with the rarest of conditions (given access to computers and the Internet) now have access to forums where they can describe and discuss both the symptoms and the progression of their illness; moreover, they can compare the type and quality of their treatments with patients experiencing the same or related conditions. Similarly, people acting as carers for patients who may be too ill to seek their own information directly can also seek support and assistance from people in similar situations.

▶ Rationale for Patient Involvement in CQI

As social and clinical relationships were changing, there was also increasing public awareness and disquiet about the incidence of medical errors. Most quality and safety practitioners and academics in the United States associate the birth of the current patient safety movement with the Institute of Medicine's *To Err Is Human* report (IOM, 2000). Although it was presenting data about error rates from a much earlier study by Brennan et al. (1991), the IOM report galvanized health care systems around the world into action; the report's metaphor of hospital errors being the equivalent of a "jumbo jet full of patients crashing every three days" drew widespread media and public attention.

Around the same time, a series of high-profile cases of negligence, incompetence, and/or medical homicide began to appear in the press. The Bristol Royal Infirmary inquiry (pediatric cardiac surgery) and Shipman inquiry (general practice) in the United Kingdom (Department of Health, 2001; Smith, 2005), the Cartwright inquiry (cervical screening) in New Zealand (Cervical Cancer Inquiry, 1988), and the Manitoba Coroner's Inquest (pediatric cardiac surgery) in Canada (Sinclair, 1994) were just some of the cases that increased public anxiety about the quality and safety of health care internationally. More recently, the Mid-Staffordshire Hospital Inquiry in the United Kingdom has shown the devastating impact of a lack of quality control (Francis, 2013). Added to these two factors were rising levels of complaints and litigation faced by health services, both public and private. The scene was set for new approaches to safeguarding patients.

Early on in the development of the patient safety movement, Vincent and Coulter (2002) asked the question "Patient safety: what about the patient?" Their argument was that "... plans for improving safety in medical care often ignore the patient's perspective" (p. 76) and that the active role of patients in the safety of their care was something that health care services and clinicians needed to acknowledge and encourage.

Patient involvement in CQI and other quality and safety strategies therefore reflects a profound change in the health service approaches to the provision of care. Health systems and clinicians now recognize that patients and their families can no longer be treated as completely passive recipients of care. In addition to the ethics involved in this traditional approach, this new perspective has a strong practical element. Patient involvement is about ensuring the accountability and transparency of services (Emanuel & Emanuel, 1997; Forrest, 2004). It is about the provision of patient-centered, as opposed to clinician-centered, care (Berntsen, 2006; Robb et al., 2006, Kitson et al., 2013), to the point more recently where health care services and clinicians have begun to work collaboratively on the codesign (Donetto et al., 2015), coproduction (Batalden et al., 2016), and redesign (Baker et al., 2016) of health care services and programs. But it is equally about joining with patients as partners in the constant vigilance and heedfulness required to protect against errors. Simply stated, practitioners, services, and managers needed to more actively listen to and engage with patients throughout the entire health care process.

▶ Methods for Involving Patients in CQI

What does patient involvement look like? The answer depends largely on the level and type of system under consideration. One way of assessing patient involvement in CQI is to focus on three levels [after Bronfenbrenner (1979)]: micro (direct clinician–patient interactions), meso (health service or system level), and macro (national or international).

Micro-Level Patient Involvement

At a micro level, patients are directly involved in the decision making and management plans associated with their individual treatment, as well as in ensuring that the intended treatment is given as planned and according to established protocols (that is, in the monitoring of

the quality and safety of their care) (Longtin et al., 2010; Peat et al., 2010). Here, terms such as *engaged, active, vigilant,* or *empowered* are applied to the patient as health services seek to assist patients in improving their health literacy and supporting them, wherever possible, to take on a self-management role (Anderson, 2007; Coulter & Elwyn, 2002; Entwistle & Quick, 2006).

Over the last decade the idea of *personalization* has been introduced and is closely associated with the CQI concept of mass customization (McLaughlin & Kaluzny, 2006). Personalization is a term that has been used in various industries, especially the computer industry. The association between personalization and mass customization is discussed in detail by Tseng and Piller (2003), who describe personalization as going beyond the traditional definition of customization by involving customers (patients) in intense communication and high levels of interaction (between customers and suppliers), including negotiating the selection of services with the customer (see Chapter 1). This terminology has begun to be adopted in medical care (Hamburg & Collins, 2010), by expanding the inclusion of patient preferences through the individualization of care and shared decision making (Barratt, 2008; Robinson et al., 2008).

Patients are increasingly involved in collaborating with clinicians to reach accurate diagnoses, decide on appropriate treatment and/or management strategies, choose a suitably experienced and safe provider, and in ensuring the appropriate administration and monitoring of, and adherence to, treatments or directions (DiGiovanni, Kang, & Manuel, 2003; Ubbink et al., 2009). At this level, patients can also contribute to reducing the inappropriate use of health care resources (such as the overuse of medications, including antibiotics), which in turn can potentially reduce health care errors (Smith, 2009) and the spread of antimicrobial resistance (McCullough et al., 2015).

Patients have increasingly been called on to identify and notify unsafe acts on the part of clinicians, including, for example, a lack of hand hygiene (Bittle & LaMarche, 2009; Seale et al., 2015). As with self-management of chronic conditions, patients are most often encouraged to participate in quality improvement programs through a combination of awareness raising, information, and educational programs (Anthony et al., 2003), including participation in social marketing programs (see Chapter 8).

Meso-Level Patient Involvement

At the meso level, patient involvement in CQI is about increasing the appropriate, effective, and safe provision of services (Bate & Robert, 2016). As consumers or customers, patients involved at this level are engaged in the planning, management, and evaluation of anything from entire health systems (Mockford et al., 2012) down to individual services (Donetto et al., 2015). Such participation can also take a variety of forms.

Individuals can be involved as members of the public, as patients, as caregivers or family members of individuals receiving care, as representatives of consumer organizations (such as advocacy and self-help groups), and as members and representatives of population groups or communities (Anderson, Shepherd, & Salisbury, 2006; Murray, 2015). The perceived effectiveness of this last type of participation has been attributed (by patients) to their own participatory behavior and the availability of institutional participatory spaces—that is, the "opening up" of CQI mechanisms to patient involvement (Delgado-Gallego & Vazquez, 2009). It is important to note that there are criticisms of the "representativeness" of consumers, in particular that the patients involved tend to be either "professional" consumers or individuals who often more closely mirror the socioeconomic and educational profiles of health care professionals than of other social groups (Coulter, 2002).

The mechanisms by which they are involved also vary. Participation can be a "one-off" involvement in a forum or workshop or attendance at a conference. Participation can occur in time-limited activities, such as membership on patient safety committees in hospitals or services, although it should be noted that there is evidence for discrepancies between the patients' and staff's expectations of this engagement process (Nathan, Johnston, & Braithwaite, 2010). Participation can also be anonymous and more passive or reactive. Feedback via patient satisfaction surveys (see Chapter 4), exit interviews, or questionnaires can contribute to quality efforts, as can involvement in focus groups or complaints and compliments letters (Ervin, 2006; Mease et al., 2007). Once again, this level of involvement may be part of a social marketing initiative, as described in Chapter 8.

Macro-Level Patient Involvement

Macro-level involvement in CQI sees the patient involved in patient safety activities at a national or international level. Various examples exist and are discussed in the following sections. The World Health Organization's (WHO) Patients for Patient Safety movement is one example of an international strategy aimed at ensuring that the patient's perspective is integrated into mechanisms to improve the quality and safety of care. The WHO's London Declaration is a pledge of partnership and a core document for its World Alliance for Patient Safety (Patients for Patient Safety, 2006).

For both publicly and privately funded health care around the world, public reporting on the quality of care remains a contested issue (Duckett et al., 2008). The argument for the publication of such data is that it will make patients (often, in this context, referred to as consumers) more active participants in their choice of providers (Utzon & Kaergaard, 2009). Effective public reporting is said to (1) engage and involve health care systems and services from the initiation of the reporting program, (2) ensure the data reported are of the highest quality, (3) provide information in a way that is accessible and appropriate to consumers, and (4) to provide clinicians with detailed information on their individual performance (Tu & Lauer, 2009). Finally, in addition to input into direct service and health system delivery issues, some countries are grappling with the involvement of consumers and the public in "upstream" areas of patient safety such as health-related research (Forsythe, 2016).

▶ # Factors Affecting Patient Involvement

What evidence is available to support the involvement of patients in the quality and safety of care? Rigorous evaluations of both educational campaigns (Schwappach, 2010) and patient involvement programs (Peat et al., 2010) were found to be lacking. Available evidence indicates that although patients tend to have a positive attitude toward the idea of being involved in their safety, their actual involvement varies both as individuals (Schwappach, 2010) and between groups, particularly in the case of "minority" groups, such as immigrants (De Freitas & Martin, 2015).

From the patients' perspective, a number of factors contribute to their willingness to participate in patient safety and quality strategies. These include their sense of self-efficacy; their acceptance of a new, more active role as patients; the perceived preventability of incidents; and the perceived effectiveness of their actions (Peat et al., 2010; Schwappach, 2010).

Health literacy is a significant factor in determining patient involvement at every level of care (Kripalani et al., 2010; Pappas et al., 2007; Peota, 2004; Rothman et al., 2009). Factors inhibiting patient involvement range from the complexity of the patient's condition (e.g., the presence of comorbidities) to a perceived lack of confidence or skills, to broader socioeconomic issues including social status

and ethnicity (Johnstone & Kanitsaki, 2009; Longtin et al., 2010). The health care setting (e.g., whether it is primary, secondary, or tertiary care, or whether the patient perceives it to be intimidating) and the actual task involved (e.g., whether "involvement" includes confronting clinicians) have also been found to contribute to patients' willingness and ability to participate in CQI-related strategies (Burroughs et al., 2005; Davis et al., 2007). Perceived power differentials between individuals from vulnerable communities and health services can cause anxiety, including fear of retribution. So too can the burden of being asked to represent the needs and concerns of an entire community, especially without adequate skills, support, or preparation (Abelson et al., 2004; Arnstein, 1969; Delgado-Gallego & Vazquez, 2009; Murie & Douglas-Scott, 2004).

The type of illness being experienced and socioeconomic factors also contribute to health workers' support of patient involvement. Clinicians' attitudes toward patient involvement are influenced by organizational issues (e.g., lack of time or training) and personal beliefs; for example, they may fear losing control or specialization, or they may perceive the "stakes" as being too high (Longtin et al., 2010). Thus, the integration of patient involvement still has some way to go before it is central to CQI and related processes.

▶ # Measuring Patient Involvement in CQI

In keeping with the London Declaration, patient satisfaction surveys have been implemented in many countries in an effort to quantify some of the many nonclinical outcomes of the patient experience and to try and increase the transparency of health and medical treatments and their associated outcomes. There is an ongoing debate about whether "satisfaction" is an adequate conceptual framework for what is at stake, and other terms such as *patient experiences* have been proposed (Hekkert et al., 2009). The use of "satisfaction" measures also indicates the influence of established models in the corporate world for gaining feedback from those paying for and/ or receiving the service in question. The type of data collected lends itself to the statistical analysis of key institutional issues against patients' demographic variables, with a prevailing assumption that objective, quantifiable data provide the necessary understanding. An important constraint is that most satisfaction surveys tend to produce relatively positive results, and institutional providers may themselves be dependent on positive indicators for funding, board approvals, and other systemic "rewards."

Thus, measuring CQI from the patient perspective is more complicated than it may initially appear. It is also clear that patient experiences, satisfaction included, can be highly individual, contextual, and fundamentally phenomenological in character—falling into the problematic "subjective" domain. Even patient responses to adverse events, up to and including disability or death, can be seen to vary enormously depending on how the health care providers respond to those errors. Consequently, the science of patient involvement generally—and patient "satisfaction" as a particular dimension of that experience—relies on a much broader understanding of what knowledge we are seeking, why we are seeking it, and how we go about acquiring the information to construct that knowledge. To rely exclusively, or even mainly, on standard quantitative measures in the highly contextualized settings that health care involves (think appendectomy vs. chemotherapy, for example) requires a richer and more sophisticated information base than generally produced from (typically) closed-ended survey instruments (see Chapter 4).

In the broader context, and given the information presented in this chapter, health care experiences do not, and realistically cannot, exist on the same level as

consumer-durable purchases and they must be seen as possessing a richer set of conceptual and psychometric properties. As a result, we need to acknowledge that our science of measurement in patient involvement and satisfaction needs to address that multilayered complexity more directly and informatively. In essence, there are many more potential opportunities for more direct patient and caregiver involvement.

▶ The M-APR Model of Patient Involvement

Drawing on the evidence base, we have developed a model of patient involvement that spans all levels and types of health care. The M-APR model of patient involvement looks at this issue across three levels—the "Ms" (e.g., micro, meso, macro) —and across two dimensions of involvement, the "APR" (e.g., active/ proactive and passive/reactive involvement). These dimensions indicate that patient, family, and public involvement and/or feedback into CQI can be more fully achieved through a variety of mechanisms.

Active participation assumes the direct and ongoing involvement of patients and their families and caregivers in CQI activities, be it direct input and decision making about patients' individual care or the determination of ethical standards for professions or services. Passive involvement sees services and systems drawing on more removed, yet still useful, sources of patient feedback. Many services are most familiar, and comfortable, with these sources, which include patient satisfaction surveys, exit interviews, patient focus groups, and more removed information provision via service report cards.

In proactive involvement, the patient is involved in attempting to actively prevent errors and directly address safety issues. These initiatives range from education and involvement in confronting potential sources of errors (e.g., addressing clinicians' hand hygiene or ensuring that the surgeon marks the appropriate limb or side of the body to be operated on), to involvement in CQI strategies and programs at service levels, to decision making about research directions at state, national, or international levels. In reactive approaches, the patient is involved in identifying the causes of errors that have *already* occurred, from the use of complaint letters to the analysis of incident reports; from involvement in root cause analysis (RCA) programs to involvement in patient safety inquiries.

M-APR is intended to be a diagnostic rather than a prescriptive model. TABLE 7.1 shows a summary of the model, along with some select examples. Examples, by necessity, reflect differences in publicly versus privately funded health systems.

Examples of Patient Involvement in CQI

In this section, we provide an overview of four very different strategies for patient involvement in CQI. These examples illustrate the different levels of the M-APR model and provide insights into mechanisms by which patients can contribute to ensuring the quality of health care for themselves and for the broader community.

Example 1: Partners in Health

For almost a decade, Kaiser Permanente in the United States has been promoting its Patients as Partners program. Led by Dr. David Sobel, this program focuses on the direct involvement of patients with long-term health conditions in their self-management and health literacy development. The concept is to reposition patients from being "consumers" of health services to being active partners in their own health treatment and management. The key concept is that patients with chronic conditions are already essentially responsible for 80% of their own diagnostic and treatment behaviors, and supporting this pattern can potentially improve care and save time, money, and resources.

This program grew out of work in the 1990s by Kate Lorig at the Stanford University Center for Research in Patient Education on a chronic disease self-management program and patient outcomes. The program at Kaiser includes the Healthwise Handbook, initially available online, and a range of other print, online, and direct, face-to-face supports. The concept of making low- and high-intensity interventions available was developed to cover a wide range of potential supports that could be adjusted to meet both patient and situational needs (e.g., clinician training, patient mailings, telephone calls, and face-to-face support groups).

Kaiser Permanente produced evidence to show that the strategy is highly effective and has lasting effects for patients as well as health service providers, including more appropriate utilization of services, improved accessibility, and measurable declines in selected types of service utilization. Satisfaction and behavioral indicators were positive, and return-on-investment measures ranged from 5:1 to 10:1 across the range of strategies. A randomized, controlled trial compared program subjects with wait-list controls. For participating patients with conditions including lung disease, heart disease, diabetes, and arthritis, the results showed improvements over 6 months in their exercise levels, their communication with physicians, self-reported health, and other measures. In addition, the program saw reductions in the number of hospital, outpatient, and emergency room admissions (Lorig et al., 1999). Although Kaiser is obviously a very large and influential health care provider, by its own estimate, up to 80% of the changes it implemented could also be implemented by smaller, less well-resourced providers where economics of scale and integration factors might not be as readily available (Sobel, 2003; Sofaer et al., 2009).

TABLE 7.1 Dimension of Patient Involvement in Quality Improvement: The M-APR Model

Dimension	Micro	Meso	Macro	Dimension	Micro	Meso	Macro
Active	Patients are involved in every aspect of decision making for their own care. Patients and their families and caregivers are directly and continuously consulted in the provision of care and are considered part of the health care team.	Patients are full1 members of hospital or service boards.	Patients are full members of health system or professional ethics committees and review boards.	**Passive**	Service utilizes existing data sources such as patient satisfaction surveys or exit interviews.	Services utilize a patient-centered approach to all planning and quality improvement mechanisms.	Data on use of services by different population groups are compared. Performance data on clinicians and services are publicly available.
Proactive	Patients and their families and caregivers are educated and encouraged to confront clinicians or services that breach patient safety standards.	Patients and their families and caregivers are involved in service-level planning, in identifying areas for improvement in the quality or safety of services, and in establishing new approaches to and design of services.	Patients are involved in patient safety campaigns and organizations at a state, national, or international level. Patients are represented on boards of system-level quality improvement and monitoring agencies, including professional registration boards and accreditation bodies.	**Reactive**	Service utilizes existing or custom-made sources of information such as complaint letters.	Services analyze incident data to identify patient characteristics and population patterns in types and distribution of errors. Patients are involved in CQI strategies developed after occurrence of errors, including root cause analysis and incident reporting.	Patients are represented on public reports and reviews of the quality of care. Patients are full members of public patient safety inquiries.

Example 2: National Patient Safety Goals in the United States

A second example of a patient involvement strategy is based on the accreditation requirements of health services and programs in the United States. The Joint Commission (TJC) has a specific National Patient Safety Goal (NPSG 13) that addresses this issue. It states that services should "encourage patients' active involvement in their own care as a patient safety strategy," with a more specific subclause (NPSG.13.01.01) that they should "define and communicate the means for patients and their families to report concerns about safety and encourage them to do so." In 2010, this goal became part of TJC's standards for accreditation of health care services. TJC published its *Patients as Partners: Toolkit for Implementing the National Patient Safety Goal* in 2007. This work grew out of the establishment of NPSG 13, which specifically addresses the idea of patients and their families and caregivers as having an important and tangible role in the identification of potential errors in patient treatment and care.

Patients as Partners has been supported by a range of related publications aimed at improving the capacity of patients and caregivers to identify patient safety issues as they see them developing. The program also involves training packages and accreditation for health service providers, including strategies for implementing, monitoring, and evaluating their performance. As with other patient safety systems around the world, being able to capture data and quantify the results of inter ventions is a crucial aspect of systemic change and program validation.

One of the key issues identified by TJC has been the diversity of patients, families, and caregivers in terms of their cultures and the variety of languages spoken and read. The focus on both English-language materials and materials for other important groups, such as Spanish speakers, has been integrated into the focus of this work. Central to this work is not simply the shifting demographics of the United States (and other immigrant-receiving countries) but also the centrality of effective communication in patient safety improvements. If patients are to be actively engaged as partners, then key communication issues such as language have to be incorporated from the beginning.

While TJC is not the only accreditation organization in the United States, it is an important organization, both nationally and internationally, in promoting patient safety and supporting the role of patients, families, and caregivers in the processes associated with patient safety's systemic development (see Chapter 12). The establishment of tangible measures of patient involvement, in addition to other indicators, means that patient involvement is more likely to occur and produce systemic change (The Joint Commission, 2010).

Example 3: Patients as Partners Program

Impact British Columbia, a not-for-profit health service provider organization specifically established to work across British Columbia's health system to support service improvement, has recently implemented a *Patients as Partners* program based on the British Columbia Primary Health Care Charter. The charter is predicated on the understanding that only 15% of the population has no engagement with the primary health care system in any given year. One of the program's goals is therefore to raise the level of patient involvement and self-management through such means as outreach programs that people can access from close to home. The training programs include patients, caregivers, and health care providers. In addition, while acute care is a major focus of the health system generally, chronic conditions contribute to a large proportion of the costs of health care and high average costs per patient, especially when patients with multiple conditions are more effectively taken into account.

The specified principles at Impact are as follows:

- People are treated with respect and dignity.
- Health care providers communicate and share complete and unbiased information with patients and families in ways that are affirmative and useful.
- Individuals and families build on their strengths through participation in experiences that enhance control and independence.
- Collaboration among patients, families, and providers occurs in policy and program development and professional education, as well as in the delivery of care.

The scope of the program aims to meet tangible goals for improving patient access to self-treatment programs, including training programs for both patients and staff on self-management programs, patient satisfaction measures, and patient and staff confidence measures in utilizing the programs. The focus is on British Columbians who are English speakers, once again acknowledging the key part that communication, more broadly, and language, in particular, play in these processes of patient engagement, empowerment, and quality improvement.

Beyond the individual level, communities are engaged in allowing providers to define their local community and its constituents. Broad targets are identified for outreach activities to community organizations and related bodies (health and nonhealth) and for the need to train health professionals in developing skills for community engagement (Impact British Columbia, 2007).

Example 4: From Partners to Owners

Historically, health services for native peoples in the United States were provided by the U.S. Indian Health Service. This did not produce successful outcomes for many groups, including the Alaskan native communities, regardless of how well-intentioned providers were. The Southcentral Foundation (SCF) and the Alaska Native Tribal Health Consortium signed an agreement in 1999 taking over the management of all Indian Health Service programs on the Alaska Native Health Campus (ANHC). These included the Alaska Native Medical Center (ANMC), the Native Primary Care Center, and the Southcentral Foundation's main administration building, as well as other facilities based in Anchorage. The realization of the goal of health service ownership by a not-for-profit organization has since seen a significant philosophical and pragmatic shift in the design and delivery of health care services to Alaskan native peoples seeking treatment at the SCF/ANHC services.

The reorientation has focused on the owners/patients as the central component in the health system's design and delivery of services. Native people were asked how they would like care to be provided, and the results have been substantial. Outcome measures were included from the outset of the change program, and key measures such as satisfaction (of patients and staff), access, quality, and utilization are all very high. The change model has also produced significant reductions in features such as patient backlogs, HIV-positive patient admissions, and emergency department admissions.

The shift from a "patient-centered" to a "patient-driven" system has produced significant and meaningful changes across the spectrum of Alaskan native health care and established a model of innovation and change management that is attracting national and international attention. The direct and practical involvement of patients has improved measures across all domains of care for both patients and providers (Eby, 2007; Gottlieb, 2007; Gottlieb, Sylvester, & Eby, 2008; The Southcentral Foundation, 2010).

▶ Conclusions

We have shown here that the involvement of patients in the health care that they receive and in CQI is no longer in question. What is also undisputed is that, despite a decade of sustained effort by governments, services, and clinicians, medical error rates have still not significantly reduced (Wachter, 2010), and a variety of disparities in both the quality and accessibility of health care persist. Determining the best way to involve consumers in reducing those errors, improving the quality of care they receive, and maximizing the benefits of that involvement, therefore remains problematic. Each health care system and service, across the world, will rightly need to take into account its unique funding and governance structures, planning strategies, and quality improvement mechanisms in deciding which patient involvement strategy is most suitable to its needs. Whatever the particulars involved, whatever method or mechanism the service chooses, it is clear that patients will have a greater level of involvement in their care and in ensuring higher quality. The years of token involvement and a "one-size-fits-all" approach are over. The question remains how health care systems will more fully integrate patients into their CQI initiatives and what actions they will take to resolve persistent quality and safety problems. Only then, we suggest, is it likely that error rates will finally reduce.

References

Abelson, J., Forest, P.-G., Eyles, J., Casebeer, A., Mackean, G., & the Effective Public Consultation Project Team. (2004). Will it make a difference if I show up and share? A citizen's perspective on improving public involvement processes for health system decision-making. *Journal of Health Services Research & Policy, 9*(4), 205–212.

Anderson, B. (2007). Collaborative care and motivational interviewing: Improving depression outcomes through patient empowerment interventions. *American Journal of Managed Care, 13*, S103–S106.

Anderson, E., Shepherd, M., & Salisbury, C. (2006). "Taking off the suit": Engaging the community in primary health care decision-making. *Health Expectatations, 9*, 70–80.

Anthony, R., Miranda, F., Mawji, Z., Cerimele, R., Davis, R., & Lawrence, S. (2003). John M. Eisenberg Patient Safety Awards. The LVHHN patient safety video: Patients as partners in safe care delivery. *The Joint Commission Journal of Quality & Safety, 29*, 640–645.

Arnstein, S. (1969). A ladder of citizen participation in the USA. *Journal of American Institutional Planners, 57*, 176–182.

Baker, G. R., Fancott, C., Judd, M., & O'Connor, P. (2016). Expanding patient engagement in quality improvement and health system redesign: Three Canadian case studies. *Healthcare Management Forum, 29*(5), 176–182.

Barratt, A. (2008). Evidence-based medicine and shared decision making: The challenge of getting both the evidence and preferences into health care. *Patient Education & Counseling, 73*, 407–412.

Bate, P., & Robert, G. (2006). Experience-based design: from redesigning the system around the patient to co-designing services with the patient. *Quality and Safety in Health Care, 15*, 307–310.

Batalden, M., Batalden, P., Margolis, P., Seid, M., Armstrong, G., Opipari-Arrigan, L., & Hartung, H. (2016). Coproduction of healthcare service. *BMJ Quality & Safety, 25*, 509–517.

Berntsen, K. J. (2006). Implementation of patient centeredness to enhance patient safety. *Journal of Nursing Care Quality, 21*, 15–19.

Betancourt, J. R., & King, R. K. (2003). Unequal treatment: The Institute of Medicine report and its public health implications. *Public Health Reports, 118*, 287–292.

Bittle, M. J., & LaMarche, S. (2009). Engaging the patient as observer to promote hand hygiene compliance in ambulatory care. *The Joint Commission Journal of Quality & Patient Safety, 35*, 519–525.

Borthwick, A. M., Short, A. J., Nancarrow, S. A., & Boyce, R. (2010). Non-medical prescribing in Australasia and the UK: The case of podiatry. *Journal of Foot & Ankle Research, 3*, 1.

Brennan, T. A., Leape, L. L., Laird, N. M., Hebert, L., Localio, A. R., Lawthers, A. G., ... Harvard Medical Practice Study I. (1991). Incidence of adverse events and negligence in hospitalized patients. Results of the Harvard Medical Practice Study I. *The New England Journal of Medicine, 324*(6), 370–376.

Bronfenbrenner, U. (1979). *The ecology of human development: Experiments by nature and design.* Cambridge, MA: Harvard University Press.

Burroughs, T. E., Waterman, A. D., Gallagher, T. H., Waterman, B., Adams, D., Jeffe, D. B., ... Fraser, V. J. (2005). Patient concerns about medical errors in emergency departments. *Academic Emergency Medicine, 12,* 57–64.

Bylund, C. L., Gueguen, J. A., D'Agostino, T. A., Li, Y., Sonet, E. (2010). Doctor-patient communication about cancer-related Internet information. *Journal of Psychosocial Oncology, 28,* 127–142.

Cervical Cancer Inquiry, Cartwright Inquiry. (1988). *The report of the Committee of Inquiry into allegations concerning the treatment of cervical cancer at the National Women's Hospital and into other related matters.* Auckland, New Zealand: Government Printing Office.

Coulter, A. (2002). Involving patients: Representation or representativeness? *Health Expectations, 5,* 1.

Coulter, A., & Elwyn, G. (2002). What do patients want from high-quality general practice and how do we involve them in improvement? *British Journal of General Practice, 52,* S22–S26.

Crouch, E., Dickes, L. A., Davis, A., & Zarandy, J. (2016). The effects of Dr. Oz on health behaviors and attitudes. *American Journal of Health Education, 47*(6), 373–378.

Davis, R. E., Jacklin, R., Sevdalis, N., & Vincent, C. A. (2007). Patient involvement in patient safety: What factors influence patient participation and engagement? *Health Expectations, 10,* 259–267.

De Freitas, C., & Martin, G. (2015). Inclusive public participation in health: Policy, practice and theoretical contributions to promote the involvement of marginalised groups in healthcare. *Social Science & Medicine, 135,* 31–39.

Delgado-Gallego, M. E., & Vazquez, M. L. (2009). Users' and community leaders' perceptions of their capacity to influence the quality of health care: Case studies of Colombia and Brazil. *Cadernos de Saude Publica, 25,* 169–178.

Dent, M. (2006). Disciplining the medical profession? Implications of patient choice for medical dominance. *Health Sociol Rev, 15,* 458–468.

Department of Health. (2001). *Learning from Bristol: The report of the public enquiry into Children's Heart Surgery at the Bristol Royal Infirmary, 1984-1995.* London: The Stationery Office.

DiGiovanni, C. W., Kang, L., & Manuel, J. (2003). Patient compliance in avoiding wrong-site surgery. *Journal of Bone & Joint Surgery, American Volume, 85-A*(5), 815–819.

Donetto, S., Pierri, P., Tsianakas, V., & Robert, G. (2015). Experience-based co-design and healthcare improvement: Realizing participatory design in the public sector. *The Design Journal, 18*(2), 227–248.

Duckett, S. J., Collins, J., Kamp, M., & Walker, K. (2008). An improvement focus in public reporting: The Queensland approach. *Medical Journal of Australia, 189*(11), 616–617.

Eby, D. K. (2007). Primary care at the Alaska Native Medical Center: a fully deployed "new model" of primary care. *International Journal of Circumpolar Health, 66,* 4–13.

Emanuel, E. J., & Emanuel, L. L. (1997). Preserving community in health care. *Journal of Health Policy Law, 22,* 147–184.

Entwistle, V. A., & Quick, O. (2006). Trust in the context of patient safety problems. *Journal of Health Organization & Management, 20,* 397–416.

Epstein, S. (1995). The construction of lay expertise: AIDS activism and the forging of credibility in the reform of clinical trials. *Science, Technology, & Human Values, 20,* 408–437.

Ervin, N. E. (2006). Does patient satisfaction contribute to nursing care quality? *Journal of Nursing Administration, 36,* 126–130.

Forrest, E. (2004). Patient-public involvement. *Health Services Journal, 114,* 26–27.

Forsythe, L. P., Ellis, L. E., Edmundson, L., Sabharwal, R., Rein, A., Konopka, K., & Frank, L. (2016). Patient and Stakeholder Engagement in the PCORI Pilot Projects: Description and Lessons Learned. *Journal of General Internal Medicine, 31,* 13–21.

Francis, R. (2013). *Report of the Mid Staffordshire NHS Foundation Trust Public Inquiry.* London: The Stationery Office.

Gottlieb, K. (2007). The family wellness warriors initiative. *Alaska Medicine, 49,* 49–54.

Gottlieb, K., Sylvester, I., & Eby, D. (2008). Transforming your practice: What matters most. *Fam Practice Manage, 15,* 32–38.

Groene, O., & Sunol, R. (2015). Patient involvement in quality management: rationale and current status. *Journal of Health Organization And Management, 29,* 556–569.

Hamburg, M. A., & Collins, F. S. (2010). The path to personalized medicine. *The New England Journal of Medicine, 363*(4), 301–304.

Hekkert, K. D., Cihangir, S., Kleefstra, S. M., van den Berg, B., & Kool, R. B. (2009). Patient satisfaction revisited: A multilevel approach. *Social Science Medicine, 69*(1), 68–75.

Hindle, D., Braithwaite, J., Travaglia, J., & Iedema, R. (2006). *Patient safety: A comparative analysis of eight inquiries in six countries.* Sydney, Australia: Centre for Clinical Governance Research in Health, University of NSW and Clinical Excellence Commission.

Illich, I. (1974). Medical nemesis. *The Lancet, 1,* 918–921.

Impact British Columbia. (2007). *Primary health care charter: A collaborative approach.* Vancouver, British Columbia: Ministry of Health.

Institute of Medicine (IOM). (2000). *To err is human: Building a safer health system.* Washington, DC: National Academies Press.

Jeong, J. S., & Lee, S. (2017, May 30). The influence of information appraisals and information behaviors on the acceptance of health information: A study of television medical talk shows in South Korea. *Health Communication*, 1–8. https://doi.org/ 10.1080 /10410236.2017.1323365. [Epub ahead of print]

Johnstone, M.-J., & Kanitsaki, O. (2009). Engaging patients as safety partners: Some considerations for ensuring a culturally and linguistically appropriate approach. *Health Policy*, *90*, 1–7.

Kitson, A., Marshall, A., Bassett, K., & Zeitz, K. (2013). What are the core elements of patient-centred care? A narrative review and synthesis of the literature from health policy, medicine and nursing. *Journal of Advanced Nursing*, *69*(1), 4–15.

Kripalani, S., Jacobson, T. A., Mugalla, I. C., Cawthon, C. R., Niesner, K. J., & Vaccarino, V. (2010). Health literacy and the quality of physician-patient communication during hospitalization. *Journal of Hospital Medicine*, *5*(5), 269–275.

Longtin, Y., Sax, H., Leape, L. L., Sheridan, S. E., Donaldson, L., & Pittet, D. (2010). Patient participation: Current knowledge and applicability to patient safety. *Mayo Clinic Proceedings*, *85*(1), 53–62.

Lorig, K. R., Sobel, D. S., Stewart, A. L., Brown, B. W., Jr., Bandura, A., Ritter, P., ... Holman, H. R. (1999). Evidence suggesting that a chronic disease self-management program can improve health status while reducing hospitalization: A randomized trial. *Medical Care*, *37*(1), 5–14.

Mak, J. C., & Faux, S. (2010). Use of complementary and alternative medicine by patients with osteoporosis in Australia. *Medical Journal of Australia*, *192*, 54–55.

McCullough, A., Parekh, S., Rathbone, J., Del Mar, C. B., & Hoffmann, T. (2015). A systematic review of the public's knowledge and beliefs about antibiotic resistance. *Journal of Antimicrobial Chemotherapy*, *71*, 27–33.

McLaughlin, C., & Kaluzny, A. (Eds.). (2006). *continuous quality improvement in health care: Theory, implementations, and applications.* Sudbury, MA: Jones & Bartlett Learning.

Mease, P., Arnold, L. M., Bennett, R., Boonen, A., Buskila, D., Carville, S., ... Crofford L. (2007). Fibromyalgia syndrome. *Journal of Rheumatology*, *34*, 1415–1425.

Mockford, C., Staniszewska, S., Griffiths, F., & Herron-Marx, S. (2012). The impact of patient and public involvement on UK NHS health care: a systematic review. *International Journal for Quality in Health Care*, *24*, 28–38.

Murie, J., & Douglas-Scott, G. (2004). Developing an evidence base for patient and public involvement. *Clinical Governance International Journal*, *9*, 147–154.

Murray, Z. (2015). Community representation in hospital decision making: a literature review. *Australia Health Reviews*, *39*, 323–328.

Nathan, S., Johnston, L., & Braithwaite, J. (2011). The role of community representatives on health service committees: staff expectations vs. reality. *Health Expectations*, *14*, 272–284.

Pappas, G., Siozopoulou, V., Saplaoura, K., Vasiliou, A., Christou, L., Akritidis, N., & Tsianos, E. V. (2007). Health literacy in the field of infectious diseases: The paradigm of brucellosis. *The Journal of Infection*, *54*, 40–45.

Patients for Patient Safety, World Health Organization World Alliance for Patient Safety. (2006). London Declaration. Geneva, Switzerland: World Health Organization. Retrieved from http://www.who.int /patientsafety/patients_for_patient/London _Declaration_EN.pdf

Peat, M., Entwistle, V., Hall, J., Birks, Y., Golder, S., & PIPS Group. (2010). Scoping review and approach to appraisal of interventions intended to involve patients in patient safety. *Journal of Health Services Research & Policy*, *15*(1), 17–25.

Peota, C. (2004). Health literacy and patient safety. *Minnesota Medicine*, *87*, 32–34.

Ramsden, I. (1993). Cultural safety in nursing education in Aotearoa New Zealand. *Nursing Praxis New Zealand*, *8*, 4–10.

Ramsden, I. (2000a). Cultural safety/Kawa Whakaruruhau ten years on: A personal overview. *Nursing Praxis New Zealand*, *15*, 4–12.

Ramsden, I. (2000b). Defining cultural safety and transcultural nursing. *Nursing New Zealand*, *6*, 4–5; author reply 5.

Robb, G., Seddon, M., & Effective Practice Informatics and Quality (EPIQ). (2006). Quality improvement in New Zealand healthcare. Part 6, keeping the patient front and centre to improve healthcare quality. *New Zealand Medical Journal*, *119*, U2174.

Robinson, J. H., Callister, L. C., Berry, J. A., & Dearing, K. A. (2008). Patient-centered care and adherence: Definitions and applications to improve outcomes. *Journal of the American Academy of Nurse Practitioners*, *20*, 600–607.

Rothman, R. L., Yin, H. S., Mulvaney, S., Co, J. P., Homer, C., & Lannon, C. (2009). Health literacy and quality: Focus on chronic illness care and patient safety. *Pediatrics*, *124*(3), S315–S326.

Schwappach, D. L. B. (2010). Review: Engaging patients as vigilant partners in safety: A systematic review. *Medical Care Research Rev*, *67*, 119–148.

Seale, H., Chughtai, A. A., Kaur, R., Crowe, P., Phillipson, L., Novytska, Y., & Travaglia, J. (2015). Ask, speak up, and be proactive: Empowering patient infection control to prevent health care-acquired infections. *American Journal of Infection Control, 43,* 447–453.

Senel, H. G. (2010). Parents' views and experiences about complementary and alternative medicine treatments for their children with autistic spectrum disorder. *Journal of Autism & Developmental Disorders, 40,* 494–503.

Shilts, R. (2007). *And the band played on: Politics, people, and the AIDS epidemic, 20th Anniversary Edition.* New York, NY: St. Martin's Griffin.

Sinclair, C. M. (1994). *Report of the Manitoba Pediatric Cardiac Surgery Inquest.* Winnipeg, Canada: Manitoba Provincial Court.

Smith, J. (2005). *Shipman: The final report.* London: HMSO.

Smith, L. H. (2009). National patient safety goal #13: Patients' active involvement in their own care: Preventing chemotherapy extravasation. *Clinical Journal of Oncology Nursing, 13,* 233–234.

Sobel, D. (2003). *Learning from Kaiser Permanente— How can the NHS make better use of its resources and improve patient care?* London: National Primary and Care Trust Development Programme.

Sofaer, S., Shaller, D., Ojeda, G., & Hibbard, J. (2009). *From patients to partners: A consensus framework for engaging Californians in their health and health care.* Berkeley, CA: California Program on Access to Care CPAC at the University of California Berkeley.

The Joint Commission. (2010). *The Joint Commission— National patient safety goals.* Oakbrook Terrace, IL: Author.

The Southcentral Foundation. (2010). *The Southcentral Foundation—about us.* Anchorage, AK: Author.

Tritter, J. Q. (2009). Revolution or evolution: The challenges of conceptualizing patient and public involvement in a consumerist world. *Health Expectations 12,* 275–287.

Tseng, M., & Piller, F. (2003). *The customer centric enterprise: Advances in mass customization and personalization.* New York, NY: Springer.

Tu, H. T., & Lauer, J. R. (2009). Designing effective health care quality transparency initiatives. *Issue Brief/Center Study Health Syst Change,* July: 1–6.

Ubbink, D. T., Knops, A. M., Legemate, D. A., et al. (2009). Choosing between different treatment options: How should I inform my patients? *Nederlands Tijdschrift voor Geneeskunde, 153,* B344.

Utzon, J., & Kaergaard, J. (2009). Publication of healthcare quality data to citizens—Status and perspectives. *Ugeskrift for Laeger, 171,* 1670–1674.

Vincent, C. A., & Coulter, A. (2002). Patient safety: What about the patient? *Quality & Safety in Health Care, 11*(1), 76–80.

Wachter, R. M. (2010). Patient safety at ten: Unmistakable progress, troubling gaps. *Health Affairs (Millwood), 29*(1), 165–173.

Wade, D. T., & Halligan, P. W. (2004). Do biomedical models of illness make for good healthcare systems? *British Medical Journal, 329,* 1398–1401.

CHAPTER 8

A Social Marketing Approach to Increase Adoption of Continuous Quality Improvement Initiatives

Carol E. Breland and Mike Newton-Ward

The aim of marketing is to know and understand the customer so well that the product or service fits him or her and sells itself.

— **Peter Drucker**

Imagine a typical scenario in which hospital management has recently implemented a continuous quality improvement (CQI) initiative to decrease the incidence of hospital-acquired conditions in their intensive care unit (ICU). Their data suggest that poor hand-washing techniques by staff and bacteria on portable equipment are to blame. The CQI plan is to provide hand-washing training, implement mandatory hand-washing for doctors when entering and leaving a patient's room, and ensure more thorough cleaning of portable X-ray machines that come into the patients' rooms.

However, patient occupancy at the hospital has increased recently due to a closure of another hospital nearby. The housekeeping staff is struggling to keep up with the demand, so staff members have responded by shortening the time they spend cleaning rooms between patients. The housekeeping personnel do not have time to measure the disinfectant product they mix with water, but do not want to run out, so they just guess at a reduced amount, resulting in a less effective cleaning product. They defer the floor mopping, reasoning that the patient is not on the floor, so its cleanliness will not matter anyway— so every time someone drops something on the floor, there is a risk of contamination. In addition, the cleaning staff has never been instructed to clean the television remote-control device and nurse call button, and thus infection-causing agents are being transferred from patient to patient via these objects.

217

Without a better understanding of these background issues, the CQI team will be disappointed in the latest data showing that infection rates have not decreased. A meeting might be held to determine how to improve the process for hand-washing and how to check for bacteria more often on equipment. Formal brainstorming, perhaps using a traditional CQI tool such as a fishbone diagram (see Chapter 4 for details) prior to the implementation phase might have led to improved outcomes. Alternatively, or as an adjunct to brainstorming, social marketing behavior theories and techniques could also have been used as a way to ensure greater success by including formative research and data gathered on multiple target audiences. Using this process, the team might have discovered that the housekeeping staff was unknowingly undermining their efforts. Through better understanding of the behavior of the housekeeping staff, a plan could be developed to remove some of the barriers to proper cleaning, such as having the disinfectant premeasured and stored nearby and having a separate designated mop team to ensure that rooms are mopped thoroughly.

Social marketing is a behavioral change methodology firmly planted in the theory and processes of commercial marketing that can be used in conjunction with other more traditional techniques to implement and help to ensure the broadest acceptance and adoption of innovations and changes, including CQI initiatives. Because it is a unique application in CQI, we will first define social marketing concepts and processes. An excellent definition of social marketing is found in Nancy R. Lee and Philip Kotler's book *Social marketing: Changing behaviors for good*: "Social marketing is a process that uses marketing principles and techniques to change target audience behaviors to benefit society as well as the individual. This strategically oriented discipline relies on creating, communicating, delivering, and exchanging offerings that have positive value for individuals, clients, partners, and society at large" (Lee & Kotler, 2016,

p. 9). Social marketing should not be confused with communication-only campaigns that rely on advertisements, public service announcements, or printed materials, but that do not address the barriers and facilitators for behaviors. Also, social marketing is sometimes confused with *social media marketing*, a term that describes the use in marketing campaigns of social media networking sites such as Facebook or Twitter (Uhrig et al., 2010). Social marketing provides a strategic framework for bringing multiple interventions to bear on a problem, while social media is a communication tactic.

The application of social marketing has evolved since the 1970s, when the term *social marketing* was first introduced by Philip Kotler and Gerald Zaltman in the *Journal of Marketing* (Kotler & Zaltman, 1971). Over the past 45 years, the field has undergone continuous growth and refinement. This evolution includes the extension of business concepts of commercial marketing, which was the traditional form of marketing prior to the 1970s, to nontraditional settings such as governmental and nongovernmental organizations and to nontraditional fields such as public health, public safety, and environmental quality. It has also included internal growth through lessons learned from ever-broadening applications within these nontraditional settings. For example, during the 1980s, some major health-related organizations, such as the Centers for Disease Control and Prevention (CDC) and the World Health Organization (WHO), began to consider implementing social marketing concepts. The ideas spread further in the 1990s when universities such as the University of South Florida in Tampa, Florida, and the University of Strathclyde in Glasgow, Scotland, began to create academic programs in social marketing (Lee & Kotler, 2016). The journal *Social Marketing Quarterly* was founded, and a pivotal text by Alan Andreasen, *Marketing social change: Changing behavior to promote health, social development, and the environment* (Andreasen, 1995) was introduced. Externally, social marketing has benefited from advances in psychology, sociology, behavioral economics, communication, and design thinking. The totality of this growth has provided social marketers with a rich set of diverse tactics for influencing behaviors that yield beneficial societal outcomes.

Social marketing has produced some well-known health behavior change campaigns, such as the anti-tobacco "Truth" campaign (Evans et al., 2002), the "VERB: It's What You Do" adolescent physical activity campaign (Wong et al., 2004), the "Save the Crabs, Then Eat 'Em" campaign for protecting the Chesapeake Bay area (Landers et al., 2006), the "Back to Sleep" campaign for sudden infant death syndrome prevention (Cotroneo, Hazel, & Chapman, 2001), and the "Click It or Ticket" campaign for seat belt use to save lives (Williams, Wells, & Reinfurt, 2002). A campaign to reduce the incidence and impact of medical errors in hospitals, the "100,000 Lives Campaign of 2004" and the subsequent "5 Million Lives Campaign" was conducted by the Institute for Healthcare Improvement from 2004 to 2008 (Berwick, Calkins, McCannon, & Hackbarth 2006; Berwick, 2014).

▶ Hallmarks of Social Marketing

It is important to note that social marketing uses the same fundamental concepts and principles as commercial marketing (Siegel & Doner, 1998). To further understand how social marketing has evolved from these roots, some understanding of traditional commercial marketing is helpful. Commercial marketers are experts at looking through the eyes of the individual and seeing what drives that person's desire for a product. Commercial marketers know, based on their audience research, that the individual will keep trying to meet some very basic human needs for acceptance and success and will want to buy their product.

Social marketers can use these same techniques to meet some of the same desires but by promoting voluntary behavior changes that encourage healthy behaviors, better health outcomes, true well-being, and a better society.

Central to all marketing is the concept of *exchange*—the idea that people perceive barriers and benefits to acting in various ways, and that they are more likely to act in ways that have fewer barriers and greater benefits. A central task of marketing, then, is to understand the perceived barriers and benefits and to effect changes that lower the barriers and increase the facilitators to action.

Commercial marketing and social marketing share other concepts but give different emphases to the concepts. The most important distinction between traditional commercial marketing and social marketing is the product or service being sold. Social marketers hope to promote (sell) a good behavior, with no real goal of financial gain, while commercial marketers are focused on selling a good or service, irrespective of its benefit to society, for financial gain. Competition for the commercial marketer is usually another similar product or company, whereas in social marketing, it is another (often unhealthy) behavior. For example, the social marketer working on an anti-smoking campaign, perhaps in a public health school or agency, is interested in decreasing smoking behavior and replacing it with a healthy behavior, such as smoking less or stopping smoking. In contrast, marketers who work for tobacco companies have a completely different goal, such as increasing use of the particular brand of cigarettes that will lead to the greatest profitability for the tobacco company, which is the ultimate goal of most commercial marketing campaigns. Commercial marketing employs a range of proven, best practice concepts that are all essential in creating an effective marketing campaign to increase the use of a product and increase the financial gain of a company. These techniques include the marketing mix (the strategies of Product, Price, Place and Promotion, known as the "four P's"), branding, exchange, audience research and segmentation, evaluation,

---

BOX 8.1 Basic Marketing Principles

Know your AUDIENCE (really!), and put them at the center of every decision you make.
It's about ACTION.
There must be an EXCHANGE.
COMPETITION always exists.
Keep the four P's of marketing (PRODUCT, PRICE, PLACE, PROMOTION) and policy in mind.

Data from Social Marketing National Excellence Collaborative. 2002. The Basics of Social Marketing: How to Use Marketing to Change Behavior. Seattle: University of Washington.

---

and monitoring. Social marketing uses the same concepts but with the goal of gaining an outcome that improves society—for example, better health in a community.

The approach is summarized in *The basics of social marketing* (Social Marketing National Excellence Collaborative, 2002), in which the authors introduce several important principles (see BOX 8.1). Although the details may vary, the goal of using social marketing to achieve behavior change is "to figure out how to make behavior change EASY, FUN, and POPULAR" (Social Marketing National Excellence Collaborative, 2002).

▶ Social Marketing Applications to CQI in Health Care

Why use social marketing, a discipline designed for influencing health behaviors, in CQI initiatives? As we have noted, there are several parallels between CQI and the approaches and methods of social marketing, but these are just a starting point for where social marketing can be applied to CQI in health care. For example, one important starting point common to CQI and social marketing is understanding customer motivation and needs. But social marketing also addresses an important next step that is sometimes overlooked in CQI; that is, understanding and

removing barriers that have led to resistance to implementing improvement initiatives, similar to the factors that thwart innovation in health care that were described in Chapter 2. Social marketing is a methodology that draws from human behavior theory; as humans are involved in endeavors to improve quality not only in industrial processes but in the provision of health services, it stands to reason that social marketing techniques can be applied to CQI initiatives that require behavior change, by internal or external "customers." Change and improvement are the fundamental basis of all CQI initiatives. As noted by Sollecito & Johnson (2019, p. 6):

CQI is simultaneously two things: a management philosophy and a management method. It is distinguished by the recognition that the customer requirements are the key to customer quality and that customer requirements ultimately will change over time because of changes in evidence-based practices and associated changes in education, economics, technology, and culture. Such changes, in turn, require continuous improvements in the administrative and clinical methods that affect the quality of patient care. ... Change is fundamental to the healthcare environment, and the organization's systems must have both a will and the way to master such change effectively.

Traditionally, CQI approaches emphasize managerial and professional processes to build a structural framework to implement changes. Individuals are needed to provide input into what changes need to be made and the best methods for changing them. In his plenary address to the First Annual European Forum on Quality Improvement in Health Care in 1996, Dr. Donald M. Berwick, then-President of the Institute for Healthcare Improvement, outlined some fundamental concepts needed for change (Berwick, 1996, p. 619). The following quotes from his address are particularly relevant to this discussion:

- "Real improvement comes from changing systems, not changing within systems."
- "To make improvement, we must be clear about what we are trying to accomplish, how we will know that a change has led to improvement, and what change we can make that will result in an improvement."
- "You win the Tour de France not by planning for years for the perfect first bicycle ride but by constantly making small improvements."

Other efforts of CQI are to deemphasize individual blame, recognize individual contributions, decentralize responsibility, and rely on hard data such as surveys, patient data, and equipment costs in making decisions.

Similarly, social marketing emphasizes first building a foundation for the change framework using behavior change theories and models such as the diffusion of innovation theory, the social norms theory, the health belief model, the theory of planned behavior, and the social cognitive theory to explore the benefits, barriers, and competition of the behavior change (Lee & Kotler, 2016). These models seek to understand the readiness of their audience to change, what perceptions they have of the desired behavior change, what the seriousness of the change is (what will happen if the change does not occur), and how they will be perceived by their peer group if they change. By considering some of these change models in implementing CQI initiatives, there is a much stronger understanding of the motivations of those who are involved in designing and implementing CQI.

The process of integration of behavior change concepts to other disciplines such as CQI is gaining momentum in the same way that other CQI processes have evolved exponentially in health care in the past several years. Nationally, social marketing has already benefited the quality improvement process. Between 2005 and 2007, the Social Marketing National Excellence Collaborative trained staff from a majority of Quality Improvement Organizations (QIOs) to apply the social marketing process to the items in their scope of work, developed by the Centers for Medicare and Medicaid Services (CMS). The collaborative conducted a series of trainings around the country. QIO staff created social marketing plans for issues such as the implementation of electronic medical records by private physician practices, reduction of pressure ulcers among nursing home patients, improved management of oral medication in home health clients, improved care of hospital patients with pneumonia, and improved validity rate of chart abstracts submitted to CMS (Rokoske, McArdle, & Schenck, 2012; Schenck, McArdle, & Weiser, 2013).

Organizational Impacts on Social Marketing Applications to CQI in Health Care

When considering the application of social marketing methods to health initiatives, it is not just individual health behaviors that can be improved by understanding and addressing the factors that produce the behavior. Improvement can also be addressed at the organization level. Lee and Kotler (2016) encourage the application of social marketing in a wide variety of settings and with upstream audiences such as policymakers, corporations, law enforcement, school districts, and non-profit organizations.

For example, if refraining from smoking in the workplace can become the standard of behavior through social marketing and public policy, then it follows that health care practices can improve, resulting in better patient outcomes, through the same methods.

To illustrate how social marketing can influence health care organizations, consider the prevalent concern about infection control. A common goal in all health care clinics is to emphasize proper hand-washing behavior to control the spread of infection (Dauer, 2007). To encourage this behavior, health care providers are regularly trained on the importance of hand-washing, and reminder messages are usually posted near sinks. Thus, health care is similar to other noncommercial settings that can be described as having standards that are based on behaviors that can be influenced (for the good) by social marketing techniques (Mah, Deshpande, & Rothschild, 2006).

Understanding the application of elements of social marketing to changes in both individual health behavior and health care practices takes some realignment of traditional attitudes toward promoting such changes. Behavior change requires more than the conviction of the agency, committee, or organization that change is needed. Social marketers seek to understand the needs of both the individuals and the organizations they are interested in and to get agreement from those individuals that change is both needed and achievable. Therefore, social marketing strategies are fundamentally consumer-focused, voluntary commercial marketing techniques that take into consideration the audience's ability and desire to change and that are designed to change behavior over time instead of all at once. One such model is the stages of change developed by Prochaska and DiClemente (1983). Parallels to CQI begin to become apparent from this definition; its focus is on consumers/customers and the ultimate goal of making gradual behavior changes (i.e., continuous improvements in health or social behaviors). Another social marketing

model/tool that is directly applicable and has similarities to CQI tools is journey mapping.

Journey Mapping

As with CQI methods and tools, the practice of social marketing is always evolving, incorporating new strategies from other fields of endeavor related to human behavior. A strategy that can be beneficial to CQI is journey mapping, borrowed from the field of human-centered design—a design process that enables designers to develop in-depth understanding about problems people encounter in doing a task, then generate creative solutions (Kelley & Kelley, 2013). A journey map graphically illustrates the steps that people go through to complete an action, such as cleaning a patient's room, or to interact with a device, such as a medication pump. The maps focus on "pain points," or the barriers people encounter, doing an action. Then they use a system of brainstorming that generates creative interventions that can be rapidly tested and implemented (IDEO, n.d.). Social marketers use insights from their audience research to create a map. A journey map for the background scenario (cleaning patient rooms) described at the beginning of the chapter might look like that in FIGURE 8.1.

Program Evaluation of Social Marketing Applications to CQI in Health Care

A key question that must be asked in all CQI initiatives is "How do we know if a change is an improvement?" (Langley et al., 2009). A logical consequence of that question is that behavior change will not always happen as quickly or as widely as it should, especially if there is disagreement about whether the change being proposed is an improvement. For example, Atul Gawande (2009) describes this concept in detail in regard to the introduction of surgical checklists. The concept is also the subject of a case study that illustrates how a

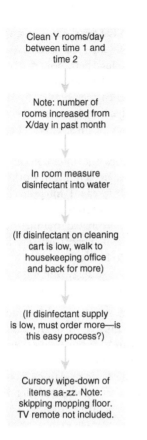

Clean Y rooms/day
between time 1 and
time 2

Note: number of
rooms increased from
X/day in past month

In room measure
disinfectant into water

(If disinfectant on cleaning
cart is low, walk to
housekeeping office
and back for more)

(If disinfectant supply
is low, must order more—is
this easy process?)

Cursory wipe-down of
items aa-zz. Note:
skipping mopping floor.
TV remote not included.

FIGURE 8.1 Journey Map for Cleaning Patient Rooms

social marketing approach can explain behaviors related to the use of surgical checklists and motivate their greater use (Breland, 2012).

Social marketing, like CQI, also relies on data when formulating the design and goals of the program and monitoring and evaluation of the program. In order to ensure greatest cost efficiency, a practical approach to gathering data is acceptable. For example, formative research for the planning stage of the initiative can be applied including the use of secondary data derived from published articles and gray literature as cost-effective supplements to primary data from focus groups, Internet and in-person surveys, social media networking, and direct observation. Formative research in social marketing aligns with the Plan, Do, Study, Act (PDSA) approach used

in CQI and, in particular, the improvement model described by Langley et al. (2009). As noted by Berwick (1996), the primary purpose of collecting and analyzing these data is learning about improvement and using the data to implement further improvements in a PDSA cycle—a direct parallel to the purpose and use of formative research in social marketing.

CQI initiatives could use these additional types of data to understand how the patients and employees may act as barriers to or may benefit from their planned program improvements. In a hypothetical example, a hospital management team might hope to improve utilization of current intensive care unit medication pumps and defer buying new equipment. The benefits that health care management would plan to obtain through CQI might be improved customer satisfaction, for both external "customers" (patients and their families) and internal "customers" (employees); more efficient use of resources, including time and equipment; and greater compliance with the CQI program. By adding social marketing methods, such as conducting formative research with the target audience, compliance with CQI implementation can be increased through better understanding barriers employees face and benefits that are important to them. For example, formative research could be conducted with a focus group of the nurses who use equipment, such as infusion pumps, to administer medications intravenously. They could provide critical information on how equipment is used and why some types of pumps seem to be in high demand when other equipment remains in the closet. Analysis of the focus group data might reveal that some pumps lack automatic drip rate calculations that introduce the possibility of error when calculating manually, and that otherwise acceptable pumps have poor display visibility, making it hard to see the readings from a distance in a darkened room. "Benefits" important to the nurses include the desire to provide a high standard of care, making their patients as comfortable as possible and quick access to the equipment. Using these data, an improvement team can address barriers to use and tie use of the pumps into the benefits that motivate the nurses, thereby obtaining better outcomes from its CQI program.

For health care service provider managers, other scenarios where social marketing theories and techniques could be used are numerous—for example, decreasing the rate of hospital readmissions for patients discharged with incisions, decreasing the rate of medication noncompliance or multi-drug interactions after hospital discharge, and improving surgical safety outcomes by implementing a simple safety checklist.

Creating a Social Marketing Strategy and Plan for CQI in Health Care

When applying social marketing methods to CQI initiatives, the same formal processes should be followed as in any social marketing campaign, beginning with a strategic marketing plan. For example, a good overview of the process is contained in the "Twelve Strategic Questions" developed by the Academy for Educational Development, a social marketing consultancy (Smith & Strand, 2008, p. 16):

1. What is the social problem I want to address?
2. Who/what is to blame?
3. What action do I believe will best address that problem?
4. Who is being asked to take that action? (audience)
5. What does the audience want in exchange for adopting this new behavior? (key benefit)
6. Why will the audience believe that anything we offer is real and true? (support)
7. What is the competition offering? Are we offering something the audience wants more? (competition)
8. What marketing mix will increase benefits the audience wants and reduce behaviors they care about?
9. What is the best time and place to reach members of our audience so that they are most disposed to receiving the intervention? (aperture)
10. How often, and from whom, does the intervention need to be received if it is to work? (exposure)
11. How can I integrate a variety of interventions to act over time in a coordinated manner to influence the behavior? (integration)
12. Do I have the resources to carry out this strategy, and if not, where can I find useful partners?

Note that answers to these questions need to be determined through audience (customer) research, not by the best guesses or the impressions of the planning team!

Once the basic questions have been considered, a more substantial detailed plan is required. A social marketing plan generally follows a specific sequence of steps, where each step is informed by the results from the previous step. Lee and Kotler (2016, pp. 50–60) outline the following (10-step) executive summary:

1. Social issue, background, purpose and focus
2. Conduct a situational analysis (SWOT: Strengths, Weaknesses, Opportunities, Threats)
3. Select target audiences
4. Set behavior objectives and target goals
5. Identify target audience barriers, benefits, and motivators; the competition; and influential others
6. Develop a positioning statement
7. Develop a strategic marketing mix (the four P's: Product, Price, Place, Promotion)
8. Develop a plan for monitoring and evaluation

9. Establish budgets and find funding sources

10. Complete an implementation plan

Once the plan is implemented, the monitoring and evaluation of data collected during and after the campaign will be critical and most often will utilize primary data. This process is directly parallel to the use of primary data collection in CQI to measure the baseline and track the impact of improvements over time—such as in a health care process—using control charts or other quantitative CQI tools, as described in Chapter 4. In social marketing settings, data for this research may be gathered from focus groups, online and in-person surveys, personal interviews, website hits and feeds, and blogs.

▶ A Scenario for How to Apply Social Marketing to a Health Care CQI Initiative

Overview

Social marketing has had numerous health applications, such as those described earlier to address automobile safety, smoking cessation, and other vital issues, but it is still relatively new in its application to CQI in health care. To illustrate how it might be applied to a significant health care issue, prevention of medical errors, the following hypothetical scenario is presented. This U.S.-based scenario utilizes a current, real-world, health care CQI initiative—a surgical safety checklist, designed and tested by the WHO to improve patient outcomes and customer satisfaction in hospitals where surgical procedures take place (Haynes et al., 2009). Checklists have long been a staple in the CQI toolbox, and are included in the list of CQI tools presented in Chapter 4, but are often overlooked due to their simplicity. However, as Gawande (2007) noted in the popular press, if a new drug was found to be as effective in saving lives as checklists are, there would be a nationwide marketing campaign urging doctors to use it. This scenario takes on that challenge.

There can be many reasons for not adopting changes and innovations in health care, and social marketing can be an effective approach not only to understand these reasons but also to change behavior. Creating a social marketing campaign for increasing the use of checklists in the reduction in surgical errors is simple to organize into basic, logical steps of planning, action, and evaluation, and provides an excellent opportunity to demonstrate how social marketing methods can be adapted to health care quality improvement. Following the executive summary steps presented earlier from Lee and Kotler's (2016) social marketing primer, the checklist utilization process is broken down into the 10 basic steps outlined earlier. Armed with the strategies just discussed, a CQI initiative using a social marketing approach can begin to take shape.

Social Marketing Strategy for the Introduction of a Surgical Safety Checklist

Step 1: Social Issue, Background, Purpose, and Focus

The first step in any social marketing initiative is to understand the background and reasons why the activity being proposed (e.g., using a surgical safety checklist), is important and beneficial. The starting point for the surgical safety checklist is a review of medical error rates. For example, prior to focusing more attention on the issue of medical errors, 44,000–98,000 deaths attributable to medical errors occurred in hospitals in the United States (AHRQ, 2000, 2012, 2013). This issue, which is also addressed in Chapters 9 and 10 of this text, has been one of several targets of CQI initiatives in health care in recent years. Several other medical publications

(Berwick, 2014; Bliss et al., 2012; Gawande, 2009; Gilkey, Earp, & French, 2008; Haynes et al., 2009; Price & Savitz, 2012; Swift et al., 2001; Thiels et al., 2015) describe the use and effectiveness of checklists as an adjunct to other improvement processes in reducing adverse outcomes in surgery; use of checklists is also discussed in Chapters 1, 2, and 4 of this text. For example, Bliss and colleagues at the University of Connecticut reported statistically significant decreases in 30-day morbidity in overall adverse events from 23.6% (historical data from the American College of Surgeons National Surgical Quality Improvement Program database) to 8.2% in cases with checklist use (Bliss et al., 2012). Although not due entirely to the use of checklists alone, improvements in quality and safety during surgery are facilitated in a formal way using a series of steps (checks) such as improving medical team communication through confirmation of specific safety checks and time outs during surgical procedures (Millat, 2012).

An example of the surgical checklist and information about implementation and outcomes is found on the WHO website (WHO, 2009). With this background information in mind, a key question that remains, as with any health care innovation or CQI initiative, is how to broaden further its adoption.

In our hypothetical scenario, hospital leadership has reviewed information on the implementation of the checklist and decided to employ a social marketing effort to encourage surgical service providers to adopt this checklist—or at least a modified version of the checklist that meets their needs, such as the Association of Perioperative Registered Nurses (AORN) Comprehensive Surgical Checklist (AORN, 2017). Social marketing can address the need to position the issue, identify the exchange being asked of affected staff, identify beliefs that promote or hinder acceptance of the checklist, identify cost-effective strategies, and set up specific, measureable goals to evaluate the outcome of the initiative.

Step 2: Conduct a Situation Analysis (SWOT)

Performing a SWOT analysis (Strengths, Weaknesses, Opportunities, and Threats) will identify any internal or external environmental influences on the initiative. Here is a list of possible issues:

- *Strengths:* Everyone on the surgical team is interested in patient safety.
- *Weaknesses:* The team is composed of various disciplines—surgeons, nurses, technologists, and anesthesiologists or nurse anesthetists who have different training backgrounds and outcome goals.
- *Opportunities:* The health care reform bills passed in 2010 in the United States have provisions to provide incentives and penalties for preventable medical errors.
- *Threats:* Other hospitals may not require the use of a checklist. The surgeon may decide to take his or her business to these other hospitals. Other members of the team may resist changing the status quo.

Step 3: Select Target Audiences

Several target audiences are involved in this initiative, and they may be in various states of readiness to change:

- *Surgeon* (a physician and the most senior-level person on the team): Does not see a need for change
- *Anesthetist* (either a physician or an advanced practitioner nurse): Is not comfortable with change
- *Cardiac perfusionist* (a surgical specialist): Is indifferent to change
- *Circulating nurse* (the surgical procedure manager): Is ready for change, as surgical errors impact outcomes, but is concerned with workflow interruptions
- *Surgical medical equipment technician* (the person responsible for equipment): Is ready for change but has feelings of powerlessness

■ *Scrub nurse* (the person responsible for assisting the surgeon): Thinks about change but does not want to disrupt the status quo

■ *Hospital administrator (the person responsible for ensuring checklist use)*: Is ready for change, as checklist implementation is his/her responsibility

Based on these characterizations of the potential target audiences, the most suitable persons to initiate change on this team are the circulating nurse and the hospital administrator. For the purposes of this scenario, the circulating nurse is chosen as the campaign leader as the person who has the most team interaction opportunities.

Step 4: Set Behavior Objectives and Target Goals

The objective of the social marketing strategy is to improve the use of the surgical safety checklist, thus increasing effective implementation of the checklist and ultimately decreasing the number of medical surgical errors and improving patient outcomes and customer satisfaction. After conducting some formative research (personal communications: Robert S. Smith, MD, and Kenneth R. Courington, MD [April 2017]) with clinicians who are surgical team members, the choice of the primary target audience is confirmed to be the circulating nurse. In deciding upon basic goals, it is critical that goals be SMART: Specific, Measurable, Attainable, Relevant, and Time-sensitive. This requires the choice of several short-term, intermediate, and long-term goals. In the following examples, the goals set will be incorporated into the monitoring and evaluation plan that will create data from the campaign, providing vital real-time sampling of the initiative, in the same way CQI methods elicit feedback. The chosen goals are as follows:

■ *Short-term goals*
  ◦ All team members will be trained on the checklist within 1 month by the quality assurance manager at the regular weekly staff meeting.
  ◦ Each surgical team will complete a checklist for one surgery per day for the 10 working days during the month, beginning on the first of the month, for a total of 10 different types of surgeries, each month for 3 months.
  ◦ The circulating nurse will receive additional training on team leadership.
  ◦ The circulating nurse will record the surgery information and report to the nurse manager and CQI team on the success or difficulties encountered at each instance, weekly.

■ *Intermediate goals*
  ◦ At the end of 6 months, each surgical team will complete a checklist on 50% of the surgeries performed during the month.
  ◦ The circulating nurse will record the surgery information and report on the success or difficulties encountered at each instance, twice a month.

■ *Long-term goals*
  ◦ At the end of 12 months, each surgical team will complete the checklist on each of the surgeries they perform.
  ◦ The circulating nurse will lead a discussion of the pros and cons of the surgical safety checklist.
  ◦ The average mortality rate will decline by 40%.
  ◦ The average complication rate will decline by 30%.

Step 5: Identify Target Market Audience Barriers, Benefits and Motivators; the Competition; and Influential Others

Understanding the reasons for current behaviors is one of the key concepts that a social marketing approach can bring to CQI. Often, the challenge is simply that changing procedures causes a disruption in the comfortable established workflow, as in this example, where the target audience is the circulating nurse. Barriers to the desired behavior change may involve a circulating nurse with a personality characteristic that makes him or her less disposed to change of any type. Teams may have worked out their group dynamics already, and the circulating nurse may be reluctant to introduce change in the group because it may cause discord or change the agreed-upon decision-making chain within the group. Surgical teams work together in close proximity in a closed environment, and change may be viewed as causing unnecessary disruption or delay in a carefully timed and orderly environment. It is important to uncover motivators for the target audience, such as pride in overseeing surgeries that avoid the embarrassment and stress of errors, and then give tools that empower the nurse with methods for improvement that are easy to perform (see Chapter 6 for more details on team processes, including motivation, empowerment, decision making and conflict resolution).

Step 6: Develop a Positioning Statement

After determining how the target audience perceives the CQI initiative, it may be necessary to reposition the behavior that is wanted. Positioning refers to how a behavior is viewed (e.g., "cool," evidence-based, desirable) compared to competing behaviors. As previously stated, the surgical safety checklist may be viewed as an unnecessary intrusion into the already tightly packed surgical procedure schedule. The circulating nurse is aware of the many times that errors have been caught at the last minute and avoided, but his or her stress and anxiety in dealing with such instances may be less intense than the stress of interrupting the established workflow during each surgery. The checklist needs to be repositioned from a

burdensome bureaucratic task to a method of enhanced communication that all team members can benefit from and that will contribute to increased patient safety, which enhances everyone's job satisfaction and decreases stress from possible situations where errors have to be caught and averted. (This latter view is consistent with the motivational goals of the Quadruple Aim as described in Chapter 2).

Step 7: Develop a Strategic Marketing Mix—The Four Ps: Product, Price, Place, Promotion

This is where the advantages of adding a combination of the commercial marketing techniques of the four P's—Product, Place, Price, and Promotion (supplemented by a fifth P, advocacy for Policy change)—enhance customization of your CQI initiative. The Product (what is being "sold") is the acceptance and use of the surgical safety checklist. Tangible activities that support adoption of the behavior might include training in the use of the checklist and blog postings from other clinicians about how they successfully incorporated use of the list. The Place, or location of the campaign, should be where the behavior is to be performed—in this case, the work environment (i.e., the surgical suite). "Costs", including time costs, are the Price for performing the behavior, such as change in the established workflow, which should already be partially determined. Any monetary incentives that might be available for adherence to the checklist, such as extra time off or a cash bonus, should also be considered here, as well as nonmonetary incentives, such as employee recognition. Other approaches that address the identified cost might include having the team discuss how they can best use the checklist to minimize disruptions or hearing from successful users of the checklist. The Promotion consists of the messages and methods for communicating to support doing the desired behavior. It may be as simple as a large laminated checklist posted in the surgical break room, daily email reminders sent to the circulating nurse's computer, or brightly colored reminder stickers or stars posted at the top of the surgical schedule clipboard.

Step 8: Develop a Plan for Monitoring and Evaluation

By identifying goals, the process for creating a plan for monitoring and evaluation has begun. A simple flowchart of inputs, outputs, and outcomes will help identify other goals and establish a system of continuous monitoring of the CQI initiative. The social media networking field has exploded, and there are numerous opportunities to use these platforms (e.g., a Facebook page) and devices (e.g., an Internet-enabled mobile phone) to gain information about attitudes and beliefs about the surgical safety checklist. A link could be set up on the hospital website leading employees to information about other hospitals' implementation of the checklist. The circulating nurse could create a blog that might be shared with other nurses on a nursing social networking website. Another link could be created on the website leading to a survey that records patient satisfaction data during the implementation of the checklist period. A sample evaluation plan is shown in TABLE 8.1. Note that this plan includes and tracks the goals defined in Step 4.

Step 9: Establish Budgets and Find Funding Sources

Monetary considerations are often a barrier when a social marketing approach is proposed, as budgets are so often tight and marketing a quality improvement initiative may seem unnecessary and expensive. The costliest parts of the process are often the marketing research activities, developing tangible products, producing communication materials (and

purchasing time, if mass media is used), and evaluation. However, much of the marketing research on the target audience may already be available commercially. Using secondary resources is often a cost-effective method for researching the target audience. Internal and external partners can often assist in developing materials or conducting evaluations. In addition, this type of campaign is very limited in scope and is generally quite inexpensive. It is important to remember that social marketing is as much a mindset and a way to think about problems and solutions as it is a series of tasks or tangible offerings that cost money.

Step 10: Complete an Implementation Plan

This final step in the plan is the actual blueprint for the campaign. Here is where formative research, objectives and goals, target audience decisions, and methods for data monitoring and evaluation come together. The implementation plan identifies who will do which activities during what timeframe. It also considers how to sustain your efforts. A unified social marketing strategy would be focused on a local target audience, the circulating nurse in the surgical department. In exchange for disrupting the comfortable established workflow, the circulating nurse gains the responsibility for leading the team in an important patient safety initiative and provides simple, effective tools for improving surgical safety. The strategy will be implemented in three distinct phases: (1) a training phase where the circulating nurse is named as the safety leader and other team members acknowledge his or her role; (2) a pilot run where the surgical checklist is only implemented in a portion of all surgeries and where the circulating nurse will record information for data analysis by the CQI team; and (3) a phase where the entire team comes together with the circulating nurse as the team leader to give feedback on the initiative to the CQI team. As a final

TABLE 8.1 Sample Evaluation Plan

Goal	Measurement Item	Method	Who Will Take Measurements
Short-Term Goals			
1. Team member training	a. Number of members trained b. Knowledge and attitude pretest c. Knowledge and attitude posttest	a. Observation (qualitative) b. Web-based survey using computers in training room c. Web-based survey using survey link	a. QA manager b. Self-administered c. Self-administered
2. Completion of checklist for 10 surgeries each month for first 3 months	a. Number completed b. Whether completed correctly c. 10 different types of surgery included d. Quality of team interaction while using checklist	a. Review of checklist data b. Review of checklist data and observation; review of surgical team data entry process using hand-held device, such as a tablet c. Review of checklist data d. Observation	a–d. QA manager
3. Circulating nurse to receive additional leadership training	a. Whether attended training b. Knowledge pretest and posttest	a. Observation b. Role-play and Web-based survey	a. QA manager b. Course trainer
4. Circulating nurse records and reports information for first 3 months	a. If recording completed b. Accuracy of record c. If report occurred weekly	a–c. Observation—data entered using secure mobile phone or hand-held device	a–c. QA manager
Intermediate Goals			
1. At the end of 6 months, team to complete a checklist on 50% of all surgeries.	a. Number completed b. If completed correctly c. Different types of surgery included and if 50% used checklist d. Quality of team interaction while using checklist	a. Review of checklist data b. Review of checklist data and observation; review of surgical team data entry process using hand-held device, such as a tablet c. Review of checklist data d. Observation	a–d. QA manager

Goal	Measurement Item	Method	Who Will Take Measurements
Intermediate Goals			
2. The circulating nurse reviews information for second 3 months and reports twice a month.	a. If recording completed b. Accuracy of record c. If report occurred biweekly	a–c. Observation—data entered using secure mobile phone or hand-held device	a–c. QA manager
Long-Term Goals			
1. At the end of 12 months, checklist will be completed on all surgeries.	a. Number completed b. If completed correctly c. Different types of surgery included and if 100% used checklist d. Quality of team interaction while using checklist	a. Review of checklist data b. Review of checklist data and observation; review of surgical team data entry process using hand-held device, such as a tablet c. Review of checklist data d. Observation	a–d. QA manager
2. The circulating nurse will lead a discussion of the pros and cons of the surgical safety checklist.	a. Team members attending b. List of pros/cons	a. Observation b. Review of data from discussion on pros/cons	a–b. QA manager
3. The average mortality rate will decrease by 40% by the end of 12 months.	Death rate due to surgical errors	Review of patient records	QA manager
4. The average complication rate will decrease by 30% by the end of 12 months.	Rate of medical complications due to surgical errors	Review of patient records	QA manager

step data evaluation and recommendations for modifications to the plan are made.

Further details and discussion of these methods and, in particular, this scenario, can be found in a case study from which this scenario has been adapted for use in this chapter (Breland, 2012).

▶ Conclusions

As with other innovations in health care, the use of social marketing as a CQI technique is evolving over time because of cross-disciplinary thinking/learning. Similar to the way that measuring patient feedback grew out of traditional commercial market research, social marketing applications have been integrated to address health and other social issues. Social marketing was built from foundations in commercial marketing and continues to grow from advances in practices and concepts in commercial marketing. There is every reason to believe that social marketing will continue to grow as a new technique and set of tools for helping to further the adoption of innovations and improvements in health care.

In this brief overview of the social marketing approach as applied to CQI, it is difficult to examine all the possibilities and uncover all nuances that the fusion of these two powerful strategies make possible. Using a scenario based on the use of the surgical safety checklist, a simple CQI method is given strength and accountability through proven social marketing methods to change behavior for the betterment of the common good of both internal and external customers—a safer surgical environment not only for patients but also for the team members performing the surgery. The use of social marketing in conjunction with CQI represents an important step in the further evolution of both fields. It is the hope that this introduction to social marketing may spark many new ideas and methods of improvement and implementation in medical environments that may be encountered by various medical specialties and situations. The use of social marketing applications not only may improve outcomes of specific CQI initiatives, but in the longer term may help to foster greater diffusion of the CQI philosophy and processes throughout the health care community.

References

Agency for Healthcare Research and Quality (AHRQ). (2000). 20 tips to help prevent medical errors. Patient fact sheet. Retrieved from http://www.ahrq.gov

Agency for Health Care Research and Quality (AHRQ). (2012). Improving the measurement of surgical site infection risk stratification/outcome detection. Final project report. Retrieved from https://www.ahrq.gov

Agency for Healthcare Research and Quality (AHRQ). (2013). Annual hospital-acquired condition rate and estimates. Retrieved from https://www.ahrq.gov

Andreasen, A. (1995). *Marketing social change: Changing behavior to promote health, social development, and the environment.* San Francisco, CA: Jossey-Bass.

Association of Perioperative Registered Nurses (AORN). (2017). AORN Comprehensive Surgical Checklist. Retrieved from https://www.aorn.org

Berwick, D. (1996). A primer on leading the improvement of systems. *British Medical Journal, 312*(7031), 619–622.

Berwick, D. M. (2014). *Promising care: How we can rescue health care by improving it.* San Francisco, CA: Jossey-Bass.

Berwick, D. M., Calkins, D. R., McCannon, C. J., & Hackbarth, A. D. (2006). The 100,000 lives campaign: Setting a goal and a deadline for improving health care quality. *Journal of the American Medical Association, 295,* 324–327.

Breland, C. (2012). Case 9: Forthright Medical Center: Social marketing and the surgical checklist. In C. P. McLaughlin, J. K. Johnson, & W. A. Sollecito (Eds.), *Implementing continuous quality improvement in health care: A global casebook.* Sudbury, MA: Jones & Bartlett Learning.

Bliss, L. A., Ross-Richardson, C. B., Sanzari, L. J., Shapiro, D. S., Lukianoff, A. E., Bernstein, B. A., & Ellner S. J. (2012). Thirty-day outcomes support implementation of a surgical safety checklist. *Journal of the American College of Surgeons, 215*(6), 766–776.

Cotroneo, S., Hazel, J., & Chapman, S. (2001). Partnering for social change: Back to Sleep—Reducing the risk of sudden infant death syndrome (SIDS). *Social Marketing Quarterly, 7*(3), 119–121.

Dauer, E. (2007). Medical errors in hospitals: Cause and prevention. Program on Health Outcomes presentation at UNC School of Public Health, Chapel Hill, North Carolina, October 5, 2007. Retrieved from http://www.sph.unc.edu

Evans, W., Wasserman, J., Bertolotti, E., & Martino, S. (2002). Branding behavior: The strategy behind the Truth^SM Campaign. *Social Marketing Quarterly, 8*(3), 17–29.

Gawande, A. (2007, December 10). The checklist. *The New Yorker*. Retrieved from https://www.newyorker.com

Gawande, A. (2009). *The checklist manifesto*. New York, NY: Metropolitan Books.

Gilkey, M. B., Earp, J. A., & French, E. A. (2008). Applying health education theory to patient safety programs: three case studies. *Health Promotion Practice, 9*(2), 123–129.

Haynes, A. B., Weiser, T. G., Berry, W. R., Lipsitz, S. R., Breizat, A. H., Dellinger, E. P., ... Safe Surgery Saves Lives Study Group. (2009). A surgical safety checklist to reduce morbidity and mortality in a global population. *The New England Journal of Medicine, 360*(5), 491–499.

IDEO. (n.d.) Design kit: Journey maps. Retrieved from http://www.designkit.org/methods/63

Institute for Healthcare Improvement—Initiatives Overview. Retrieved from http://www.ihi.org/Engage/Initiatives /Pages/default.aspx

Kelley, T., & Kelley, D. (2013). *Creative confidence: Unleashing the creative potential within us all*. New York, NY: Crown Business.

Kotler, P., & Zaltman, J. (1971). Social marketing: An approach to planned social change. *Journal of Marketing, 35*, 3–12.

Landers, J., Mitchell, P., Smith, B., Lehman, T., & Conner, C. (2006). "Save the crabs, then eat 'em": A culinary approach to saving the Chesapeake Bay. *Social Marketing Quarterly, 12*(1), 15–18.

Langley, G. L., Moen, R. D., Nolan, K. M., Nolan, T. W., Norman, C. L., & Provost, L. P. (2009). *The improvement guide: A practical approach to enhancing organizational performance*, 2nd ed. San Francisco, CA: Jossey-Bass.

Lee, N. R., & Kotler, P. (2016). *Social marketing: Changing behaviors for good*, 5th ed. Thousand Oaks, CA: Sage Publications.

Mah, W. M., Deshpande, S., & Rothschild, M. L. (2006). Social marketing: A behavior change technology for infection control. *American Journal of Infection Control, 34*, 452–457.

Millat, B. (2012).The check list: a useful tool for the entire operation room team. *Journal of Visceral Surgery, 149*(6), 369–370.

Price, C. S., & Savitz, L. A. (2012). Improving the measurement of surgical site infection risk stratification/outcome detection. Final report (prepared by Denver Health and its partners under contract no. 290-2006-00-20). AHRQ Publication No. 12-0046-EF. Rockville, MD: Agency for Healthcare Research and Quality.

Prochaska, J. O., & DiClemente, C. C. (1983). Stages and processes of self-change of smoking: Toward an integrative model of change. *Journal of Consulting and Clinical Psychology, 51*(3), 390–395.

Rokoske, F., McArdle, J., & Schenck, A. (2012). Case 3: Clemson's nursing home: Working with the state quality improvement organization's restraint reduction initiative. In C. P. McLaughlin, J. K. Johnson, & W. A. Sollecito (Eds.), *Implementing continuous quality improvement in health care: A global casebook*. Sudbury, MA: Jones & Bartlett Learning.

Schenck, A., McArdle, J., & Weiser, R. (2013). Quality improvement organizations and continuous quality improvement in Medicare. In W. A. Sollecito & J. K. Johnson (Eds.), *McLaughlin & Kaluzny's continuous quality improvement in health care*, 4th ed. Burlington, MA: Jones & Bartlett Learning.

Siegel, M., & Doner, L. (1998). *Marketing public health: Strategies to promote social change*. Gaithersburg, MD: Aspen Publishers.

Smith, W. A., & Strand, J. (2008). Social marketing behavior: A practical resource for social marketing professionals [Electronic version]. Washington, DC: Academy for Educational Development. Retrieved from http://www.drexel.edu

Social Marketing National Excellence Collaborative. (2002). *The basics of social marketing*. [Electronic version]. Seattle: University of Washington. Retrieved from http://www.turningpointprogram.org

Sollecito, W. A., & Johnson, J. K. (2019). The global evolution of continuous quality improvement: From Japanese manufacturing to global health services. In J. K. Johnson & W. A. Sollecito (Eds.), *McLaughlin & Kaluzny's continuous quality improvement in health care*, 5th ed. Burlington, MA: Jones & Bartlett Learning.

Swift, E. K., Koepke, C. P., Ferrer, J. A., & Miranda, D. (2001). Preventing medical errors: Communicating a role for medicare beneficiaries. *Health Care Financing Review, 23*(1), 77–85.

Thiels, C., Lal, T., Nienow, J., Pasupathy, K. S., Blocker, R. C., Aho, J. M., ... Bingener, J. (2015). Surgical never events and contributing human factors. *Surgery, 158*(2), 515–521.

Uhrig, J., Bann, C., Williams, P., & Evans, W. D. (2010). Social marketing websites as a platform for disseminating social marketing. *Social Marketing Quarterly*, *16*(1), 2–20.

Williams, A., Wells, J., & Reinfurt, D. (2002). Increasing seat belt use in North Carolina. In R. C. Hornik (Ed.), *Public health communication: Evidence for behavior change* (pp. 85–96). Mahwah, NJ: Lawrence Erlbaum Associates.

Wong, F., Huhman, M., Asbury, L., Bretthauer-Mueller, R., McCarthy, S., Londe, P. (2004). VERB™—A social marketing campaign to increase physical activity among youth. *Preventing Chronic Disease*, *1*(3), A10.

World Health Organization. (2009). Safe surgery/surgical safety checklist. Retrieved from http://www.who.int

CHAPTER 9

Assessing Risk and Preventing Harm in the Clinical Microsystem

Paul Barach and Julie K. Johnson

To err is human, to cover up is unforgivable, and to fail to learn is inexcusable.

— **Sir Liam Donaldson**

The framework of health care delivery is shifting rapidly. Capital budgets and operational efficiency are critical in this time of shrinking reimbursement, increasing share of risk, and evolving models of care delivery. Modern medical care is complex, expensive, and at times dangerous. Across the world, hospital patients are harmed 9.2% of the time, with death occurring in 7.4% of these events. Furthermore, it is estimated that 43.5% of these harm events are preventable (de Vries et al., 2008; Landrigan et al., 2010). As illustrated in FIGURE 9.1, medical error is now the third-leading cause of death, following heart disease and cancer (Makary & Daniel, 2016). The rates could be debated, as they depend on the methods used in the studies as well the levels of underreporting; however, what is clear is that

we need to change and improve our health care systems dramatically. Most significantly, the study of patient safety has identified the need to design better systems—ones that make sense to providers and respect their work—to prevent errors from causing patient harm (Barach & Phelps, 2013). From all perspectives—patients' and providers' as well as the health care system's—the current level of avoidable harm is unacceptable and financially ruinous.

The goal of this chapter is to discuss how to develop reliability and resilience in health care systems while embedding a vision of zero avoidable harm into the culture of health care. Achieving this vision requires a risk management strategy that includes: (1) *identifying risk*—finding out what is going wrong; (2) *analyzing risk*—collecting data and using appropriate methods to understand what it means; and (3) *controlling risk*—devising and implementing strategies to better detect, manage, and prevent the problems that produce harm (Dickson, 1995).

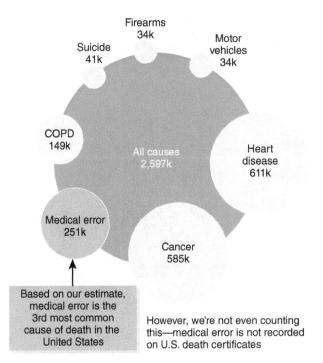

FIGURE 9.1 Leading Causes of Death

Reproduced from Makary, M. A. & Michael, D. Medical error—the third leading cause of death in the US. *BMJ, 353,* i2139.

This chapter begins with the background and definitions of risk management. We discuss the universal ingredients of individual accidents, organizational accidents, and human error. We then discuss models of risk management, focusing on how to address the barriers to creating an effective culture of safety and engagement and present strategies for applying concepts to clinical microsystem settings. The chapter concludes with a discussion on the role of disclosure of adverse events as part of a comprehensive risk management strategy.

▶ Risk Management— Background and Definitions

Traditionally, risk has been seen as exposure to events that may threaten or damage the organization (Walshe, 2001). Essentially, risk is the chance of something happening that will have an impact on key elements. It can be measured in terms of consequences and likelihood. The task of risk management, therefore, becomes balancing the costs and consequences of risks against the costs of risk reduction. The goal in clinical risk management should be to improve care and protect patients from harm; however, a perverse incentive for the organization as well as for those who work within the organization is that risk management may become a financially driven exercise that is at odds with the clinical mission of the organization (Vincent, 1997). Clinical risk management is the culture, process, and structures that are directed toward the effective management of potential opportunities and adverse events. We measure risk in terms of the likelihood and consequences of something going wrong, which is in contrast to how we measure quality (i.e., the extent to which a service or product achieves a desired result or outcome). Quality is commonly measured by whether a product or service is safe, timely, effective, efficient, equitable, and patient-centered (IOM, 2001).

There is substantial evidence that the majority of harm caused by health care is avoidable and the result of systemic problems rather than poor performance or negligence by individual providers. The past several years have seen an increase in proposed or operative legislation, including a near-miss reporting system, changes in mandated reporting systems, and the creation of state agencies dedicated to the coordination of patient safety research and implementation of change. There is clear policy guidance and a compelling ethical basis for the disclosure of adverse events to patients and their families. Mechanisms have been developed to involve all stakeholders—the government, health care professionals, administrators and planners, providers, and consumers—in ongoing, effective consultation, communication, and cultural change. These cultural and regulatory devices have helped engender more trust, which is an essential element in developing and sustaining a culture of safety.

Accidents

Research in managing risk has focused on the culture and structure of the organization. Perrow (1984) advanced the Normal Accidents Theory, which describes accidents as inevitable in complex, tightly coupled systems such as chemical plants and nuclear power plants. These accidents occur irrespective of the skill and intentions of the designers and operators; hence, they are normal and difficult to prevent. Perrow further argues that as the system gets more complex, it becomes opaque to its users, so that people are less likely to recognize and fear potential adverse occurrences. There are three universal ingredients of accidents:

1. *All human beings, regardless of their skills, abilities, and specialist training, make fallible decisions and commit unsafe acts.* This human propensity for committing errors and violating safety procedures can be moderated by selection, training, well-designed equipment, and good management, but it can never be entirely eliminated.

2. *All man-made systems possess latent failures to some degree.* This is true no matter how well designed, constructed, operated, and maintained a system may be. These unseen failures are analogous to resident pathogens in the human body that combine with local triggering factors (e.g., life stress, toxic chemicals) to overcome the immune system and produce disease. Adverse events such as cancers and heart attacks in well-defended systems do not arise from single causes but from multifactorial hits that overwhelm the system's natural defenses. The adverse conjunction of such factors, each necessary but insufficient alone to breach the defenses, are behind the majority of adverse events.

3. *All human endeavors involve some measure of risk.* In many cases, the local hazards are well understood and can be guarded against by a variety of technical or procedural countermeasures. No one, however, can foresee all the possible adverse scenarios, so there will always be defects in this protective armor.

These three ubiquitous accident ingredients reveal something important about the nature of making care safer (Bernstein, 1996). We can mitigate the risk of adverse events by process improvement, standardization, and an in-depth understanding of the safety degradations in systems, but we cannot prevent all risk. Embracing this uncertainty and implementing the training and curriculum to cope with it, as opposed to focusing solely on minimizing it, is essential in high-risk, highly coupled industries.

Outside health care, the most obvious impetus for the renewed interest in human error and impact of the organizational dynamics has been the growing concern over the terrible costs of human errors that led to disasters. Examples include the Tenerife runway collision in 1977 (540 fatalities), the Three Mile Island nuclear disaster in 1979, the Bhopal methyl isocyanate tragedy in 1984, the Challenger space shuttle accident in 1986 (Vaughn, 1996), the Chernobyl nuclear disaster in 1986 (Reason, 1997), and the Deepwater Horizon disaster in 2010 (Ingersoll, Locke, & Reavis, 2012). There is nothing new about tragic accidents caused by human error, but in the past, the injurious consequences were usually confined to the immediate vicinity of the disaster. Today, the nature and scale of highly coupled, potentially hazardous technologies in society and hospitals means that human error can have adverse effects far beyond the confines of the individual provider and patient settings. For example, *Pseudomonas aeruginosa* contamination of a single damaged bronchoscope potentially infected dozens of patients (DiazGranados et al., 2009). In recent years, there has been a noticeable spirit of *glasnost* (openness) within the medical profession concerning the role played by human error in causing medical adverse events (Millenson, 1997).

The Organizational Accident

Certain systems have been designed and redesigned with a wide variety of technical and procedural safeguards (e.g., operating rooms), yet they are still subject to accidents and adverse events (e.g., fire in the operating room, wrong-patient procedure, drug errors). These types of accidents and adverse events have been termed *organizational accidents* (Perrow, 1984; Reason, 1997). Organizational accidents are mishaps that arise not from single errors or isolated component breakdowns, but from the insidious culture change due to

an accumulation of failures occurring mainly within the managerial and organizational spheres. Such latent failures may subsequently combine with active failures and local triggering factors by errant but well-meaning providers to penetrate or bypass the system defenses. In his classic study of surgical teams, *Forgive and remember*, Bosk (1979) demonstrates how the underlying culture acts to acculturate newcomers, encourage normalized deviance, and suppress external views for change while enabling substandard practices to go unchecked. Systemic flaws set up good people to fail (Vaughn, 1999). People often find ways of getting around processes that seem to be unnecessary or that impede the workflow. This accumulated and excepted acceptance of cutting corners or making work-arounds poses a great danger to health care over time. By *deviance*, we mean organizational behaviors that deviate from normative standards or professional expectations (e.g., low hand-washing compliance before patient contact, minimal consultant oversight of hospital care on weekends, suppressing information about poor care, and so forth). Once a professional group normalizes a deviant organizational practice, it is no longer viewed as an aberrant act that elicits an exceptional response; instead, it becomes a routine activity that is commonly anticipated and frequently used (Weick, 2009). A permissive ethical climate, an emphasis on financial goals at all costs and an opportunity to act amorally or immorally, all can contribute to managerial and clinician decisions to initiate deviance (Barach & Phelps, 2013).

The etiology of an organizational accident can be divided into five phases (Perrow, 1984):

1. Organizational processes giving rise to latent failures;
2. Conditions that produce errors and violations within workplaces (e.g., operating room, pharmacy, intensive care unit);

3. The commission of errors and violations by "sharp end" individuals (the "sharp end" refers to the personnel or parts of the health care system in direct contact with patients. In contrast, the "blunt end" refers to the many layers of the health care system that affect the individuals at the sharp end. These colloquial terms are more formally known as "active errors," which occur at the point of contact between a human and some aspect of a larger system, and "latent errors," which are the less apparent failures of the organization);

4. The breaching of defenses or safeguards;

5. Outcomes that vary from a "free lesson" to a catastrophe.

Viewed from this perspective, the unsafe acts of those in direct contact with the patient are the end result of a long chain of events that originate higher up in the organization. One of the basic principles of error management is that the transitory mental states associated with error production—momentary inattention, distraction, preoccupation, forgetting—are the least-manageable links in the error chain because they are both unintended and largely unpredictable (Hollnagel, Woods, & Leveson, 2006). These errors have their cognitive origins in highly adaptive mental processes (Sagan, 1993). Such states can strike health care providers at any time, leading to slips, forgetfulness, and inattention. The system must be designed with in-depth defenses to mitigate the impact of these momentary lapses in awareness and to maintain the integrity of patient care.

Human Error and Performance Limitations

Although there was virtually no research in the field of safety in medicine and health care

delivery until the mid-1980s, in other fields, such as aviation, road and rail travel, nuclear power, and chemical processing, safety science and human factor principles have been applied to understand, prevent, and mitigate the associated adverse events (e.g., crashes, spills, and contaminations). The study of human error and of the organizational culture and climate, as well as intensive crash investigations, have been well developed for several decades in these arenas (Rasmussen, 1990; Sagan, 1993). The presumption of the non-linear and increasing risk in health care, associated with an apparent rise in the rate of litigation in the 1980s and attributable to the media's amplified attention to the subject, has brought medical adverse events to the attention of both clinicians and the general public (Kasperson et al., 1988).

In parallel with these developments, researchers from several disciplines have developed increasingly sophisticated methods for analyzing all incidents (Turner & Pidgeon, 1997). Theories of error and accident causation have evolved and are applicable across many human activities, including health care (Reason, 1997). These developments have led to a much broader understanding of accident causation, with less focus on the individual who commits an error at the "sharp end" of the incident and more on preexisting organizational and system factors that provide the context in which errors and patient harm can occur. An important consequence of this has been the realization that rigorous and innovative techniques of accident analysis may reveal deep-rooted, latent, and unsafe features of organizations. James Reason's "Swiss cheese" model captures these relationships very well (Reason, 1990). Understanding and predicting performance in complex settings requires a detailed understanding of the setting, the regulatory environment, and the human factors and organizational culture that shapes and influence this performance.

▶ Models of Risk Management

Risk management deals with the fact that adverse events, however rare, do continue to occur. Furthermore, risk management as a concept means that we should never ignore the possibility or significance of rare, unpredictable events. Using a creative analogy, Nassim Nicholas Taleb (2010) argues that before Europeans discovered Australia, there was no reason to believe that swans could be any color but white. However, when they discovered Australia, they found black swans. Black swans remind us that things do occur that we cannot possibly predict. Taleb continues the analogy to say that his "black swan" is an event with three properties: (1) the probability is low based on past knowledge, (2) the impact of the occurrence is massive, and (3) it is subject to hindsight bias; that is, people do not see it coming, but after its occurrence, everyone recognized that it was likely to happen.

In general, risk management models take into consideration the probability of an event occurring, which is then multiplied by the potential impact of the event. FIGURE 9.2 illustrates a simple risk management model that considers the probability of an event (low, medium, or high) and the impact of the consequences (limited/minor, moderate, or significant). Assigning an event in one of the cells is not an exact science, but the matrix offers a guideline to an appropriate organizational response to the risk. The individual unit or organization would need to determine how to translate each cell into action (e.g., what is required for "extensive management" of events with a significant negative impact and high likelihood of occurring).

▶ Engineering a Culture of Safety

How do we create an organizational climate in health care that fosters safety? What are the ingredients and key values of a safety culture? While national cultures arise largely out of shared norms and values, an organizational culture is shaped mainly by shared practices. And practices can be shaped by the implementation and enforcement of rules. Culture can be defined as the collection of individual and group values, attitudes, and practices that guide the behavior of group members (Helmreich &

	Probability		
	Low	**Medium**	**High**
Significant	Considerable management required	Substantial management and monitoring of risks	Extensive management crucial
Moderate	May accept risks but monitor them	Management effort worthwhile	Management effort required
Limited/Minor	Accept risks	Accept but monitor risks	Manage and monitor risks

FIGURE 9.2 Risk Management Model

Merritt, 2001). Acquiring a safety culture is a process of organizational learning that recognizes the inevitability of error and proactively seeks to identify latent threats. Characteristics of a strong safety culture include (Pronovost et al., 2003):

1. A commitment of the leadership to discuss and learn from errors
2. Communications founded on mutual trust and respect
3. Shared perceptions of the importance of safety
4. Encouragement and practice of teamwork
5. Incorporation of nonpunitive systems for reporting and analyzing adverse events

Striving for a safety culture is a process of collective learning. When the usual reaction to an adverse incident is to write another procedure and to provide more training, the system will not become more resistant to future organizational accidents. In fact, these actions may deflect the blame from the organization as a whole. There is a long tradition in medicine of examining past practices to understand how things might have been done differently. However, morbidity and mortality conferences, grand rounds, and peer reviews share many of the same shortcomings, such as a lack of human factors and systems thinking, a narrow focus on individual performance that excludes analysis of the contributory team factors and larger social issues, retrospective bias (a tendency to search for errors as opposed to the myriad system causes of error induction), and a lack of multidisciplinary integration into the organization-wide culture (Cassin & Barach, 2017).

If clinicians at the sharp end are not empowered by managerial leadership to be honest and reflective on their practice, rules and regulations will have a limited impact on enabling safer outcomes. Health care administrators need to understand the fundamental dynamics that lead to adverse events. Employing tools such as root cause analysis and failure mode and effects analysis can help clinicians and others better understand how adverse events occur, but only if done in an open and safe manner (Dekker, 2004). Collecting and learning from near-misses is essential. Definitions vary somewhat, but we define a near-miss as any error that had the potential to cause an adverse outcome but did not result in patient harm (Barach & Small, 2000). It is indistinguishable from a full-fledged adverse event in all but outcome (March, Sproull, & Tamuz, 2003). Near-misses offer powerful reminders of system hazards and retard the process of forgetting to be afraid of adverse events. A comprehensive effort to record and analyze near-miss data in health care has, however, lagged behind other industries (e.g., aviation, nuclear power industry) (Small & Barach, 2002). Vital but underappreciated studies suggest that near-misses are quite common. In a classic study, Heinreich (1941) estimated there are approximately 100 near-misses for every adverse event resulting in patient harm.

A focus on learning from near-misses offers several advantages (Barach & Small, 2000):

1. Near-misses occur 3–300 times more often than adverse events, enabling quantitative analysis.
2. There are fewer barriers to data collection, allowing analysis of interrelations of small failures.
3. Recovery strategies can be studied to enhance proactive interventions and to deemphasize the culture of blame.
4. Hindsight bias is more effectively reduced.

If near-misses and adverse events are inevitable, how do we learn from them once they occur? The next section discusses an approach for learning from events using a microsystem framework.

▶ # Applying Risk Management Concepts to Improving Quality and Safety Within the Clinical Microsystem

The clinical microsystem as a unit of research, analysis, and practice is an important level at which to focus patient safety interventions. A clinical microsystem has been defined as a small team of providers and staff providing care for a defined population of patients (Mohr, 2000; Mohr & Batalden, 2002; Mohr, Batalden, & Barach, 2004). Most patients and caregivers meet and work at this system level, and it is here that real changes in patient care can (and must) be made. Errors and failure occur within the microsystem, and ultimately it is the well-functioning microsystem that can prevent or mitigate errors and failure to avoid causing patient harm. Safety is a property of the clinical microsystem that can be achieved only through a systematic application of a broad array of process, equipment, organization, supervision, training, simulation, and teamwork changes. The scenario included in **EXHIBIT 9.1** illustrates a patient safety event in an academic clinical microsystem and how the resulting analysis enables a microsystem to learn from the event. Throughout the story, as told from the perspective of a senior resident physician in pediatrics, there are many process and system failures.

EXHIBIT 9.1 Patient Safety Scenario—Interview with a Third-Year Pediatrics Resident

Resident: I had a patient who was very ill. He was 12 years old and was completely healthy up until 3 months ago, and since then has been in our hospital and two other hospitals pretty much the entire time. He has been in respiratory failure, he's had mechanical ventilation (including oscillation), he's been in renal failure, he's had a number of ministrokes, and when I came on service he was having diarrhea—3 to 5 L/day—and we still didn't know what was going on with him. We thought that an abdominal CT would be helpful, and it needed to be infused.

He was a very anxious child. Understandably, it's hard for the nurses, and for me, and for his mother to deal with. He thought of it as pain, but it was anxiety, and it responded well to anxiolytics.

When I came in that morning, it hadn't been passed along to nursing that he was supposed to go to CT that morning. I heard the charge nurse getting the report from the night nurse. I said, "You know that he is supposed to go for a CT today." She was already upset because they were very short staffed. She heard me and then said that she was not only the charge nurse, but also taking care of two patients, and one had to go to CT. She went off to the main unit to talk to someone. Then she paged me and said, "If you want this child to have a scan, you have to go with him." I said, "OK." Nurses are the ones who usually go. But it didn't seem to be beyond my abilities . . . at the time.

So, I took the child for his CT and his mom came with us. We gave him extra ativan on the way there, because whenever he had a procedure he was extra anxious. When we got there, they weren't ready. We had lost our spot from the morning. My patient got more and more anxious and was actually yelling at the techs, "Hurry up!" We went into the room. He was about 5 or 6 hours late for his study, and we had given him contrast enterally. The techs were concerned that he didn't have enough anymore and wanted to give him more through his G-tube. I said, "That sounds fine." And they mixed it up and gave it to me to give through his G-tube. I went to his side and—not registering that it was his central line—I unhooked his central line, not only taking off the cap but unhooking something, and I pushed 70 cc of the gastrografin in. As soon as I had finished the second syringe I realized I was using the wrong tube. I said, "Oh no!" Mom was right there and said, "What?" I said, "I put the stuff in the wrong tube. He looks OK. I'll be right back, I have to call somebody."

I clamped off his intravenous line and I called my attending and the radiologist. My attending said that he was on his way down. The radiologist was over by the time I had hung up the phone. My patient was stable the whole time. We figured out what was in the gastrografin that could potentially cause harm. We decided to cancel the study. . . . I sent the gastrografin—the extra stuff in the tubes—for a culture just in case he grew some kind of infection and then we would be able to treat it and match it with what I had pushed into the line. I filled out an incident report. I called my chiefs and told them. . . . They said, "It's OK. He's fine, right?" I said, "Yes." They came up later in the evening just to be supportive. They said, "It's OK. It's OK to make a mistake."

Interviewer: What was your attending's response?

Resident: The attending that I had called when I made the mistake said, "I'm sorry that you were in that situation. You shouldn't have been put in that situation." Another attending the next day was telling people, "Well, you know what happened yesterday," as if it were the only thing going on for this patient.

I thought it was embarrassing that he was just passing on this little tidbit of information as if it would explain everything that was going on. As opposed to saying, "Yes, an error was made, it is something that we are taking into account." And he told me to pay more attention to the patient. Yes, I made the mistake, but hands-down, I still—and always did—know that patient better than he did. I just thought that was mean and not fair. And the only other thing I thought was not good was the next morning when I was prerounding, some of the nurses were whispering, and I just assumed that was what they were whispering about. I walked up to them and said, "I'm the one who did it. I made a mistake. How is he doing?" I tried to answer any questions they had and move on.

Interviewer: How did the nurses respond when you said that you made a mistake?

Resident: The nurse that had sent me down with him told me, "It's OK, don't worry about it." The others just listened politely and didn't say anything.

Interviewer: How did the mother respond to you the next day?

Resident: The next day, I felt really bad. I felt very incompetent. I was feeling very awkward being the leader of this child's care—because I am still at a loss for his diagnosis. And after the event, when the grandma found out—she was very angry. I apologized to the mom, and I thought it would be overdoing it to keep saying, "I am so sorry." So, the next day, I went into the room and said to the mom, "You need to have confidence in the person taking care of your son. If my mistake undermines that at all, you don't have to have me as your son's doctor, and I can arrange it so that you can have whoever you want." She said, "No. No, it's fine. We want you as his doctor." Then we just moved on with the care plan. That felt good. And that felt appropriate. I couldn't just walk into the room and act like nothing had happened. I needed her to give me the power to be their doctor. So, I just went and asked for it.

Many methods are available to explore the causal system at work (Dekker, 2002; Reason, 1995; Vincent, 2003; Vincent, Taylor-Adams, & Stanhope, 1998), and they all suggest the importance of holding the entire causal system in our analytic frame, not just seeking a "root" cause. One method that we have found to be useful for systematically looking at patient safety events builds on William Haddon's (1972) overarching framework on injury epidemiology (Mohr et al., 2003). Haddon, as the first Director of the National Highway Safety Bureau (1966–1969), is credited with a paradigm change in the prevention of road traffic deaths and injuries moving from an "accidental" or "pre-scientific" approach to an etiologic one. Haddon was interested in the broader issues of injury and system failures that results from the transfer of energy in such ways that inanimate or animate objects are damaged. The clinical microsystem offers a setting in which this injury can be studied. According to

Haddon (1970), there are a number of strategies for reducing losses:

- Prevent the marshaling of the energy.
- Reduce the amount of energy marshaled.
- Prevent the release of the energy.
- Modify the rate or spatial distribution of release of the energy.
- Separate in time and space the energy being released and the susceptible structure.
- Use a physical barrier to separate the energy and the susceptible structure.
- Modify the contact surface or structure with which people can come in contact.
- Strengthen the structure that might be damaged by the energy transfer.
- When injury does occur, rapidly detect it and counter its continuation and extension.
- When injury does occur, take all necessary reparative and rehabilitative steps.

All these strategies have a logical sequence that is related to the three essential phases of injury control relating to preinjury, injury, and postinjury.

Haddon developed a 3 × 3 matrix with factors related to an auto injury (human, vehicle, and environment) heading the columns and phases of the event (preinjury, injury, and postinjury) heading the rows. FIGURE 9.3 demonstrates how the Haddon Matrix can be applied to analyze an auto accident (Haddon, 1972). The use of the matrix focuses the analysis on the interrelationship between the factors and phases. A mix of countermeasures derived from Haddon's strategies is necessary to minimize injury and loss. Furthermore, the countermeasures can be designed for each phase—pre-event, event, and postevent—similar to designing mechanisms to preventing patient harm. This approach confirms what we know about adverse events in complex health care environments—it takes a variety of strategies to prevent and/or mitigate patient harm. Understanding injury in its larger context helps us recognize the basic nature of "unsafe" systems and the important work of humans to mitigate the inherent hazards (Dekker, 2002).

We can also use the Haddon Matrix to guide the analysis of patient safety adverse events. Adapting this tool from injury epidemiology to patient safety, we have revised the matrix to include phases labeled *pre-event*, *event*, and *postevent* instead of *preinjury*, *injury*, and *postinjury*. The revised factors, *patient–family*, *health care professional*, *system*,

		Factors		
		Human	**Vehicle**	**Environment**
Phases	**Preinjury**	Alcohol intoxication	Braking capacity of motor vehicles	Visibility of hazards
	Injury	Resistance to energy insults	Sharp or pointed edges and surfaces	Flammable building materials
	Postinjury	Hemorrhage	Rapidity of energy reduction	Emergency medical response

FIGURE 9.3 Haddon Matrix Used to Analyze Auto Accident

Haddon, W. A. (1972). Logical framework for categorizing highway safety phenomena and activity. *J Trauma, 12*(2), 197.

		Factors			
		Patient/Family	**Health Care Professional**	**System**	**Environment**
Phases	**Pre-Event**	• Consent (process, timing) • Anxiety • Patient lines • Mother's presence	• Not familiar with procedure • Lack of MD–RN communication • Focus on anxiety and not on procedure • Assumed roles, made assumptions • Arrogance/respect	• Several lines in patient • Silos	• Nurse shortage • Scheduling delays • Manufacturing (performance shaping factors, human factors) • Lack of process for risk analysis
	Event	• Anxiety (patient's and parent's) • No shared expectations • No active participation	• Fatigue • Aware of limitations • Training	• Work hours • Protocols • Standardization • Double-checking	• Work hours for residents • Rushed • No other clinician
	Post-Event	• Lack of explanation • Disclosure • Who should talk to family?	• Guilt • Lack of confidence • Loss of face	• Lack of understanding of errors/ systems • Lack of supportive environment for resident • Incidence report morbidity and mortality • Analysis of event	• Regulatory

FIGURE 9.4 Completed Patient Safety Matrix

and *environment*, replace *human, vehicle*, and *environment*. Note that we have added a fourth factor, *system*, to refer to the processes and systems that are in place for the microsystem. This addition recognizes the significant contribution that systems and teams make toward harm and error in the microsystem.

"Environment" refers to the context (enablers and barriers) that the microsystem exists within. **FIGURE 9.4** shows a completed matrix using the pediatric case. The next step in learning from errors and adverse events is to develop and execute countermeasures to address the issues in each cell of the matrix. **FIGURE 9.5** provides a list of tools that would be appropriate to assess each "cell" of the matrix as part of a microsystems risk assessment framework.

Microsystems and Macrosystems

Health care organizations are composed of multiple, differentiated, variably autonomous microsystems. These interdependent small systems exhibit loose and tight coupling (Weick & Sutcliffe, 2001). Several assumptions

		Factors		
		Patient/Family	**Health Care Professional**	**Systems/Environment**
Phases	**Pre-Event**	• Orientation to the process (process mapping)	• Probablistic risk assessment • Scenario building • Hazard analysis • Checklists	• Failure modes effects analysis • Human factors engineering
	Event	• Interview	• Crew resource management • Checklists	• Root cause analysis
	Post-Event	• Interview • Focus group interviews	• Microsystem analysis • Morbidity and mortality conference	• Root cause analysis • Artifact analysis

FIGURE 9.5 Patient Safety Matrix with Tools for Assessing Risk and Analyzing Events

are made about the relationship between these microsystems and the macrosystem (Nelson et al., 2002):

1. Bigger systems (macrosystems) are made of smaller systems.
2. These smaller systems (microsystems) produce quality, safety, and cost outcomes at the front line of care.
3. Ultimately, the outcomes from macrosystems can be no better than the microsystems of which they are formed.

These assumptions suggest that it is necessary to intervene within each microsystem in the organization if the organization as a whole wants to improve. A microsystem cannot function independently from the other microsystems it regularly works with or its macrosystem. From the macrosystem perspective, senior leaders can enable an overall patient safety focus with clear, visible values, expectations, and recognition of "deeds well done." They can set direction by clearly expecting that each microsystem will align its mission, vision, and strategies with the organization's mission, vision, and

strategies. Senior leadership can offer each microsystem the flexibility needed to achieve its mission and ensure the creation of strategies, systems, and methods for achieving excellence in health care, thereby stimulating innovation and building knowledge and capabilities. Finally, senior leaders can pay careful attention to the questions they ask as they nurture meaningful work and hold the microsystem's leadership accountable to achieve the strategic mission of providing safer care.

TABLE 9.1 builds on the research of high-performing microsystems (Mohr, 2000; Mohr & Batalden, 2002; Mohr, Batalden, & Barach, 2004) and provides specific actions that can be further explored to apply patient safety concepts to understanding the impact and performance of clinical microsystems. It also provides linkages to the macrosystem's ongoing organization-centered and issue-centered quality efforts, which can either support or conflict with this approach, as discussed in greater detail in Chapter 13. **BOX 9.1** provides a set of accountability questions that senior leaders should ask as they work to improve the safety and quality of the organization.

TABLE 9.1 Linkage of Microsystem Characteristics to Patient Safety

Microsystem Characteristics	What This Means for Patient Safety
1. Leadership	▪ Define the safety vision of the organization ▪ Identify the existing constraints within the organization ▪ Allocate resources for plan development, implementation, and ongoing monitoring and evaluation ▪ Build in microsystems participation and input to plan development ▪ Align organizational quality and safety goals ▪ Engage the board of trustees in ongoing conversations about the organizational progress toward achieving safety goals ▪ Recognition for prompt truth-telling about errors or hazards ▪ Certification of helpful changes to improve safety
2. Organizational support	▪ Work with clinical microsystems to identify patient safety issues and make relevant local changes ▪ Put the necessary resources and tools in the hands of individuals
3. Staff focus	▪ Assess current safety culture ▪ Identify the gap between current culture and safety vision ▪ Plan cultural interventions ▪ Conduct periodic assessments of culture ▪ Celebrate examples of desired behavior, for example, acknowledgment of an error
4. Education and training	▪ Develop patient safety curriculum ▪ Provide training and education of key clinical and management leadership ▪ Develop a core of people with patient safety skills who can work across microsystems as a resource
5. Interdependence of the care team	▪ Build PDSA* cycles into debriefings ▪ Use daily huddles to debrief and to celebrate identifying errors *PDSA: Plan, Do, Study, Act
6. Patient focus	▪ Establish patient and family partnerships ▪ Support disclosure and truth around medical error
7. Community and market focus	▪ Analyze safety issues in community, and partner with external groups to reduce risk to population
8. Performance results	▪ Develop key safety measures ▪ Create feedback mechanisms to share results with microsystems
9. Process improvement	▪ Identify patient safety priorities based on assessment of key safety measures ▪ Address the work that will be required at the microsystem level
10. Information and information technology	▪ Enhance error-reporting systems ▪ Build safety concepts into information flow (e.g., checklists, reminder systems)

BOX 9.1   Questions Senior Leaders Could Ask About Patient Safety

What information do we have about errors and patient harm?
What is the patient safety plan?
How will the plan be implemented at the organizational level and at the microsystem level?
What type of infrastructure is needed to support implementation?
What is the best way to communicate the plan to the individual microsystems?
How can we foster reporting—telling the truth—about errors?
How will we empower microsystem staff to make suggestions for improving safety?
What training will staff need?
Who are the key stakeholders?
How can we build linkages to the key stakeholders?
What stories can we tell that relate the importance of patient safety?
How will we recognize and celebrate progress?

Promoting System Resilience Across and Between the Microsystems

Microsystems usually coexist with multiple other microsystems within the organization. Patients are aware of the gaps and handoffs between microsystems as they navigate the health care system, such as when they transfer from inpatient care back into the community. Patients are aware of the challenges of "synthesizing" knowledge across the various microsystems they encounter. Models developed by Zimmerman and Hayday (1999) for understanding and supporting work on the relationships across microsystems offer insight into the generative work of interdependence. Understanding the dynamics of effective organizational relationships can be helpful in thinking about how to foster relationships between microsystems within the same organization and across differing organizations. These cross-microsystem relationships are fundamentally related to improving handoffs, but this inquiry can also provide opportunities for learning about systemic problems within the institution and interventions to improve quality and safety (Groene et al., 2012). An effective collaborative relationship is based on the underlying assumption that collaboration is a more effective approach to achieve a goal than multiple individual efforts (Toccafondi et al., 2012).

Weick suggests that leaders today need to develop groups that are also respectful of the interactions that hold the group together (Weick, 1993, 1995). Resilient groups have respectful interactions that are founded on three major elements (Weick, 1996):

1. *Trust*—a willingness to base beliefs and actions on the reports of others
2. *Honesty*—reporting so that others may use one's observations in developing and enhancing their own beliefs
3. *Self-respect*—integrating one's perceptions and beliefs with the reports of others without depreciating them or oneself

Four aspects of the relationship can help generate creative responses to the diagnosed challenges facing entities needing to work better together (Zimmerman & Hayday, 1999):

1. The separateness or differences of the two microsystems
2. The talking–listening–tuning opportunities that the two microsystems have
3. The action opportunities that the two entities have

4. The reasons they have to work together

Balanced attention to each of these aspects enables creative work.

The conditions also must be present for relationships to develop across organizations (Kaluzny, 1985). For voluntary interactions—which may be quite different than those mandated by an external power—several conditions must be met. There must be an internal need for resources, a commitment to an external problem, and the opportunity to change. In addition, there must be a consensus regarding both the external problem(s) facing the organizations and the specific goals and services for developing a joint effort. The Institute of Medicine report *To err is human* (IOM, 2000) brought patient safety to the forefront of the agenda and set the stage for discussing specific goals and strategies for achieving those goals.

Mitchell and Shortell (2000) provide a synthesis of the literature on the success of community health partnerships that suggests several factors that influence the success of interorganizational relationships. These factors are:

- Context
- Strategic intent
- Resource base
- Membership heterogeneity
- Coordination of skills
- Response to accountability

Context refers to the environment in which the partnership exists—the internal and external stakeholders, their historical relationships and influence, the presence or absence of human and financial resources, the political environment, public sentiments, and the current challenges facing the community. Strategic intent—a similar concept to a consensus on the external problem(s) facing the organizations—refers to the reasons the interorganizational relationship is formed. A diversified resource base helps ensure that the collaborative is able to pursue the strategic intent without getting sidetracked by pursuing the goals of a single funding agency. Membership heterogeneity

refers to the balance of the participating members in regard to the number and types of participants. Informal as well as formal communication mechanisms ensure that the collaborators meet their own goals and are held accountable to demonstrate their progress internally and externally.

▶ Role of Risk Management and Patient Disclosure

When patients seek medical care, they entrust their health to us. Health care providers have a responsibility or "fiduciary duty" to act in the best interests of the patient (Kraman & Hamm, 1999). Properly assessing the type of procedure planned (e.g., invasive vs. noninvasive), patient risk factors, type of drug to use (e.g., hypnotic vs. analgesic), and type of team and level of support are all critical. When assessing the level of risk of the procedure, we should ask, *What are the desired clinical effects? How quickly are effects desired? What is the desired duration of effects? And are there any adverse "other" clinical effects?*

Injured patients and their families want to know the cause of their bad outcomes, especially if the adverse event was caused by an error (Studdert, Mello, & Brenna, 2004). The most important factor in the decision to file lawsuits is not negligence but ineffective communication between patients and providers (Wu et al., 1997). Malpractice suits often result when an unexpected adverse outcome is met with no effort to apologize, with a lack of empathy from physicians and a perceived or actual withholding of essential information (Barach, 2005; Wu et al., 1997).

Studies consistently show that health care providers are understandably reticent about discussing errors, believing they have no appropriate assurance of legal protection (LeBlang & King, 1984). This reticence, in turn, impedes systemic and programmatic efforts to prevent medical errors. A growing initiative in health care has been to encourage open and frank discussion with patients and their families after an adverse event; this initiative has met with salutary effects. The lack of evidence that disclosure adversely impacts claims, case resolution, and patient and family perceptions is changing organizational practices.

Evidence from the University of Michigan supports an aggressive disclosure policy (Clinton & Obama, 2006). In 2002, the University of Michigan Health System launched a program with three components: (1) acknowledge cases in which a patient was hurt because of medical error and compensate these patients quickly and fairly, (2) aggressively defend cases that the hospital considers to be without merit, and (3) study all adverse events to determine how procedures and systems can be improved.

Disclosing an adverse event should occur when the adverse event (1) has a perceptible effect on the patient that was not discussed in advance as a known risk, (2) necessitates a change in the patient's care, (3) potentially poses an important risk to the patient's future health, even if that risk is extremely small, and (4) involves providing a treatment or procedure without the patient's consent (Cantor et al., 2005). From an ethical perspective, the disclosure process should begin at the time of discussing the consent form and interventions with the patients (Barach & Cantor, 2007).

▶ Conclusions

The health care system has begun to approach patient safety in a more systematic way, but we continue to tolerate an extraordinary level of risk and preventable harm. There is a clear need to improve the safety of care, as patients still suffer harm from medical care at alarmingly high rates. Strong leadership is needed to change organizational cultures to achieve a vision of zero tolerance of preventable harm. The application of safety science and reliability principles, methods, and analytical tools in

the health sector promises the development of a coherent bundle of interrelated strategies for change. Reliability principles include methods of evaluating, calculating, and improving the overall reliability of a complex system—have been used effectively in industries such as manufacturing to improve both safety and the rate at which a system consistently produces appropriate outcomes. Even the most advanced health care organizations acknowledge that they are on a journey to achieving high reliability and need to address four essential building blocks: (1) a culture devoted to quality; (2) responsibility and accountability of staff; (3) optimizing and standardizing processes; and (4) constant measurement of performance.

Much organizational and leadership work is needed to change the mental model of clinicians and providers toward a system-based change. The traditional approach within medicine and health care was to emphasize the individual's responsibility for errors and to encourage the belief that the way to eliminate adverse events was for individual clinicians to perfect their practices. This simplistic approach fails to address the important and complex systematic flaws that contribute to the genesis of adverse events, and also perpetuates a myth of infallibility that is a disservice to both clinicians and their patients. The focus on the actions of individuals as the sole cause of adverse events inevitably results in continued system failures, resulting in the injury and death of patients and the tendency for clinicians to blame themselves for this harm. The efforts of the innumerable government bodies around the world to align external financial, regulatory, and educational incentives are beginning to have an impact on clinicians' and providers' interest in embracing the safety themes described in this chapter.

Cultural and process changes require profound alterations in management thinking, staff empowerment, and communications skills within and across disciplines. Attributing errors to system failures does not absolve clinicians of their duty of care or their fiduciary duty to act in the best interests of their patients. In fact, acknowledging system failures adds to that duty a responsibility to admit errors, investigate them collaboratively, and participate in redesign for a safer system. One way to achieve this is to deconstruct errors and

failures at the front lines of health care as a way to assess risk and develop further strategies for managing risk. Such understanding and corrective efforts can be made to embed quality and safety into the microsystem.

References

Barach, P. (2005). The unintended consequences of Florida Medical Liability Legislation. *Perspectives on patient safety.* Retrieved from http://www.webmm.ahrq.gov/

Barach, P., & Cantor, M. (2007). Adverse event disclosure: Benefits and drawbacks for patients and clinicians. In S. Clarke & J. Oakley (Eds.), *Informed consent and clinician accountability: The ethics of report cards on surgeon performance.* Cambridge, UK: Cambridge University Press.

Barach, P., & Phelps, G. (2013). Clinical sensemaking: a systematic approach to reduce the impact of normalised deviance in the medical profession. *Journal of the Royal Society of Medicine, 106*(10), 387–390.

Barach, P., & Small, S. (2000). Reporting and preventing medical mishaps: Lessons from non-medical near miss reporting systems. *British Medical Journal, 320,* 759–763.

Bernstein, P. (1996). *Against the gods. The remarkable story of risk.* New York, NY: Wiley.

Bosk, C. (1979). *Forgive and remember: Managing medical failure.* Chicago: University of Chicago Press.

Cantor, M. D., Barach, P., Derse, A., et al. (2005). Disclosing adverse events to patients. *The Joint Commission Journal of Quality & Patient Safety, 31*(1), 5–12.

Cassin, B., & Barach, P. (2017). How not to run an incident investigation. In J. Sanchez, P. Barach, H. Johnson, & J. Jacobs (Eds.), *Perioperative patient safety and quality: Principles and practice.* New York, NY: Springer.

Clinton, H. R., & Obama, B. (2006). Making patient safety the centerpiece of medical liability reform. *The New England Journal of Medicine, 354*(21), 2205–2208.

Dekker, S. (2002). *The field guide to human error investigations.* Aldershot, UK: Ashgate Publishing Limited.

Dekker, S. (2004). *Ten questions about human error: A new view of human factors and system safety.* Mahwah, NJ: Erlbaum.

de Vries, E., Ramrattan, M., Smorenburg, S. M., et al. (2008). The incidence and nature of in-hospital adverse events: A systematic review. *Quality & Safety in Health Care, 17,* 216–223.

DiazGranados, C. A., Jones, M. Y., Kongphet-Tran, T., White, N., Shapiro, M., Wang, Y. F., Ray, S. M., & Blumberg, H. M. (2009). Outbreak of *Pseudomonas aeruginosa* infection associated with contamination of a flexible bronchoscope. *Infection Control & Hospital Epidemiology, 30*(6), 550–555.

Dickson, G. (1995). Principles of risk management. *Quality Healthcare, 4,* 75–79.

Groene, R. O., Orrego, C., Suñol, R., Barach, P., & Groene, O. (2012). "It's like two worlds apart": an analysis of vulnerable patient handover practices at discharge from hospital. *BMJ Quality & Safety, 21*(Suppl 1), i67–i75.

Haddon, M. (1970). On the escape of tigers: An ecologic note. *American Journal of Public Health 60*(12), 2229–2234.

Haddon, W. J. (1972). A logical framework for categorizing highway safety phenomena and activity. *Journal of Trauma, 12*(2), 193–207.

Heinreich, H. (1941). *Industrial accident prevention.* New York, NY: McGraw-Hill.

Helmreich, R., & Merritt, A. (2001). *Culture at work in aviation and medicine.* Burlington, VT: Ashgate.

Hollnagel, E., Woods, D. D., & Leveson, N. (Eds.). (2006). *Resilience engineering: Concepts and precepts.* Aldershot, UK: Ashgate.

Ingersoll, C., Locke, R. M., & Reavis, C. (2012). BP and the Deepwater Horizon disaster of 2010. MIT Sloan School of Management: Ethics, Values and Voice Module 10-110, Rev. April 3, 2012. Retrieved from https://mitsloan.mit.edu/LearningEdge/CaseDocs/10%20110%20BP%20Deepwater%20Horizon%20Locke.Review.pdf

Institute of Medicine (IOM). (2000). *To err is human: Building a safer health system.* Washington, D.C.: National Academies Press.

Institute of Medicine (IOM). (2001). *Crossing the quality chasm: A new health system for the 21st century.* Washington, D.C.: National Academies Press.

Kaluzny, A. (1985). Design and management of disciplinary and interdisciplinary groups in health services: Review and critique. *Medical Care Reviews, 42*(1), 77–112.

Kasperson, R., Renn, O., Slovic, P., Brown, H., Emel, J., Goble, R., Kasperson J. X., & Ratick, S. (1988). Social amplification of risk: A conceptual framework. *Risk Analysis, 8*(2), 177–187.

Kraman, S. S., & Hamm, G. (1999). Risk management: Extreme honesty may be the best policy. *Annals of Internal Medicine, 131*(12), 963–937.

Landrigan, C. P., Parry, G. J., Bones, C. B., et al. (2010). Temporal trends in rates of patient harm resulting from medical care. *The New England Journal of Medicine, 363*(22), 2124–2134.

LeBlang, T., & King, J. L. (1984). Tort liability for nondisclosure: The physician's legal obligations to disclose patient illness and injury. *Dickinson Law Rev*, *89*, 1–18.

Makary, M. A., & Daniel, M. (2016). Medical error—the third leading cause of death in the US. *British Medical Journal*, *353*, i2139.

March, J., Sproull, L., & Tamuz, M. (2003). Learning from samples of one or fewer. *Quality & Safety in Health Care*, *12* (6), 465–472.

Millenson, M. (1997). *Demanding medical excellence: Doctors and accountability in the information age*. Chicago, IL: The University of Chicago Press.

Mitchell, S. M., & Shortell, S. M. (2000). The governance and management of effective community health partnerships. *The Milbank Quarterly*, *78*(2), 241–289.

Mohr, J. (2000). *Forming, Operating, and Improving Microsystems of Care*. Hanover, NH: Center for the Evaluative Clinical Sciences, Dartmouth College.

Mohr, J., Barach, P., Cravero, J. P., Blike, G. T., Godfrey, M. M., Batalden, P. B., & Nelson, E. C. (2003). Microsystems in health care: Part 6. Designing patient safety into the microsystem. *The Joint Commission Journal of Quality & Safety*, *29*(8), 401–408.

Mohr, J., & Batalden, P. (2002). Improving safety at the front lines: The role clinical microsystems. *Quality & Safety in Health Care*, *11*(1), 45–50.

Mohr, J., Batalden, P., & Barach, P. (2004). Integrating patient safety into the clinical microsystem. *Quality & Safety in Health Care*, *13*(2), ii34–ii38.

Nelson, E., Batalden, P., Huber, T. P., Mohr, J., Godfrey, M. M., Headrick, L. A., & Wasson, J. H. (2002). Microsystems in health care: Part 1. Learning from high-performing front-line clinical units. *The Joint Commission Journal of Quality Improvement*, *28*(9), 472–493.

Perrow, C. (1984). *Normal accidents, living with high-risk technologies*. New York, NY: Basic Books.

Pronovost, P., Weast, B., Holzmueller, C. G., Rosenstein, B. J., Kidwell, R. P., Haller, K. B., . . . Rubin, H. R. (2003). Evaluation of the culture of safety: Survey of clinicians and managers in an academic medical center. *Quality & Safety in Health Care*, *12*, 405–410.

Rasmussen, J. (1990). The role of error in organising behaviour. *Ergonomics*, *33*, 1185–1199.

Reason, J. (1990). *Human Errors*. New York: Cambridge University Press.

Reason, J. (1995). Understanding adverse events: Human factors. In C. Vincent, (Ed.), *Clinical risk management: Enhancing patient safety* (pp. 31–54). London: BMJ Publications.

Reason, J. (1997). *Managing the risks of organizational accidents*. Aldershot, UK: Ashgate.

Sagan, S. D. (1993). *The limits of safety*. Princeton, NJ: Princeton University Press.

Small, D., & Barach, P. (2002). Patient safety and health policy: A history and review. *Hematology/Oncology Clinics of North America*, *16*(6), 1463–1482.

Studdert, D. M., Mello, M. M., & Brenna, T. A. (2004). Medical malpractice. *The New England Journal of Medicine*, *350*(3), 283–292.

Taleb, N. N. (2010). *The black swan: The impact of the highly improbable*. New York, NY: Random House.

Toccafondi, G., Albolino, S., Tartaglia, R., Guidi, S., Molisso, A., & Venneri, F. The collaborative communication model for patient handover at the interface between high-acuity and low-acuity care. *BMJ Quality & Safety*, *21*(Suppl 1), i58–i66.

Turner, B., & Pidgeon, N. (1997). *Man-made disasters*. London: Butterworth and Heinemann.

Vaughan, D. (1996). *The Challenger launch decision: Risky technology, culture, and deviance at NASA*. Chicago, IL: University of Chicago Press.

Vaughan, D. (1999). The dark side of organizations: mistake, misconduct and disaster. *Annual Review of Sociology*, *25*, 271–305.

Vincent, C. (1997). Risk, safety, and the dark side of quality. *British Medical Journal*, *314*, 1775–1776.

Vincent, C. (2003). Understanding and responding to adverse events [see comment]. *The New England Journal of Medicine*, *348*(11), 1051–1056.

Vincent, C., Taylor-Adams, S., & Stanhope, N. (1998). Framework for analysing risk and safety in clinical medicine. *British Medical Journal*, *316*(7138), 1154–1157.

Walshe, K. (2001). The development of clinical risk management. In C. Vincent, (Ed.), *Clinical risk management: Enhancing patient safety*. London: BMJ Books.

Weick, K. E. (1993). The collapse of sensemaking in organizations: The Mann Gulch disaster. *Administrative Science Quarterly*, *38*, 628–652.

Weick, K. E. (1995). *Sensemaking in organizations*. Thousand Oaks, CA: Sage.

Weick, K. E. (1996). Prepare your organization to fight fires. *Harvard Business Review*, *74*(3), 143–148.

Weick, K. E. (2009). Emergent change as a universal in organizations. In: K. E. Weick (Ed.), *Making sense of the organization* (Vol. 2). Chichester, UK: Wiley.

Weick, K., & Sutcliffe, K. (2001). *Managing the unexpected: Assuring high performance in an age of complexity*. Ann Arbor, MI: University of Michigan Business School.

Wu, A. W., Cavanaugh, T. A., McPhee, S. J., Lo, B., & Micco, G. P. (1997). To tell the truth: Ethical and practical issues in disclosing medical mistakes to patients. *Journal of General Internal Medicine*, *12*(12), 770–775.

Zimmerman, B., & Hayday, B. (1999). A board's journey into complexity science. *Group Decision Making & Negotiating*, *8*, 281–303.

CHAPTER 10

Classification and the Reduction of Medical Errors

Donna Woods

Human fallibility is like gravity, weather, and terrain, just another foreseeable hazard.

— **J. T. Reason** (1997, p. 25)

The publication of the Institute of Medicine's report, *To err is human*, highlighted that 44,000 to 98,000 deaths occurred each year from the care patients receive for a particular condition, rather than the condition itself (IOM, 2000). In fact, updated error incidence findings from the 2010 Office of the Inspector General's Report on Adverse Events in Hospitalized Medicare Beneficiaries (Levinson, 2010) now estimate that 180,000 deaths occur in hospitals per year in people over 65 years of age. Without even including the remainder of the population, this made medical errors the third-leading cause of death after cardiovascular disease and cancer.

Given this considerable excess mortality and harm, one of the key foci of the field of patient safety is to understand the underlying attributes, vulnerabilities, and causes in the systems and processes of care leading to errors and harm. If the mechanisms and causes are well understood, interventions to address these can be developed in order to prevent or mitigate harm.

When errors occur in high-risk environments, such as health care (IOM, 2000), there is a greater potential for harm. *Health care is very complex, and an effective system of classification should accurately represent this level of complexity.* By understanding human error, we can plan for likely, and potentially predictable, error scenarios and implement barriers to prevent or mitigate the occurrence of potential errors. This chapter will discuss the definitions, theories, and existing systems of classification that are used improve our understanding of the mechanisms of errors and patient safety events in order to apply this knowledge to reduce harm. Common definitions are essential to a standardized classification system. See TABLE 10.1 for some common definitions of some important terms in the field of patient safety.

TABLE 10.1 Terms and Definitions

Terms	Definitions
Error	"Error is defined as the failure of a planned action to be completed as intended or the use of a wrong plan to achieve an aim." (IOM, 2000; QuIC, 2000)
	Errors can occur in both the planning and execution stages of a task. Plans can be adequate or inadequate, and actions (behavior) can be intentional or unintentional. If a plan is adequate, and the intentional action follows that plan, then the desired outcome will be achieved. If a plan is adequate, but an unintentional action does not follow the plan, then the desired outcome will not be achieved. Similarly, if a plan is inadequate, and an intentional action follows the plan, the desired outcome will again not be achieved (IOM, 2000; QuIC, 2000).
	"An act of commission (doing something wrong) or omission (failing to do the right thing) leading to an undesirable outcome or significant potential for such an outcome." This definition highlights the fact that an error while it can lead to harm does not need to lead to harm to be so assessed (IOM, 2000; QuIC, 2000).
Adverse Event	"An adverse event is defined an injury that was caused by medical management (rather than the underlying disease) and that prolonged the hospitalization, produced a disability at the time of discharge, or both." (Thomas et al., 2000)
Preventable Adverse Event	A preventable adverse event is defined "as an adverse event that could have been prevented using currently available knowledge and standards." (Thomas et al., 2000)
Sentinel Event	A sentinel event is a Patient Safety Event that reaches a patient and results in any of the following: ■ Death ■ Permanent harm ■ Severe temporary harm and intervention required to sustain life (TJC, 2017).
Never Events	National Quality Forum described 29 serious events also called Serious Reportable Events, "which are extremely rare medical errors that should never happen to a patient." (AHRQ, 2017b)
Incident	"An *unplanned, undesired* event that hinders completion of a task and may cause injury, illness, or property damage or some combination of all three in varying degrees from minor to catastrophic. Unplanned and undesired do not mean *unable to prevent*. Unplanned and undesired also do not mean *unable to prepare for*. Crisis planning is how we prepare for serious incidents that occur that require response for mitigation." (Ferrante, 2017b)
Near Miss	"A near miss is defined as event that could have had adverse consequences but did not and was indistinguishable from fully fledged adverse events in all but outcome. In a **near miss**, an error was occurred, but the **patient** did not experience clinical harm, either through early detection or sheer luck." (AHRQ, 2017a)

▶ Why Classify Safety Events?

A key component of improving patient safety is to conduct an assessment of safety incidents or events that occur, and through these assessments, to gain an understanding of the vulnerabilities that exist in the related systems and processes. Risk assessment is the science of risks and their probability (Haimes, 2004). This commonly involves error or event classification. A patient safety error/event classification is a method for standardizing language, definitions, and conceptual frameworks for optimal discussion, improvement, and dissemination of knowledge on patient safety (IOM, 2004; Woods et al., 2005). A classification system can be used within a reporting system or used to analyze events. Through the classification of events, trends can be assessed. The use of an effective system of classification is an important part of risk assessment and helps to group "like" (similar) risks and safety events as well as to distinguish characteristics in similar but "unlike" events for more effective and nuanced intervention development.

Event classification is a standardized method by which the event, contributors and causes of the event, including the root causes, are grouped into categories (Woods et al., 2005). Accident classification was initially used in nuclear power and aviation and has expanded into use in health care (Barach & Small, 2000). Additionally, by analyzing many events and applying the same standardized classification scheme, patterns can be detected in how these events develop and occur (Woods et al., 2008). An understanding of the different error types is critical for the development of effective error prevention and mitigation tools and strategies (Vincent, 2006). A variety of these tools and strategies must be implemented to target the full range of error types if they are to be effective. There are several different systems of classifications of error that describe differing characteristics of an error. Many of these systems of classification are built on the prevailing theoretical framework of Reason's Swiss Cheese Model of accident occurrence (Reason, 2000).

▶ Skill-, Rule-, and Knowledge-Based Classification

James Reason posited a classification of human error (Reason, 1990). Errors result from a variety of influences however, believed the underlying mental processes that lead to error are consistent, allowing for the development of a human error typology. The terms *skill-, rule-,* and *knowledge-based information processing* refer to the degree of conscious control exercised by the individual over his or her activities. Failures of action, or unintentional actions, were classified as skill-based errors. This error type is categorized into slips of action and lapses of memory. Failures in planning are referred to as mistakes, which are categorized as rule-based mistakes and knowledge-based mistakes (Reason, 1990):

- Skill-based errors—slips and lapses—when the action made is not what was intended.
  Examples of skill-based errors in daily life and health care include:
  - Daily life—a skilled driver stepping on the accelerator instead of the brake.
  - Health care—an experienced nurse administering the wrong medication by picking up the wrong syringe.
- Rule-based mistakes—actions that match intentions but do not achieve their intended outcome due to incorrect application of a rule or inadequacy of the plan. Examples of rule-based mistakes in daily life and in health care include:
  - Daily life—using woodworker's glue to mend a broken plastic eyeglasses frame.
  - Health care—proceeding with extubation before the patient is able to breathe independently, because of incorrect application of guidelines.

■ Knowledge-based mistakes—actions which are intended but do not achieve the intended outcome due to knowledge deficits. Examples of knowledge-based mistakes in daily life and in health care include:

• Daily life—a failed cake because a novice baker mistakenly thought baking soda could be used in place of baking powder.
• Health care—prescribing the wrong medication because of incorrect knowledge of the drug of choice.

Slips, Lapses, Mistakes, and Violations

Reason's human error typology was further elaborated to describe slips as attentional failures and lapses as memory failures as depicted in **FIGURE 10.1** (Reason, 1990). Violations were added as intended actions with further break-down into common, routine accepted violations (e.g., work-arounds, short cuts, potentially risky actions, movement into the margin of error) and exceptional violations

that are not accepted (i.e., alcohol or drug use while providing patient care).

Planning and Execution

Error types can be further classified into whether the error involved taking an action or inaction. If a needed action is omitted, it is considered an error of omission. For active errors, there is a further breakdown into whether the error was the use of a wrong plan—an error of planning; or whether the plan was good, but the error was in the execution of the plan—an error of execution. An example of an error of planning would be a decision to order a medication that was wrong for a patient's condition (e.g., an antiviral medication ordered for a person with a bacterial infection). An example of an error of execution would be administering a medication to one patient that was intended for a different patient.

Furthermore, these elements of error classification can interact with the classification of slips, lapse, mistakes, and violations described above and as seen in Figure 10.1.

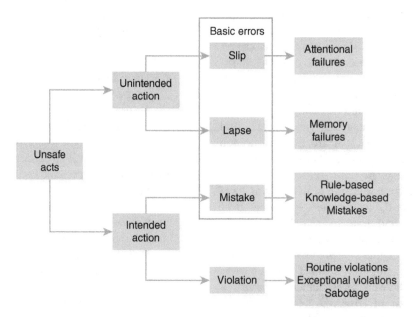

FIGURE 10.1 Generic Error Modeling System (GEMS)

Reproduced from Reason, J. *Human Error*. Cambridge University Press, Cambridge, UK. 1990.

Runciman and colleagues conducted a review of adverse events in a random selection of admissions in Australia and developed a classification system called the Quality in Australia Health Care Study (QAHCS) (Wilson et al., 1995; Runciman et al., 2009). Risk classification has been an important tool for risk reduction and safety improvement in high risk high reliability industries such as nuclear power, aviation, chemical manufacturing and others. Valid and reliable classifications of risk and details of hazards and risks is a very important tool for exploring risk.

Reason hypothesized that most accidents can be traced to one or more of four failure domains: organizational influences, supervision, preconditions, and specific acts. For example, in aviation, preconditions for unsafe acts include fatigued air crew or improper communications practices. Unsafe supervision encompasses for example, pairing inexperienced pilots on a night flight into known adverse weather. Organizational influences encompass such things as organizational budget cuts in times of financial austerity.

The Swiss Cheese Model

James Reason (1990) proposed the Swiss Cheese Model as a theory of accident occurrence, which has become the dominant paradigm of accident occurrence in health care. Reason's "Swiss Cheese" model describes four levels within which active failures and latent failures may occur during complex operations.

In the Swiss Cheese Model, an organization's defenses against failure are modeled as a series of barriers, represented by slices of cheese. The holes in the cheese slices represent weaknesses in individual parts of the system and are continually varying in size and position across the slices. The system produces failures when a hole in each slice momentarily aligns, permitting (in Reason's words) "a trajectory of accident opportunity," so that a hazard passes through holes in all of the slices, leading to a failure (Reason, 1990). The Swiss Cheese model, as Reason conceived of it, includes both active and latent failures. Active failures encompass the unsafe acts that can be directly linked to an accident, such as human error. This is not about blame for the action, it is intended to depict the actions taken most proximal to the event whether a violation or an error. Latent failures include contributory factors that may lie dormant for days, weeks, or months until they contribute to the accident. Latent failures span the first three domains of failure in Reason's (1990) model (FIGURE 10.2).

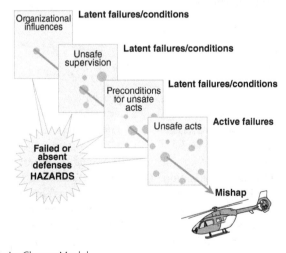

FIGURE 10.2 Reason's Swiss Cheese Model

Human Factors Analysis and Classification System (HFACS)

In the early 2000s, Wiegmann and Shappell were tasked by the U.S. Navy with developing a classification of risks to reduce the high rate of error. They developed the Human Factors Analysis and Classification System (HFACS). HFACS was designed as a broad human error framework heavily based on Reason's Swiss Cheese Model and was used initially by the U.S. Navy to identify active and latent failures that combine to result in an accident with the goal of understanding the causal factors that led to the accident (Weigmann & Shappell, 2000, 2003).

The HFACS framework describes human error at each of four levels of failure (FIGURE 10.3):

1. Unsafe acts of operators (e.g., aircrew)
2. Preconditions for unsafe acts
3. Unsafe supervision
4. Organizational influences

Within each HFACS level, causal categories were developed that identify the active and latent failures that occur. In theory, at least one failure will occur at each level leading to an adverse event. If one of the failures is corrected at any time leading up to the adverse event, it is thought that the adverse event would be prevented.

As can be seen in Figure 10.3, the HFACS classification further defines an incident in relation to Reason's categories of Errors and Violations, with *skill-based errors, decision errors*, and *perceptual errors* under the Errors classification and *routine violations* and *exceptional violations* under the Violations classification. Likewise, further defining each of the four primary classifications. Using the HFACS framework for accident investigation, organizations are able to identify the breakdowns within the entire system that allowed an accident to occur and provide insight for the development of potential interventions for improvement.

While the HFACS classification system was developed by the U.S. Navy, the HFACS framework has been used to assess root causes within the military, commercial, and general aviation sectors to systematically examine underlying human causal factors and to improve aviation accident investigations as well as in many other high-risk industries such as rail, construction, and mining and has demonstrated acceptable to high reliability. Studies have shown that the results from the HFACS classification system are reliable in capturing the nature of, and relationships among, latent conditions and active failures. The kappa statistic is reported in these studies to assess agreement (kappa is a standard statistical measure of inter-rater agreement that ranges from 0.00–1.00). In one study, a post-hoc analysis was conducted on a sample National Transportation Safety Board (NTSB) serious incident reports and achieved an inter-rater reliability kappa of 0.85. In another study in the biopharmaceutical industry, three pairs of coders used the HFACS classification system to code a sample of 161 reports of "upstream" incidents, "downstream" incidents, and incidents in "operational services." In this study, they achieved an overall agreement of 96.66 with a 0.66 kappa, suggesting that this classification system has reasonable reliability for use (Cintron, 2015).

The Joint Commission Patient Safety Event Taxonomy

Improvement in patient safety involves risk assessment to understand the attributes of a safety incident. The Joint Commission (TJC) encouraged hospitals to conduct risk assessments on events that occurred in hospitals, particularly serious adverse events or "sentinel events" to reduce harm. To support and facilitate the conduct of hospital safety risk assessments, in 2005 TJC developed the Patient Safety Event Taxonomy to put forward a standardized terminology and classification

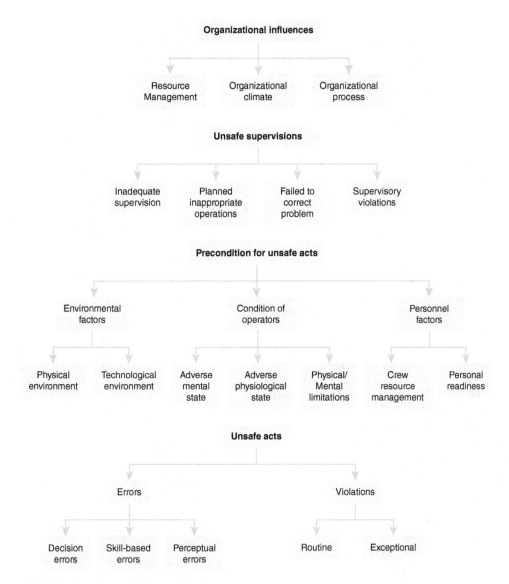

FIGURE 10.3 Depiction of HFACS Classification System

Reproduced from Patterson J, Shappell SA. Operator error and system deficiencies: Analysis of 508 mining incidents and accidents from Queensland, Australia using HFACS. *Accident Analysis and Prevention.* 42 (2010) 1379–1385.

schema for near miss and adverse events to develop a common language and definitions (Chang et al., 2005). This taxonomy was developed through application of the results from a systematic literature review, evaluation of existing patient safety terminologies and classifications, assessment of the taxonomy's face and content validity, patient safety expert review and comment, and assessment of the taxonomy's comparative reliability. Five root nodes were proposed based on the review of other classification schemes. The root nodes include: impact, type, domain, cause, and prevention and mitigation (Chang et al., 2005).

The taxonomy was applied qualitatively to reports submitted to TJC's Sentinel

Event Program. According to the developers, the taxonomy incorporated works by Reason (1990), Rasmussen (1986), Runciman (1998, 2002), and Hale (1997) as well as contributions from aviation and other high-risk/high-reliability industries. Root nodes were divided into 21 subclassifications, which were then subdivided into more than 200 coded categories and an indefinite number of noncoded text fields to capture narrative information about specific incidents.

World Health Organization International Classification for Patient Safety (ICPS)

The Patient Safety Event Taxonomy was disseminated internationally through TJC International and then in response to the growth in the recognition of the magnitude of excess morbidity and mortality from patient safety, the World Health Organization (WHO) launched the World Alliance for Patient Safety to "'pay the closest possible attention to the problem of patient safety and to establish and strengthen science-based systems necessary for improving patients' safety and quality of care" (WHO, 2002). Concurrent with the development of TJC (then JACHO) Patient Safety Event Taxonomy, since 2005, WHO was tasked with developing global norms and standards to support and inform the development of effective patient policies and practices. Runciman et al. (2009) drafted the International Classification for Patient Safety (ICPS), drawing on many sources and terms including TJC Patient Safety Taxonomy. The accumulated terms were analyzed and assessed through responses to a Delphi process, with the focus on patient safety classification (Thomson, 2009). The conceptual framework for the ICPS, consisting of 10 high level classes (FIGURE 10.4) (WHO, 2009):

1. Incident type
2. Patient outcomes
3. Patient characteristics
4. Incident characteristics
5. Contributing factors/hazards
6. Organizational outcomes
7. Detection
8. Mitigating factors
9. Ameliorating actions
10. Actions taken to reduce risk

According to the conceptual framework for the ICPS, "A *patient safety incident* in this context is an event or circumstance that could have resulted, or did result, in unnecessary harm to a patient. A patient safety incident can be a *near miss*, a *no harm incident* or a *harmful incident* (adverse event). The class, *incident type*, is a descriptive term for a category made up of incidents of a common nature grouped because of shared, agreed features, such as "clinical process/procedure" or "medication/ IV fluid" incident. Although each concept is clearly defined and distinct from other concepts, a patient safety incident can be classified as more than one incident type. A *patient outcome* is the impact upon a patient, which is wholly or partially attributable to an incident. Patient outcomes can be classified according to the type of harm, the degree of harm and any social and/or economic impact. Together, the classes *incident type* and *patient outcomes* are intended to group patient safety incidents into clinically meaningful categories" (The World Alliance for Patient Safety Drafting Group, 2009).

In an NIH-funded research study, the author of this chapter tried to classify the Incident Types and the Contributing Factors through application of the WHO ICPS for clinician described incidents that occurred during the course of surgical care, which included operating room set-up, the surgery itself, and anesthesia management. We developed a web-based confidential Debriefing Tool, which would proactively collect issues, challenges, problems, incidents, near misses, and preventable adverse events from everyone involved in specific surgeries. The web-based

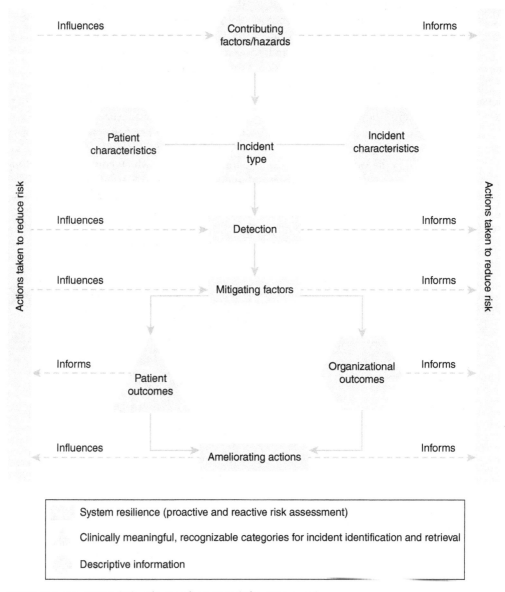

FIGURE 10.4 International Classification for Patient Safety Framework

Reproduced from The World Alliance For Patient Safety Drafting Group, Sherman H, Castro G, Martin Fletcher M on behalf of The World Alliance for Patient Safety, Hatlie M, Hibbert P, Jakob R, Koss R, Lewalle P, Loeb J, Perneger T, Runciman W, Thomson R, Van Der Schaaf T, Virtanen1 M. Towards an International Classification for Patient Safety: the conceptual framework. *Int J Qual Health Care*. 2009 Feb; 21(1): 2–8

tool is emailed to all of those involved in the procedure immediately following the procedure with 2 reminders within 3 days if needed. Both open-ended questions and specific prompts are used. We sought to develop a method which would overcome many of the barriers to incident reporting in a surgical context, including developing a method that would be perceived as safe for all involved, to report anything that occurred, large or small, without fear of personal reprisal or reprisals for others on the team. The web-based Debriefing Tool was deployed across four large transplant centers. See examples of reported incidents and the application, function, and results of the use of the WHO ICPS system of classification to classify emblematic incidents reported from the surgical care teams below.

Unlike the HFACS which can model the complexity of multiple causal inputs to an accident, as represented by the Swiss Cheese Model of accident causation, the WHO ICPS is represented as a linear hierarchical system of classification that requires reviewers to select one sole Incident Type and one sole Contributing Factor. Within the Incident Type classification, there are 13 primary Incident Type classifications. However, the requirement to select only one classification created forced choices. For example, for an incident in which the consent was not available, the primary Incident Type classification could be either or both Clinical Administration and/or Documentation, where both could actually be true error types related to this incident. Furthermore, each Primary Incident Type has different downstream classification options which could stunt resulting understanding of the event. Selecting one or the other will lead the classification down very different paths where the secondary classification would be very different. See TABLE 10.2 for a representation of this challenge.

TABLE 10.2 Depiction of WHO Classification Challenges

Reported Incident	Primary Incident Type	Secondary Incident Type	Tertiary Incident Type
Consent was not available at the time of the surgery in the OR suite	Clinical Administration	Consent	Not Performed when indicated and/or incomplete/ inadequate
	Documentation	Document Involved—Forms Certificates	Document Missing or Delay in accessing document
Could not get x-ray into the OR, disrupted surgical case, attending unscrubbed to get an x-ray tech	Medical Device/ Equipment	X-ray machine	Lack of availability (there is no code for could not fit into room)
	Clinical Process/ Procedure	Diagnosis/ Assessment	Unavailable (there is no code for accessing was disruptive)
	Resources/ Organizational Management	Bed/service availability adequacy	

Unfamiliar scrub for case, not all equipment immediately available	Resources/ Organizational management	Matching of Workload Management	
		Service adequacy	
		Organization of Teams/people	
	Clinical Process/ Procedure	Procedure	Incomplete/ Inadequate
The anesthesia team seemed so overwhelmed that they did not pay attention with the time out and needed to be repeatedly reminded to pay attention.	Behavior	Staff	Noncompliant/ Uncooperative/ Obstructive
	Resources/ Organizational Management	Matching workload management	
		Human Resources/ Staff adequacy	
		Protocols/ Policy Procedure Guidelines	
	Clinical Process/ Procedure	Procedure/ Treatment/ Intervention	Incomplete/ Inadequate

For example, for Documentation, the secondary classification choices would be, Document Involved—Forms/Certificates, and the Problem classification could be Document Missing or Delay in Accessing Document as compared with Clinical Administration where the secondary classification of the Process would be Consent and the Problem could be either Not Performed When Indicated and/or Incomplete/Inadequate. When a classification system allows only exclusive classification where the classification of the same event could be accurately classified as involving multiple codes, information in the classification results of the incident will be lost and as well the results will likely lack strong reliability and accuracy which can confuse the development of interventions to improve care and can lead to loss of important information. Likewise, the primary incident type for ABO Incompatibility can be classified as Documentation, Clinical Administration, or Blood Products; Incorrect counts or a lost needle can be classified as a Clinical Process/Procedure or as Medical/Device, Equipment/Property. In our study, we developed a more specific set of definitions that created a forced choice selection of one of the classification pathways for similar events, but this was somewhat arbitrary, lacked precision and lost potentially important information about the incident. The linear nature of the classification patterns limited the classification of incidents, as it did not accurately reflect the reality of the emergence of the incidents (McElroy, 2016; Khorzad, 2015; Ross, 2011)

Similarly, in the classification of contributing factors and hazards, an incident reviewer must choose between the included factors, even though frequently many of the listed factors can contribute to the occurrence of an incident (McElroy, 2016; Khorzad, 2015; Ross, 2011). The listed primary classifications for contributing factors in the ICPS are:

1. Staff Factors
2. Patient Factors
3. Work Environment Factors
4. Organizational Service Factors
5. External Factors
6. Other

Assigning a single contributing factor in many cases oversimplifies the classification of an incident and is not an accurate representation of the complexity of the interacting components of these types of events. In many safety incidents, patient factors are interacting with staff factors in the context of work environment factors, and organizational factors. There can be plural factors related to each component. The requirement in the ICPS to select one Contributing Factor also sets up a false choice for the individual conducting the classification, reliability is compromising reliability, and introducing subjective bias to the process of classification.

Systems Engineering Initiative for Patient Safety (SEIPS)

Vincent, a leading thought leader in the field of human error and safety, described seven elements that influence safety (Vincent, Taylor-Adams, & Stanhope, 1998; Vincent, 2006):

1. Organization and management factors
2. Work environment factors
3. Team factors
4. Task factors
5. Individual factors
6. Patient characteristics
7. External environment factors

Building upon Vincent's model of human error and safety related elements, Carayon and colleagues proposed a Systems Engineering Initiative for Patient Safety (SEIPS) model for human error and design in health care (Carayon et al., 2006, 2014; Carayon & Wood, 2010). In the SEIPS classification model, components of the system are helpfully depicted with intersecting arrows that illustrate how these components in the system can interact with one another, representing the emergent properties of simultaneously interacting risks depicted through the Swiss Cheese Model. In the SEIPS 2.0 Framework, shown in **FIGURE 10.5**, accidents arise from the interaction among humans, machines, and the environment in the sociotechnical system. Similar to Vincent's seven elements that influence safety, in the SEIPS Model 2.0 (Holden, 2013) the five interacting elements within the work system include:

- People—patient and clinical professionals
- Tasks
- Technology and tools
- The organization
- External environment

This framework is able to represent the dynamic work system and work system risks to effectively model the complexity of medical work. This framework and depiction facilitates the ability to understand the characteristics and specific patterns of the simultaneous interactions of activities and systems leading to risk and an incident. This depiction enables the representation of both safety and risk as dynamic, not static, and represents an incident as having not just one input but

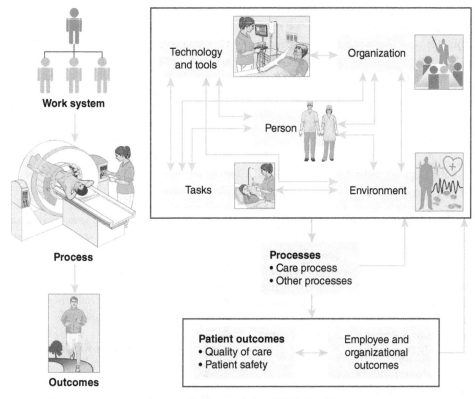

FIGURE 10.5 Systems Engineering Initiative for Patient Safety (SEIPS) Model 2.0

Reproduced from Carayon P, Hundt AS, Karsh B, et al. Work system design for patient safety: The SEIPS model. *Qual Safe Health Care*. 2006;15(Suppl I):i50–i58.

multiple inputs to creates a pattern, a perfect storm, that is frequently hard to foresee prospectively. This form of classification is then represented as patterns of interactions of the components in the system and can then provide a fuller, more complete characterization of the incident. Johnson, Haskell, and Barach (2016) portray actual patient safety cases to provide an exercise using this framework for readers to conduct an analysis of the Lewis Blackwell case.

Carayon and colleagues (2006, 2014) apply this kind of incident classification and analyses and portrayed this in what they call the configural work systems concepts and configural diagrams, which provide a more nuanced and more accurate representation of the incident. This method for incident analysis and classification enables modeling of both proximal factors (sharp end) as well as latent factors (blunt end) and can provide insights regarding how they interact as well as the specific impact.

By using the configural work system diagram for incident analysis, it is possible to investigate the types of incidents that occurred when a particular work system factor (e.g., excessive workload) or combination of factors (e.g., workload and worker fatigue) were an active part of the configuration. The diagram can also be used to analyze and compare how two or more units or organizations have configured their work system, by design or otherwise, for the same process or processes. Ideal types of configurations could be identified for improved safety and resilience and safety planning. For example, as Holden (2013) notes, "If we introduce technology A versus technology B, which new interactions will become relevant between each of those technologies and the work system's people, task, other tool and technology, organization, internal environment and external environment factors?"

Using Error Classification for Mitigation and Safety Improvement

High Reliability Organizations

A high reliability organization (HRO) is an organization that has succeeded in avoiding catastrophes in an environment where normal accidents can be expected due to *risk* factors and complexity. In studying these organizations, Weick and Sutcliffe (2015) found several common features across these industries that they called HRO principles:

- Preoccupation with Failure
- Reluctance to simplify
- Sensitivity to operations
- Commitment to resilience
- Deference to expertise

These principles are very important to safety risk reduction and mitigation and apply well to the task of error classification. HROs do not ignore failures no matter how small as well as how things could fail. Error reporting systems are designed to collect this type of information (adverse events, preventable adverse events, near-misses, etc.) for classification and analysis. In the analysis of these events, it is important not to overly simplify what has occurred and to represent the complexity of interactions within the system that lead to an event not only from the perspective of the clinician but also the perspective of the patients and their families (Travaglia & Robertson, 2013). In the recommendation to be sensitive to operations is the encouragement to understand real processes and their inputs as they actually occur as opposed to

relying on an idealized process or operation that may not include various work-arounds. This is also important for error classification and risk mitigation. Through a commitment to resilience there is also attention to the potential of unintended consequences even while applying interventions to improve care based on an analysis of events. Deference to expertise rather than authority in the context of classification means that the person with the most information about an incident or a process to provide relevant contextual knowledge.

In order to effectively improve the safety of processes in health care and reduce harm, it is necessary to accurately represent the complexity of the incident, various contributors and contextual circumstances. HRO Principles are very helpful for this. Establishing a culture of safety with these principles will increase the number of events reported and the use of these events to inform safety improvement (Sollecito & Johnson, 2013).

The SEIPS framework is effective at representing the appropriate complexity, contributors, and inputs in the occurrence of an incident or event such that an intervention can address the actual problems. There have been numerous studies in which the SEIPS framework was used to improve health care design and safety, for example, a study of the timeliness of follow-up of abnormal test results in outpatient settings (Singh et al., 2009); a study on the safety of the Electronic Health Record (EHR) technology (Sittig & Singh, 2009); a study improving electronic communication and alerts (Hysong et al., 2009); characterizing patient safety hazards in cardia surgery (Gurses et al., 2012); and a study to improve patient safety for radiotherapy (Rivera & Karsh, 2008). The SEIPS framework has been used effectively to examine patient safety in multiple care settings (Intensive Care Units, pediatrics, primary care, outpatient surgery, cardiac surgery, and transitions of care). Many studies that applied the SEIPS framework not only to demonstrate its effectiveness for understanding error and incident causation but also for how to apply this learning to safety improvement and safety planning.

▶ Conclusions

Safety events are very frequent in health care. In this chapter, several systems of classification in use have been described. Some are descriptive and others a based on the psychology of error, and the strengths and weakness of each have been presented. When the nature of the system of classification can represent the varying patterns of incident occurrence, it can be used as an important and effective tool for risk reduction and safety improvement. These are frameworks of event classification that can be used in Incident Reporting Systems and to provide a framework for analysis of incidents capture trends and inform quality and safety improvement. The value of event classification has been demonstrated by numerous other high risk, high reliability industries as well as in health care, that systems of error

and risk classification are important to understanding patient safety risks in health care to improve safety (Weigmann & Shappell, 2003; Carayon et al., 2014; Busse & Johnson, 1999). We further understand that High Reliability Organizations apply the practice of "Reluctance to Simplify Operations" (Weick & Sutcliffe, 2007). However, if the system for classification does not accurately describe the nature and patterns of medical work and the resulting specific risks or over simplifies the understanding of the interactions of elements of medical work or risks in the work system, important information will be lost and attempts at using the resulting information for safety improvement will be flawed. In this review of systems of error and incident classification, the HFACS and the SEIPS frameworks, both of which rely heavily on the theoretical underpinnings of Reason's work, have effectively enabled classification systems that model the complexity of health care and error occurrence and have demonstrated their use for effective risk identification and safety improvement in health care.

References

Agency for Healthcare Research and Quality (AHRQ). (2017a). Patient safety primer: Adverse events, near misses, and errors. Retrieved from https://psnet.ahrq.gov

Agency for Healthcare Research and Quality (AHRQ). (2017b). Patient safety primer: Never events. Retrieved from https://psnet.ahrq.gov

Barach, P., & Small, S. (2000). Reporting and preventing medical mishaps: lessons from non-medical near miss reporting systems. *British Medical Journal, 320*(7237), 759–763.

Busse, D., & Johnson, C. (1999). Identification and analysis of incidents in complex, medical environments. *Proceedings of the First Workshop on Human Error and Clinical Systems,* pp. 101–120. Glasgow Accident Analysis Group.

Carayon, P., Hundt, A. S., Karsh B.-T., Gurses, A., Alvarado, C. J., Smith, M., & Brennan, P. F. (2006). Work system design for patient safety: The SEIPS model. *Quality & Safety in Health Care, 15*(Suppl 1), i50–i58.

Carayon, P., Wetterneck, T., Rivera-Rodriguez, A. J., Hundt, A. S., Hoonakke, P., Holden, R., & Gurses, A. (2014). Human factors systems approach to healthcare

quality and patient safety. *Applied Ergonomics, 45*(1), 14–25.

Carayon, P., & Wood, K. (2010). Patient safety: the role of human factors and systems engineering. *Studies in Health Technology & Informatics, 153,* 23–46.

Chang, A., Schyve, P. M., Croteau, R. J., O'Leary, D. S., & Loeb, J. M. (2005). The JAHCO patient safety event taxonomy: A standard terminology and classification schema for near misses and adverse events. *International Journal for Quality in Health Care, 17*(2), 95–105.

Cintron, R. (2015). Human factors analysis and classification system interrater reliability for biopharmaceutical manufacturing investigations. (Doctoral dissertation, Walden University). Retrieved from https://scholarworks.waldenu.edu/dissertations/194/

Ferrante, P. (2011, September 6). Incident vs. accident: What's the difference? Retrieved from safety.blr.com

Gurses, A. P., Kim, G., Martinez, E. A., Marsteller, J., Bauer, L., Lubomski, L. H., Pronovost, P. J., & Thompson D. (2012). Identifying and categorising patient safety hazards in cardiovascular operating rooms using an interdisciplinary approach: A multisite study. *BMJ Quality & Safety, 21,* 810–818.

Haimes, Y. Y. (2004). *Risk modeling, assessment, and management*. Hoboken, NJ: John Wiley & Sons, Inc.

Hale, A., Wilpert, B., & Freitag, M. (1997). *After the event: From accidents to organizational learning*. Kidlington, Oxford, UK: Elsevier Science.

Holden, R., Carayon, P., Gurses, A., Hoonakker, P., Hundt, A., Ozok, A., & Rivera-Rodriguez, A. J. (2013). SEIPS 2.0: A human factors framework for studying and improving the work of healthcare professionals and patients. *Ergonomics 56*(11), https://doi.org/ 10.1080/00140139.2013.838643

Hysong, S., Sawhney, M., Wilson, L., Sittig, D., Esquivel, A., Watford, M., ... Singh, H. (2009). Improving outpatient safety through effective electronic communication: a study protocol. *Implementation Science, 4*, 62.

Institute of Medicine (IOM). (2000). *To err is human: Building a safer health system*. Washington, D.C.: National Academy Press.

Institute of Medicine (IOM) Committee on Data Standards for Patient Safety. (2004). *Patient safety: Achieving a new standard for care*. Washington, D.C.: National Academies Press.

Johnson, J. K., Haskell, H., & Barach, P. (2016). *Case studies in patient safety: Foundations for core competencies*. Burlington, MA: Jones & Bartlett Learning.

Khorzad, R., Woods, D. M., Pomfret, E., Simpson, M. A., Guarrera, J., Fisher, R., ... Ladner, D. (2015). Patient safety in living donor liver transplantation: Equipment & supply incidents. ASTS.

Levinson, D. R. (2010). Adverse events in hospitalized Medicare patients. *Report no. OEI-06-09-00090*. Washington, D.C.: US Department of Health and Human Services, Office of the Inspector General.

McElroy, L., Woods, D. M., Yanes, A., Skaro, A., Daud, A., Curtis, T., Wymore E., ... Ladner D. (2016). Applying the WHO conceptual framework for the International Classification for Patient Safety to a surgical population. *International Journal for Quality in Health Care, 28*(2), 166–174.

Patterson, J., & Shappell, S. A. (2010). Operator error and system deficiencies: Analysis of 508 mining incidents and accidents from Queensland, Australia using HFACS. *Accident Analysis and Prevention, 42*, 1379–1385.

Quality Interagency Coordination Task Force (QuIC). (2000). Understanding medical errors. In *Doing what counts for patient safety: Federal actions to reduce medical errors and their impact*. Report of the Quality Interagency Coordination Task Force (QuIC) to the President, February 2000. Retrieved from archive.ahrq.gov

Rasmussen, J. (1986). *Information processing and human-machine interaction*. Amsterdam: North-Holland.

Reason, J. (1990). *Human error*. Cambridge, UK: Cambridge University Press.

Reason, J. (2000). Human error: models and management. *British Medical Journal, 320*(7237): 768–770.

Rivera, A. J., & Karsh, B. T. (2008). Human factors and systems engineering approach to patient safety for radiotherapy. *International Journal of Radiation Oncology, Biology, & Physics, 71*, S174–S177.

Ross, O., Skaro, A., Lyuksemburg, V., Lakhoo, K., Woods D., Torricelli, A., ... Ladner, D. (2011). Safety issues identified by proactive liver transplant safety debriefing. American Transplant Congress 2011 Abstract #221. *American Journal of Transplantation, 11*(4), 97.

Runciman, W. B., Edmonds, M. J., Pradhan, M. (2002). Setting priorities for patient safety. *Quality & Safety in Health Care, 11*, 224–229.

Runciman, W. B., Helps, S. C., Sexton, E. J., Malpass, A. (1998). A classification for incidents and accidents in the health-care system. *Journal of Quality in Clinical Practice, 19*, 199–211.

Runciman, W., Hibbert, P., Thomson, R., Van Der Schaaf, T., Sherman, H., & Lewalle, P. (2009). Towards an International Classification for Patient Safety: Key concepts and terms. *International Journal for Quality in Health Care, 21*(1), 18–26.

Singh, H., Thomas, E. J., Mani, S., Sittig, D. F., Arora, H., Espadas, H., & Petersen, L. A. (2009). Timely follow-up of abnormal diagnostic imaging test results in an outpatient setting: Are electronic medical records achieving their potential. *Archives of Internal Medicine, 169*(17), 1578–1586.

Sittig, D. F., & Singh, H. (2009). Eight rights of safe electronic health record use. *Journal of the American Medical Association, 302*(10), 1111–1113.

Shappell, S. A., Wiegmann, D. A. (2000). The Human Factors Analysis and Classification System—HFACS. DOT /FAA/AM-00/7. U.S. Department of Transportation Federal Aviation Administration.

The Joint Commission (TJC). (2017, June 29). Sentinel event policy. Retrieved from https://www .jointcommission.org

The World Alliance for Patient Safety Drafting Group, Sherman H., Castro, G., Martin F., World Alliance for Patient Safety, Hatlie, M., ... Virtanen, M. (2009). Towards an international classification for patient safety: the conceptual framework. *International Journal for Quality in Health Care, 21*(1), 2–8.

Thomas, E. J., Studdert, D. M., Burstin H. R., Orav E. J., Zeena, T., Williams, E. J., Howard, K. M., ... Brennan, T. A. (2000). Incidence and types of adverse events and negligent care in Utah and Colorado. *Medical Care, 38*(3), 261–271.

Thomson, R., Lewalle, P., Sherman H., Hibbert, P., Runciman, W., & Castro, G. (2009). Towards an international classification for patient safety: A Delphi survey. International Journal for Quality in Health Care, 21(1), 9–17.

Travaglia, J., & Robertson, H. (2013). The role of the patient in continuous quality improvement. In W. Sollecito & J. K. Johnson (Eds.), *Continuous quality improvement in healthcare* (4th ed.). Burlington, MA: Jones & Bartlett Learning.

Vincent, C. (2006). *Patient safety.* London: Elsevier.

Vincent, C., Taylor-Adams, S., & Stanhope N. (1998). Framework for analysing risk and safety in clinical medicine. *British Medical Journal, 316,* 1154–1157.

Wachter, R. (2012). *Understanding patient safety.* New York, NY: McGraw-Hill, Inc.

Weick, K., & Sutcliffe, K. (2007). *Managing the unexpected: resilient performance in an age of uncertainty.* San Francisco, CA: Jossey-Bass.

Weick, K., & Sutcliffe, K. (2016). *Managing the unexpected: Sustained performance in a complex world* (3rd ed.). Hoboken, NJ: Wiley and Sons.

Wiegmann, D., & Shappell, S. (2003). *A human error approach to aviation accident analysis: The human factors analysis and classification system.* Burlington, VT: Ashgate Publishing, Ltd.

Wilson, R. M., Runciman, W. B., Gibberd, R. W., Harrison, B. T., & Hamilton, J. D. (1995). The quality in Australian health care study. *Medical Journal of Australia, 163*(9), 458–471.

Woods, D. M., Holl, J., Young, J., Reynolds, S., Schwalenstocker, E., Wears, R., Barnathan, J., & Amsden, L. (2008). Leveraging Existing Assessments of Risk Now (LEARN) safety analysis: A method for extending patient safety learning. In K. Henriksen, J. B. Battles, M. A. Keyes, & M. L. Grady (Eds.), *Advances in patient safety: New directions and alternative approaches (vol. 1: Assessment).* AHRQ Publication No.: 08-0034-1. Rockville, MD: Agency for Healthcare Research and Quality.

Woods, D. M., Johnson, J., Holl, J. L., Mehra, M., Thomas, E. J., Ogata, E. S., & Lannon, C. (2005). Anatomy of a patient safety event: A pediatric patient safety taxonomy. *Quality & Safety in Health Care, 14*(6), 422–427.

World Health Organization (WHO). (2002). *Fifty-fifth world health assembly.* Geneva, Switzerland: Author. Retrieved from http://apps.who.int/iris/bitstream/handle/10665/259364/WHA55-2002-REC1-eng.pdf.

World Health Organization (WHO). (2009). *Conceptual framework for the international classification for patient safety version 1.1: Final Technical Report.* Retrieved from http://www.who.int/patientsafety/taxonomy/icps_full_report.pdf

CHAPTER 11

Continuous Quality Improvement in U.S. Public Health Organizations: Widespread Adoption and Institutionalization

Sara E. Massie, Charlotte E. Randolph, and Greg D. Randolph

Without change, there is no innovation, creativity, or incentive for improvement. Those who initiate change will have a better opportunity to manage the change that is inevitable.

—William Pollard

International health statistics demonstrate that the United States trails other developed nations in many public health indicators. A recent survey of 11 high-income nations found that the United States is an outlier among surveyed countries in regard to ensuring access to health care, revealing that roughly one-third (33%) of American adults went without recommended care, declined to see a doctor when they were sick, or did not fill a prescription due to cost (Osborn et al., 2016). Regarding both infant and maternal mortality, the United States has continuously ranked poorly in past decades when compared to other developed nations (United Health Foundation, 2016). This trend has endured in recent years, with the United States ranking 26th in infant deaths among 29 Organisation for Economic Co-operation and Development (OECD) nations, with 6.1 deaths per 1,000 live births (compared to 2.3 deaths per 1,000 live births in the top-ranked nation, Finland) (MacDorman et al., 2014). Furthermore, although the United States is by far the highest among 39 OECD nations in health expenditures, the country ranks near the bottom in life expectancy at birth—landing at 26th for men and 29th for women (Organisation for Economic Co-Operation and Development, 2014). With rankings such as these, it is evident that we need to improve public health services and outcomes in the United States.

Over the past three decades, U.S. public health organizations have increasingly undertaken a variety of efforts to ensure and improve the quality of their services. In recent years, accreditation has become part of a national focus to advance the quality and performance of public health. At the same time, public health agencies have been implementing quality improvement using proven methods, such as the Model for Improvement, Lean, and Plan, Do, Study, Act (PDSA) cycles described throughout this text and elsewhere (Deming, 2000; Langley et al., 2009; Smith et al., 2012). Efforts such as these indicate that public health is moving beyond a series of projects and tools toward adopting continuous quality improvement (CQI) as a means of achieving a public health system that is effective, efficient, and in step with other industrialized nations around the world.

Objectives

In this chapter, we provide an overview of the adoption and institutionalization of CQI in U.S. public health organizations. We begin by providing a brief history of CQI in public health. We then describe current efforts to promote CQI and explore the opportunities, challenges and progress of public health organizations in the adoption and institutionalization of CQI, including the important role of accreditation. Finally, we conclude with a practical example/case study of how a public health agency has applied quality improvement methods and tools and their steps toward institutionalizing CQI.

▶ Clarifying Key Terms

In public health, *quality* has been defined as "the degree to which policies, programs, services, and research for the population increase the desired health outcomes and conditions in which the population can be healthy" (U.S. DHHS, 2008, p. 2). *Quality assurance* is the systematic monitoring and evaluation of the performance of an organization or its programs to ensure that standards (usually set by public health experts) of quality are being met. *Quality improvement* involves using formal methods and tools in designing and redesigning systems to meet customers' needs by testing and implementing ideas from evidence-based strategies, front-line staff, and customers. In public health, quality improvement has been described as a "distinct management process and set of tools and techniques that are coordinated to ensure that departments [local public health agencies] consistently meet their communities' health needs and strive to improve the health status of their populations" (Riley et al., 2010, p. 5).

Continuous quality improvement (CQI) in public health organizations is a structured organizational infrastructure and culture for involving staff in planning and executing a continuous flow of improvements to provide quality that meets or exceeds the expectations of communities. It focuses on systems change and generally includes these characteristics: a link to the organization's strategic plan, a quality council made up of the organization's top leadership, quality improvement training programs for staff, a mechanism for prioritizing quality improvement projects and launching quality improvement teams, and staff support and motivation for quality improvement activities. An organization that is committed to CQI may have both quality improvement and quality assurance processes, but the predominant focus is on quality improvement.

▶ History of Actions to Promote CQI in Public Health

In 1988, an Institute of Medicine (IOM) report, *The future of public health,* declared that the United States "has lost sight of its public health goals and has allowed the system of public health to fall into disarray" (p. 1). Following the 1988 IOM report, public health experts and analysts promoted a variety of methods and frameworks for changing the public health system and improving performance. By the mid-1990s, the IOM, the Centers for Disease Control and Prevention (CDC), the American Public Health Association, and the National Association of County and City Health Officials (NACCHO) adopted the 10 essential public health services framework that describes the key public health activities that all communities should address.

Using that framework, the National Public Health Performance Standards Program developed three assessment instruments to help state and local public health agencies identify gaps in achieving optimal performance and inform quality improvement efforts (CDC, 2015).

During this time of standards development, the Turning Point initiative, jointly funded by the Robert Wood Johnson Foundation (RWJF) and the W. K. Kellogg Foundation and directed by NACCHO, sought to transform U.S. public health systems into more community-based and collaborative organizations working to prevent disease and injury, protect the public from threats to their health, and promote healthy behaviors (Turning Point, 2006). Turning Point emphasized the use of performance standards in conjunction with measurement and reporting as well as the institution of quality improvement methods to manage change and achieve quality.

Over time, public health organizations became increasingly interested in standardizing and ensuring quality public health services,

which led to a focus on national public health accreditation (Stone & Davis, 2012).

In late 2004, the RWJF established the Exploring Accreditation Steering Committee to develop recommendations for implementing a voluntary national accreditation program, and, in 2005, launched the Multi-State Learning Collaborative (MLC) to explore the feasibility of voluntary national public health agency accreditation and collect data on existing accreditation practices (Beitsch et al., 2006; Russo, 2007). In the first phase of the MLC, five states with mature accreditation or assessment programs received 1-year grants to enhance their existing performance assessment and share information with the Steering Committee and one another. Following that phase, the Steering Committee recommended a national model for accreditation, which was subsequently endorsed by NACCHO and the Association of State and Territorial Health Organizations (ASTHO), among others.

In 2007, the second phase of the MLC began and 10 states received 1-year grants to focus on quality improvement in the context of accreditation and assessment. The states explored ways to improve their own accreditation and assessment programs, shared their tools and resources, conducted training in quality improvement, initiated quality improvement practices, and informed the planning for the national public health accreditation program (Gillen et al., 2010).

The third phase began in 2008, when 16 states received 3-year grants to prepare for national voluntary accreditation, support the Public Health Accreditation Board (PHAB) in the development of the national voluntary accreditation program, and bolster use of quality improvement methods in local and state health departments through mini-collaboratives in each state (Joly et al., 2010). The mini-collaboratives—teams of local and state health department representatives and other partners—implemented quality improvement projects targeting public health processes (e.g., developing a community health profile) and outcomes in specific topic areas (e.g., tobacco, immunizations) (Gillen et al., 2010; Joly et al., 2010).

Also in 2008, the U.S. Department of Health and Human Services (U.S. DHHS) released the *Consensus Statement on Quality in the Public Health System*, which, for the first time, framed a clear, uniform definition of quality for the public health system: "the degree to which policies, programs, services, and research for the population increase the desired health outcomes and conditions in which the population can be healthy" (p. 2). The *Consensus Statement* also identified nine quality aims for the public health system: *population-centered, equitable, proactive, health promoting, risk reducing, vigilant, transparent, effective,* and *efficient* (Honoré et al., 2011; U.S. DHHS, 2008).

Providing a national quality framework through the *Consensus Statement* was deemed necessary to facilitate consistent implementation of quality improvement in the daily routines of public health practitioners and their organizations. Another purpose of the *Consensus Statement* was to demonstrate a national commitment to quality improvement application throughout all parts of the public health system, including finance, programs, management, governance, and education (Honoré, 2009; Honoré et al., 2011). After the release of the *Consensus Statement*, U.S. DHHS charged the IOM with developing quality measures for the 12 leading health indicator priorities and 26 leading health indicators in Healthy People 2020 (IOM, 2013). The report provides suggestions for how government, communities, funders, hospitals, and other health care organizations could use the quality measures to guide decisions related to population health.

In 2010, the CDC Office for State, Tribal, Local and Territorial Support began what became a 4-year National Public Health Improvement Initiative (NPHII) to support health departments to address performance improvement, accelerating public health accreditation readiness activities, and sharing

practice-based evidence. The initiative supported 73 state, tribal, local, and territorial public health organizations via the Prevention and Public Health Fund of the Affordable Care Act. By the end of the second year of the program, "[a]pproximately 26% of awardees had completed an organizational PHAB self-assessment, 72% had established at least 1 of the 4 components of a performance management system, and 90% had conducted QI activities focused on increasing efficiencies and/or effectiveness" (McLees et al., 2014, p. 29).

▶ Factors Affecting the Ongoing Adoption and Institutionalization of CQI in Public Health

Accreditation Programs

Accreditation programs at the state and national level have served as major drivers of the promotion and adoption of CQI among state and local public health departments. State accreditation programs were instrumental in guiding the development of a national accreditation program, in addition to helping drive CQI in health departments. North Carolina has been one of the leaders at the state level. Indeed, North Carolina was the first state to pilot a state accreditation program as well as the first to mandate accreditation for all of its local health departments (Reed et al., 2009). All 84 North Carolina local health departments have gone through initial accreditation and have also been re-accredited as of July, 2018 (A. Thomas, personal communication, July 12, 2018).

The North Carolina program has clearly demonstrated the potential to drive CQI in health departments. A case study by Stone and Davis (2012) illustrates the link between CQI and public health accreditation in local public health agencies in North Carolina. Today, there are three ongoing state accreditation programs in North Carolina, Michigan, and Missouri. Michigan's statewide program has many similarities to North Carolina's, and Missouri's program is currently being updated and revised (D. Stone, personal communication, March 4, 2017).

Building on the early accreditation experience in states, the PHAB was established in 2007 to manage and promote a national voluntary accreditation program for state, local, territorial, and tribal public health departments (PHAB, 2013). The PHAB program has been very successful in engaging health departments across the United States. As of March 2017, PHAB has accredited 179 state, local, and tribal health departments (23, 155, and 1, respectively), and there are an additional 158 health departments currently in the PHAB accreditation process pipeline (PHAB, 2017).

Accreditation, whether in public health, in other areas of health care, or in related industries, has traditionally been primarily a quality assurance strategy focused on meeting standards set by external experts. In some industries, such efforts have not been particularly successful or popular; of note, they are often unpopular with workers because of the focus on human error, rather than systems, as the source of most problems. However, Bender and Halverson (2010) describe the approach to PHAB accreditation as follows: "Unlike some health-related agencies and services that are accredited or otherwise regulated, the PHAB board of directors has set the public health accreditation work solidly on the cornerstone of CQI. In other words, accreditation is a means to an end, not an end unto itself" (p. 80).

Due to PHAB's rapidly expanding reach, and its focus on CQI, PHAB accreditation has been a major driver of adoption of CQI in all public health settings. Further, PHAB requirements also foster institutionalization of CQI, especially its annual report process for accredited health departments, wherein the accredited health department is required to report on the elements of CQI that it has implemented, and plans to implement in the coming

year. Indeed, recent evaluation data from the PHAB program reveals that 92% of PHAB participants agree or strongly agree that the PHAB accreditation process led to a "strong QI culture." Further, focus groups revealed that PHAB accreditation changed CQI use in their health department from periodic to more institutionalized (Kronstadt et al., 2016).

For a further discussion of the role of accreditation in health care quality, on a local and global scale, readers are referred to Chapter 12 of this text.

Governmental and Nonprofit Organizations

Numerous governmental and nonprofit organizations are providing substantial leadership in promotion of CQI in the U.S. public health system. These well-respected organizations have the visibility and influence to advance CQI in public health and have been doing so over the past decade. We have already mentioned some of the most influential: ASTHO, NACCHO, CDC, U.S. DHHS, PHAB, and RWJF. Other influential groups that provide technical assistance, training, and visibility/promotion include the National Network of Public Health Institutes (NNPHI), the Public Health Foundation (PHF), and Population Health Improvement Partners, an organization that helps health-focused organizations and coalitions build organizational and community capacity to improve and sustain population health. Population Health Improvement Partners has provided local and national organizations with continuous improvement expertise and support since 2009 (Population Health Improvement Partners, 2017). **TABLE 11.1** lists some of the resources these key organizations offer.

For example, NNPHI has taken on leading an ongoing "spin off" of the MLC, convening the RWJF-funded Open Forum for Quality Improvement, a biannual national meeting to showcase CQI application and learnings in public health practice to support the ongoing community of practice started through the MLC.

TABLE 11.1 Several Key Organizations and Resources That Support CQI in Public Health	
National Network of Public Health Institutes http://www.nnphi.org	**Public Health Improvement Training** Search "Public Health Improvement Training" on the NNPHI homepage for more information. **Open Forum for Quality Improvement** Search "Open Forum" on the NNPHI homepage for more information.
Population Health Improvement Partners https://www.improve partners.org/	**CQI eLearning** Visit the Improvement Partners homepage and select "eLearning" from the navigation menu to view the online modules, tools, and templates.
Public Health Foundation http://www.phf.org	**Public Health Improvement Resources Center** Search for "PHIRC" on the PHF homepage for more information. **Performance Improvement Services** Search for "Performance Improvement Services" on the PHF homepage to learn more.

NNPHI also provides quality improvement training via the CDC's Public Health Improvement Training (PHIT). PHF provides a free searchable database for CQI resources and offers a multitude of training and technical assistance programs to help public health departments learn and apply CQI. Population Health Improvement Partners offers numerous training and technical assistance programs to help public health departments and their community partners learn and apply CQI. In addition, Population Health Improvement Partners provides a free online set of resources that includes a step-by-step guide for executing a quality improvement project, online learning modules, and a database of examples of quality improvement projects. Both PHF and Population Health Improvement Partners have published extensively about their CQI work and related lessons learned in public health settings.

Evidence-Based Strategies and Programs

To improve public health, it is increasingly acknowledged that the field has to generate, and more effectively, apply evidence-based strategies, interventions, and programs, while avoiding investment in those that have uncertain benefit (other than in research and evaluation activities) or have been proven to have no effect. The evidence base for public health interventions is limited in some areas, and additional funding for research on developing new approaches and documenting the effectiveness of current public health interventions is necessary (U.S. DHHS, 2009). However, many evidence-based strategies, interventions, and programs for improving health and preventing disease in communities are available and catalogued in free online resources, such as those as shown in **TABLE 11.2**.

To be effectively implemented, resources such as these must also be available in a user-friendly and comprehensively described format with support for selection of community/population appropriate interventions and programs, as well as providing comprehensive support and resources for how to implement them to support public health organizations involved in improvement efforts at the community level. The Healthy North Carolina Improvement App (IMAPP) is specifically designed to bolster support for selection and

TABLE 11.2 Resources for Community-Based Strategies, Interventions and Programs

Evidence-based Practice for Public Health http://library.umassmed.edu/ebpph/	University of Massachusetts Medical School
Guide to Community Preventive Services http://www.thecommunityguide.org/index.html	Centers for Disease Control and Prevention
Healthy NC Improvement App (IMAPP) https://www.ncimapp.org/	Population Health Improvement Partners
What Works for Health Visit http://www.countyhealthrankings.org/ and search "What Works for Health"	Robert Wood Johnson Foundation

implementation, however, most of the interventions are currently focused on a single state's priorities. Fortunately, Population Health Improvement Partners is partnering with the Institute for Healthcare Improvement (IHI) to develop a national version of IMAPP to support the 100 Million Healthier Lives campaign (IHI, 2017). More research and development is needed to increase the availability and usability of evidence-based approaches; likewise, more educational and training opportunities are needed to ensure the effective application of these approaches.

Innovative Partnerships

Local and state public health agencies alone cannot address many important public health problems, such as the increasing burden of chronic diseases. There is growing recognition that a coalition of partners from complementary organizations is often necessary. Public–private and other innovative partnerships will likely become increasingly important, especially as resources for public health continue to contract in many states. Local partnerships can be an excellent way to leverage limited public health resources.

One major opportunity for innovative partnerships is the 2014 changes in IRS requirements of nonprofit hospitals (78% of U.S. hospitals) through the Affordable Care Act (ACA), which mandates that they conduct a Community Health Needs Assessment (CHNA) every 3 years and collaborate with their local health department to do so, including developing strategies to address the priorities (James, 2016).

An excellent example of this type of collaboration in action is Western North Carolina (WNC) Healthy Impact. WNC Healthy Impact is a partnership and coordinated process between hospitals, public health agencies, and key regional partners in western North Carolina, working toward a vision of improved community health. Collectively, these entities work together locally and regionally across 16 counties on a community health improvement process to assess health needs, develop collaborative plans, take coordinated action, and evaluate progress and impact.

This locally-led and implemented initiative supports and enhances regional efforts by:

- Standardizing and conducting data collection and analysis
- Creating reporting and communication templates and tools
- Encouraging collaboration and peer learning
- Providing training and technical assistance (including Results Based Accountability™ and scorecards)

- Supporting regional priorities
- Sharing evidence-based and innovative practices

This innovative regional partnership, supported by financial and in-kind contributions from hospitals, public health agencies, and partners, is housed and coordinated by WNC Health Network, Inc., an alliance of hospitals and partners in western North Carolina that works to improve health and health care.

Private foundations have been another major force driving innovative partnerships. The RWJF Culture of Health effort is a well-known national example, as is the Healthy People, Healthy Carolinas Initiative. The Duke Endowment, a private foundation focused on improving health and well-being in North Carolina and South Carolina communities, has partnered with Population Health Improvement Partners and the South Carolina Alliance for Health to empower community health improvement efforts by strengthening and supporting local coalitions to improve health in their communities. This initiative aims to stimulate innovation in local partnerships and improve community health by focusing on supporting the implementation of evidence-based interventions targeting nutrition, physical activity, and prevention of chronic disease. The initiative currently involves 10 local partnerships and plans to expand to a total of 35 partnerships by 2020.

Finally, numerous states have used innovative partnerships to enhance the adoption and institutionalization of CQI in public health settings. For example, Population Health Improvement Partners, the North Carolina Division of Public Health, the North Carolina Association of Local Health Directors, the North Carolina Area Health Educations Centers, and the North Carolina Institute for Public Health partnered to provide basic and advanced CQI training for all local health departments and all state health programmatic areas, beginning in 2009. To date, nearly all of North Carolina's 84 local health departments have been trained, as have

dozens of state health department programs, yielding impressive improvements and return on investment (Davis et al., 2016; Crawley-Stout et al., 2016). The Rhode Island Department of Health has used multiple funding sources and initiatives, such as its Home Visiting Collaborative Improvement & Innovation Network (COIIN), to provide CQI training for numerous state maternal and child health programs and their staff and all of its local partner agencies in collaboration with Population Health Improvement Partners.

Financing of Public Health Organizations

In many states, governmental public health agencies have been under substantial financial strain related to governmental austerity, even during an expanding economy. In fact, the CDC's budget (nearly three-fourths of which funds state and local communities) has declined by over $1.5 billion (15%) in the past decade (Segal & Martín, 2017). New and innovative approaches to financing local and state public health agencies are greatly needed and can help improve the population's health as governmental funding is shrinking. For instance, public health organizations could benefit from testing and adapting financial approaches that have been successful in other industries, such as economic impact and return on investment analyses.

CQI relates to these financial challenges in at least three ways. First, implementing CQI should help reduce overall costs while increasing quality, just as it has in many other industries and organizations (Spear & Bowen, 1999). Reducing costs and inefficiencies can help increase capacity and allow for a greater focus on population health improvement. Indeed, the CDC and other U.S. DHHS agencies are beginning to tie incorporation of CQI into their grants to state and local public health agencies and programs. Second, if the financing of public health services remains focused on funding specific services and programs rather than infrastructure and other more flexible uses, then public health agencies will likely have great difficulty investing in the infrastructure needed for CQI. Lesneski (2012) presents a case study describing the link between quality management and the analysis of financial indicators in a local health department. Finally, and perhaps most importantly, we believe the increasing focus on *value* (higher quality at a lower cost) in the ongoing health care transformation in the United States, which is largely driven by the ACA, and the need to control the rapid increases in health care costs, will drive health systems to have a greater focus on improving the health of the populations they serve. U.S. DHHS has set a goal of linking 50% of Medicare fee-for-service payments to quality or value through alternative payment models by 2018 (CMS, 2017). An unhealthy population will have much higher health care costs, thus opening the door for innovative funding models between public health and health care entities as they strive for the mutually beneficial goal of improving the health of a population to create higher health care value. (See Chapter 14 for further discussion of the importance of focusing on value in health care and CQI).

🔍 CASE STUDY: INSTITUTIONALIZATION OF CONTINUOUS QUALITY IMPROVEMENT

This case study presents an example of a local public health agency that adopted and institutionalized continuous quality improvement. As you read through the case, refer to the NACCHO Roadmap to a Culture of Quality Improvement (NACCHO, 2013) and consider these questions:

- According to the NACCHO Roadmap, which elements of a CQI culture are present and which appear to be lacking?
- What could the organization do to address elements that appear to be lacking?
- What are three additional steps the organization could take to ensure sustainability of their CQI efforts?

CQI in a Local Public Health Agency: Macon County, North Carolina

After becoming accredited through North Carolina's accreditation program in 2008, the Macon County, North Carolina, Public Health Department began to focus on changing its quality culture. They established a QI council and part-time position for a quality program manager and began to implement a quality improvement program. Over the course of 2 years, they trained staff and leadership in quality improvement tools and methods, including Lean (see Chapters 4 and 5).

During this time, staff members completed small quality improvement projects, which helped them apply the concepts they were learning and secure buy-in throughout the organization. After staff were trained and had completed a few successful small-scale projects, the health department began focusing on "projects that would have a greater impact on the organization's overall performance, improve patient/customer service outcomes, and achieve demonstrable cost savings." One such project aimed to improve the appointment scheduling process by seeing all patients within 72 hours of requesting an appointment, while also improving patient and staff satisfaction. The team participated in a rapid cycle improvement event (or, *kaizen* event) that involved using Lean and Plan-Do-Study-Act cycles, performing a *gemba* walk (direct observation of the work), creating work flow diagrams and detailed process maps, and generating and testing change ideas. Soon after, the clinics were scheduling patients for visits in less than 72 hours. Their no-show rates decreased, visit numbers increased, staff downtime decreased, and both patient and staff satisfaction increased.

Leveraging this success, the health department began to spread quality improvement initiatives to other areas of the organization and focused on projects related to the client feedback process, child health visit flow, and vaccine storage and management among others. To keep staff informed of the organization's quality improvement work, as well as foster ongoing staff engagement, the health department keeps an electronic directory of their work (including project aim statements, meeting notes, process maps and flow diagrams, as well as other team-related communication) and highlights activities and results in the hallways of their organization. They also reinvest cost savings from the projects into other vital activities of the health department. Overall, the health department's continuous improvement efforts have led to organizational efficiency as well as improved care and patient experience (Bruckner, See, & Randolph, 2013).

▶ Conclusions

The need to improve the public's health in the United States is evident. Although public health organizations are still early in the process of institutionalizing CQI compared to organizations in many other industries, they have made remarkable progress and adoption in the second decade of the 21st century, particularly with the support of accreditation locally and nationally. The increased attention placed on the adoption of CQI in public health is both timely and encouraging. Numerous factors are presented to explain the growth of CQI in public health and, most important, the substantial progress that has been made toward true institutionalization of CQI in public health. Among those factors is accreditation, with similarities to the impact accreditation has had on health care globally (see Chapter 12). Continuing to use accreditation efforts to promote CQI and learning from health care and other industries will help accelerate widespread adoption and institutionalization of CQI. Public health organizations that adopt CQI to help employees work as a team, address gaps in performance by analyzing and redesigning processes, and encourage innovation to meet the needs of communities hold the promise for a healthier future, both in the United States and throughout the world.

References

Beitsch, L. M., Thielen, L., Mays, G., Brewer, R. A., Kimbrell, J., Chang, C., ... Landrum, L. B. (2006). The multistate learning collaborative, states as laboratories: Informing the national public health accreditation dialogue. *Journal of Public Health Management & Practice, 12*, 217–231.

Bender, K., & Halverson, P. K. (2010). Quality improvement and accreditation: What might it look like? *Journal of Public Health Management & Practice, 16*(1), 70–82.

Bruckner, J., See, C. H., & Randolph, G. D. (2013). Case study: Quality improvement in the Macon County Health Department. *North Carolina Medical Journal 74*(2), 138–139.

Centers for Disease Control and Prevention (CDC). (2015, January). National Public Health Performance Standards Program. Retrieved April 21, 2017, from https://www.cdc.gov/nphpsp/

Centers for Medicare & Medicaid Services (CMS). (2017). Health Care Payment Learning and Action Network. Retrieved April 21, 2017, from https://innovation.cms.gov

Crawley-Stout, L. A., Ward, K. A., See, C. H., & Randolph, G. (2016). Lessons learned from measuring return on investment in public health quality improvement initiatives. *Journal of Public Health Management & Practice, 22*(2), e28–e37.

Davis, M. V., Cornett, A. C., Mahanna, E., See, C. H., & Randolph, G. (2016). Advancing quality improvement in public health departments through a statewide training program. *Journal of Public Health Management & Practice, 22*(2), e21–e27.

Deming, W. E. (2000). *The new economics for industry, government, and education,* 2nd ed. Cambridge, MA: MIT Press.

Gillen, S. M., McKeever, J., Edwards, K. F., & Thielen, L. (2010). Promoting quality improvement and achieving measurable change: The lead states initiative. *Journal of Public Health Management & Practice, 16*(1), 55–60.

Honoré, P. (2009). Quality in the public health system. Presentation at the 137th Annual Meeting of the American Public Health Association, Philadelphia, PA.

Honoré, P., Wright, D., Berwick, D. W., Clancy, C. M., Lee, P., Nowinski, J., & Koh, H. K. (2011). Creating a framework for getting quality into the public health system. *Health Affairs (Millwood), 30*(4), 737–745.

Institute of Medicine (IOM). (1988). *The future of public health.* Washington, D.C.: National Academies Press.

Institute of Medicine (IOM). (2013). *Toward quality measures for population health and the leading health indicators.* Washington, D.C.: The National Academies Press.

Institute for Healthcare Improvement (IHI). (2017). 100 Million healthier lives. Retrieved from http://www.ihi.org

James, J. (2016, February 25). Health policy brief: Nonprofit hospitals' community benefit requirements. *Health Affairs/RWJF Policy Brief.* Retrieved from https://www.rwjf.org

Joly, B. M., Shaler, G., Booth, M., Conway, A., & Mittal, P. (2010). Evaluating the multi-state learning collaborative. *Journal of Public Health Management & Practice, 16*(1), 61–66.

Kronstadt, J., Meit, M., Siegfried, A., Nicolaus, T., Bender, K., & Corso, L. (2016). Evaluating the impact of national public health department accreditation— United States, 2016. *Morbidity and Mortality Weekly Report, 65*(31), 803–806.

Langley, G. L., Moen, R. D., Nolan, K. M., Nolan, T. W., Norman, C. L., & Provost, L. P. (2009). *The improvement guide: A practical approach to enhancing organizational performance.* San Francisco, CA: Jossey-Bass.

Lesneski, C. D. (2012). Financial analysis and quality management in Patriot County, Ohio. In C. P. McLaughlin, J. K. Johnson, & W. A. Sollecito (Eds.), *Implementing continuous quality improvement in health care: A global casebook.* Sudbury, MA: Jones & Bartlett Learning.

MacDorman, M. F., Mathews, T. J., Mohangoo, A. D., & Zeitlin, J. (2014). International comparisons of infant mortality and related factors: United States and Europe, 2010. *National Vital Statistics Reports, 63*(5). Hyattsville, MD: National Center for Health Statistics.

McLees, A. W., Thomas, C. W., Nawaz, S., Young, A. C., Rider, N., & Davis, M. (2014). Advances in public health accreditation readiness and quality improvement: Evaluation findings from the national public health improvement initiative. *Journal of Public Health Management & Practice, 20*(1), 29–35.

National Association of County & City Health Organizations (NACCHO). (2013). Foundational elements of a QI culture. Retrieved from http://qiroadmap.org

Organisation for Economic Co-Operation and Development. (2014). *OECD Health Statistics 2014: How does the United States compare?* [Fact Sheet]. Retrieved from https://www.oecd.org

Osborn, R., Squires, D., Doty, M. M., Sarnak, D. O., & Schneider, E. C. (2016). In new survey of eleven countries, U.S. adults still struggle with access to and affordability of health care. *Health Affairs (Millwood) 35*(12), 2327–2336.

Population Health Improvement Partners. (2017). Retrieved July 10, 2017, from https://www.improvepartners.org

Public Health Accreditation Board (PHAB). (2013). Public Health Department Accreditation Background. Retrieved from http://www.phaboard.org

Public Health Accreditation Board (PHAB). (2017). Accreditation activity as of March 31, 2017. Retrieved from http://www.phaboard.org

Reed, J., Pavletic, D., Devlin, L., Davis, M. V., Beitsch, L. M., & Baker, E. L. (2009). Piloting a state health department accreditation model: The North Carolina experience. *Journal of Public Health Management & Practice, 15*(2), 85–95.

Riley, W. J., Moran, J. W., Corso, L. C., Beitsch, L. M., Bialek, R., & Cofsky, A. (2010). Defining quality improvement in public health. *Journal of Public Health Management & Practice, 16*(1), 5–7.

Russo, P. (2007). Accreditation of public health agencies: A means, not an end. *Journal of Public Health Management & Practice, 13*(4), 329–331.

Segal, L. M., & Martín, A. (2017). *A funding crisis for public health and safety: State-by-state public health funding and key health facts, 2017.* Retrieved from http://healthyamericans.org/assets/files/TFAH-2017-FundingCrisisRpt-FINAL.pdf

Smith, G., Poteat-Godwin, A., Harrison, L. M., & Randolph, G. D. (2012). Applying Lean principles and Kaizen rapid improvement events in public health practice. *Journal of Public Health Management & Practice, 18*(1), 52–54.

Sollecito, W. A., & Johnson, J. K. (2013). *McLaughlin and Kaluzny's continuous quality improvement in health care.* Burlington, MA: Jones & Bartlett Learning.

Spear, K., & Bowen, H. K. (1999). Decoding the DNA of the Toyota production system. *Harvard Business Review, 77*, 96–106.

Stone, D., & Davis, M. V. (2012). North Carolina Local Health Accreditation Program: Case 15. In C. P. Mc Laughlin, J. K. Johnson, & W. A. Sollecito (Eds.), *Implementing continuous quality improvement in health care: A global casebook.* Sudbury, MA: Jones & Bartlett Learning.

Turning Point. (2006). *About turning point.* Retrieved January 29, 2010, from http://www.turningpointprogram.org

United Health Foundation. (2016). *America's health rankings health of women and children report*. Retrieved from http://assets.americashealthrankings.org

U.S. Department of Health and Human Services. (2008, August). Consensus statement on quality in the public health system. Retrieved from http://www.dhhs.gov

U.S. Department of Health and Human Services. (2009). Evaluating sources of knowledge for evidence-based actions in public health. Retrieved from http://www.healthedpartners.org

WNC Health Network. (2013). *WNC healthy impact*. Retrieved from http://www.wnchealthyimpact.com/

CHAPTER 12

Health Service Accreditation: A Strategy to Promote and Improve Safety and Quality

David Greenfield and Marjorie Pawsey

Healthcare organizations have a mandate to provide the highest standard of care for patients and their families. While it may be difficult to empirically demonstrate that an organization provides a high standard of care using basic outcomes such as mortality, the foundations of both measuring and improving healthcare quality include consideration of adequate structures and processes of care with proven relationships to better outcomes.

—Andre Amaral and Brian Cuthbertson (2016, p. 824)

how accreditation programs have become a common strategy to improve health organizations and care, including examining the requirements and motivations to participate. The chapter also considers the impact of continuous quality improvement within accreditation programs on organizations and care delivered. Accreditation agencies, standards and surveyor reliability are reviewed, with public health accreditation programs in the United States as a practical example.

The accreditation of health care services remains a key regulatory mechanism employed by many governments, at both national and state levels, to monitor and improve safety and quality. The objective of this chapter is to provide an overview of health service accreditation programs, outline health service accreditation, including explaining the current model of accreditation, and review

▶ An Overview of Accreditation

Health care organizations, services within them, and individual professionals, can all be accredited. Health care organizations are accredited for the management and provision of their services, including hospitals, general practices, geriatric care facilities, and public health (Accreditation Canada, 2016a; Ingram et al., 2014; The Joint Commission, 2017). Within health care organizations, specialized health services can be accredited, such as tissue banks (American Association of Tissue Banks, 2017), pharmacies (American College of Health-System Pharmacists, 2017), and *aeromedical* transportation services (Commission on Accreditation of Medical Transport Systems, 2017). Additionally, programs or individual professionals from medical (American Academy of Neurology, 2017), nursing (American Academy of Nurse Practitioners, 2017), and allied health fields (American Occupational Therapy Association, 2017; Council on Podiatric Medical Education, 2017), and administrators, including medical administrators (American Academy of Medical Management, 2018), are increasingly required to be certified. Whether it is the organization, service or individual focused upon, accreditation is the action whereby they have demonstrated competency, authority, or credibility to meet a predetermined set of standards. When successfully undertaken they are awarded the status of being "accredited" by a recognized, credible, designated authority. In short, a health service accreditation program is a mechanism that reviews and assesses an organization's quality improvement initiatives and ongoing efforts to demonstrate that minimum safety and quality standards are being achieved (Almasabi & Thomas, 2017; Carman & Timsina, 2015; Devkaran & O'Farrell, 2015; Haj-Ali et al., 2014; Hinchcliff, Greenfield, Westbrook, et al., 2013; Jaafaripooyan, 2014; Lanteigne & Bouchard, 2016; Teymourzadeh et al., 2016; Yan & Kung, 2015).

Current Model of Health Service Accreditation

The model of health service accreditation, enacted by many health accreditation agencies, is similar. A breakdown of the process typically involved in this model is as follows: An organization seeking to be accredited develops, implements, and continuously reviews its quality improvement plan and self-assesses progress against the standards of the accreditation program. It concludes this task by providing a written self-assessment report to the accrediting agency. The accrediting agency assesses the organization's report and dispatches an accreditation survey team, comprised of peer reviewers, to visit and assess the organization on site. The visit comprises observations of facilities, interviews with staff, and a review of documentation. The survey team during and at the conclusion of the survey provides verbal feedback to the organization. The accrediting agency receives a written report from the survey team a short time after the visit. The report summarizes the survey team's assessment of the organization's progress in achieving the standards and makes recommendations or commendations as appropriate. Following the correction of any errors of fact by the organization, the report is then considered by the accrediting agency. The agency assesses the report and decides whether to award accreditation status or not.

Accreditation is in effect for a defined period, typically for 3 to 5 years. It is common for accrediting agencies to send survey teams to reassess an organization during the accreditation period. The survey team reviews the organization's continual progress against the updated quality plan and accreditation standards. The surveyors provide verbal feedback, and, after endorsement by the accrediting agency, a written report is provided to the organization. The improvement cycle continues, with the organization using the report to initiate further reflection and examination of its structures, processes, and practices to identify and drive areas for ongoing improvement.

▶ Accreditation: A Common Strategy to Improve Health Organizations and Care

Accreditation in health was first initiated in the United States through the work of the American College of Surgeons, which in 1917 developed the Minimum Standards for Hospitals. This organization subsequently collaborated with colleges and associations from the United States and Canada to create, in 1951, the Joint Commission on Accreditation of Hospitals, which is now referred to as The Joint Commission (TJC). From this beginning, health care accreditation has spread to be practiced across the world (Agrizzi, Agyemang, & Jaafaripooyan, 2016; Devkaran & O'Farrell, 2015; Shaw, 2015; Teymourzadeh et al., 2016; Triantafillou, 2014). Accreditation is now in more than 70 countries, including: Australia (ACSQHC, 2016; Greenfield, Hinchcliff et al., 2016; Mumford, Reeve, et al., 2015), Canada (Accreditation Canada, 2016a; Mitchell et al., 2015), France (Haute Autorité de Santé, 2015); Iran (Agrizzi, Agyemang, & Jaafaripooyan, 2016; Mohebbifar et al., 2017), Lebanon (Haj-Ali et al., 2014); Pakistan (Sax and Marx, 2014), Saudi Arabia (Aboshaiqah, Alonazi, & Patalagsa, 2016; Almasabi & Thomas, 2016), Taiwan (Yan and Kung, 2016), United Arab Emirates (Devkaran & O'Farrell, 2015), and the United States (The Joint Commission, 2016, 2017).

In the United States, TJC accredits more than 4,000 organizations, or 88% of the hospitals in the country (The Joint Commission, 2016). The Haute Autorité de Santé (HAS) accredits all acute health care organizations in France, which total more than 700 hospitals (Haute Autorité de Santé, 2015). Accreditation Canada (Accreditation Canada, 2016b) and the Australian Council on Healthcare Standards (ACHS) (ACHS, 2016) each accredit more than 1,000 and 800 organizations, respectively.

These, and many other major health care accreditation agencies, are independent, not-for-profit, nongovernment agencies.

The uptake of accreditation has been, in part, driven by governments (Agrizzi, Agyemang, & Jaafaripooyan, 2016; Devkaran & O'Farrell, 2015; Sax & Marx, 2014; Shaw, 2015; Teymourzadeh et al., 2016; Thielen et al., 2014; Triantafillou, 2014; Yan & Kung, 2015). They have used accreditation programs and other regulation strategies to attempt abatement or control of risks to society by indirect means (Agrizzi, Agyemang, & Jaafaripooyan, 2016; Sparrow, 2000). Accreditation programs reflect a shift in philosophy by governments whereby they have sought to provide a framework for the governance of services rather than to provide those services themselves. Accreditation is an element in a network of activities that seeks to regulate conduct in the health sector. Health organizations are networked together, and their behavior is assessed by independent bodies through accreditation programs, standards, and quality indicators. Regulation via this network has been called "nodal governance" (Shearing & Wood, 2003); that is, organizations, services, and professional behavior in health care are shaped by an increasing variety of government and nongovernment bodies related to but independent of each other (Triantafillou, 2014). A further factor shaping organizational behavior is the public disclosure of accreditation information and results (Greenfield et al., 2013). The idea has widespread support from governments, health care organizations, and consumers, and is implemented in practice by many agencies; however, the production of information that is meaningful and useable by consumers remains a challenge. The main impact of the public disclosure of accreditation information is to stimulate a positively reinforcing cycle of transparency encouraging organizational accountability and further improvement (Agrizzi, Agyemang, & Jaafaripooyan, 2016; Greenfield et al., 2013).

There is an international agency, the International Society for Quality in Health Care (ISQua), that accredits the accreditors

(ISQua, 2018). As of October 2016, ISQua had accredited 68 accrediting organizations, 146 accreditation standards, and 30 surveyor training programs (ISQua, 2018). ISQua promotes self-governance through their accrediting of accreditation agencies. That is, ISQua members, themselves drawn from accrediting bodies, provide guidelines, support, and assessment of accreditation and surveyor training programs to one another. Furthermore, the self-governance modality is reinforced through ISQua's encouragement of participation in its organization and the international health quality and safety conferences it convenes. Consequently, the work of ISQua has evoked an international convergence of understanding about, and similarity in the enactment of, health accreditation programs.

The evidence base for health service accreditation programs continues to strengthen. There have been calls, over many years, for increased research, transparency, and innovation into accreditation (Devkaran & O'Farrell, 2015; Greenfield & Braithwaite, 2009; Hinchcliff, Greenfield, Moldovan, et al., 2013). Research organizations and accrediting agencies have responded, particularly in the last few years, undertaking an increasing number of studies (Agrizzi, Agyemang, & Jaafaripooyan, 2016; Devkaran & O'Farrell, 2015; Hinchcliff, Greenfield, Moldovan, et al., 2013; Teymourzadeh et al., 2016). This includes those involving HAS, TJC, Accreditation Canada, the ACHS, the Italian Society for Quality of Health Care, the Irish Health Services Accreditation Board, and the Spanish accrediting agency, Fundación Avedis Donabedian.

Requirements and Motivations to Participate in a Health Service Accreditation Program

There are external requirements and internal motivations that drive health care organizations to seek accreditation (Greenfield & Braithwaite, 2008; Sax & Marx, 2014). An external

requirement comes from governments, insurers, and consumers demand that organizations undertake efforts that demonstrate outcomes that advance high-quality and safer health care (Accreditation Canada, 2016c; Agrizzi, Agyemang, & Jaafaripooyan, 2016; Shaw, 2015; The Joint Commission, 2017). Individually, and collectively, they seek to be reassured that organizations are making efforts to achieve published standards or address safety and quality. The internal impetus comes from health professionals. They report a desire to improve their services and the care they provide (Greenfield & Braithwaite, 2008). Together these two motivations, which are mutually reinforcing, have combined to draw many health care organizations under the umbrella of accreditation.

The external pressures and explicit regulatory requirements which necessitate participation in an accreditation program means the distinction between voluntary and mandatory accreditation programs is increasingly difficult to separate. The "choice" many organizations have is not whether to participate but with which accrediting agency and program they will be associated. In effect, health service accreditation, in many countries, has become a requirement in practice if not in name. Research contrasting two programs, one mandated and the other voluntary, found that both programs incorporated compulsory and flexible elements. There were positive impacts from both the mandated and voluntary programs, and that there was a convergence of the two approaches (Greenfield, Hinchcliff et al., 2016; Shaw, 2015).

▶ Accreditation: A Process Promoting Continuous Quality Improvement

Accreditation programs now require that organizations have structures and processes that promote safety and quality, and also that they are functioning effectively. These requirements represent a philosophical shift from *quality assurance* to *continuous quality improvement* (Greenfield, Hinchcliff et al., 2016). The former is regarded as a program that strives to improve quality through defining and measuring it. The latter incorporates both retrospective and prospective assessments, and is aimed at developing strategies to make things better and to create systems to prevent errors (Lanteigne & Bouchard, 2016). While the continuous quality improvement model is the dominant accreditation model for health care organizations, there is an alternative, more generic model that can be described as an "audit model." In this model, an external reviewer, with or without health care experience, uses a generic set of quality standards to assess the presence or absence of organizational quality activities. This model is endorsed by the International Organization for Standardization, which accredits organizations in many diverse industries, including health (see the International Organization for Standardization website).

In simple terms, continuous quality improvement involves health professionals constantly asking themselves, "Despite having the 'right' things in place to do the 'right' things, what are we doing now that we can do better?" Furthermore, accreditation is about answering the question posed by external assessors: "What systems have you implemented, how do they work, and can you show me how you are planning to do things better?" The shift can be illustrated by an example concerning patient satisfaction surveys. An accreditation program promoting a quality assurance approach would focus on a patient satisfaction survey and how it is developed and administered. In contrast, an accreditation program with a quality improvement philosophy would focus on the response rate of the surveys, the issues identified by the patients, the organization's actions, and confirmation of improvement in subsequent surveys.

There is still much to be learnt about under what circumstances and how an accreditation program fosters quality improvement

and learning (Devkaran & O'Farrell, 2015; Hinchcliff, Greenfield, Moldovan, et al., 2013; Jaafaripooyan, 2014; Melo, 2016; Riley et al., 2012; Shaw, 2015; Yan & Kung, 2015). With each revision of standards, there remains debate about whether we keep raising the bar to stimulate efforts to improve—or will this strategy promote adverse behaviors? Knowing how best to stimulate improvements in quality and safety in health systems facing significant cost pressures and increasing demands is a challenge for governments, health care organizations, and professionals. Many health professionals, whether they participate in accreditation activities directly, indirectly, or not at all, seem to hold strong opinions about the value and benefits, or lack thereof. The topic generates polarized views. Professionals who do and do not participate in accreditation efforts can perceive the efforts as external bureaucratic reporting mechanisms (Agrizzi, Agyemang, & Jaafaripooyan, 2016; Jaafaripooyan, 2014). Conversely, participating in accreditation cultivates communication and cooperation among individuals and teams, and promotes a positive quality and safety culture, thereby promoting change in an organization (Beatty et al., 2015; Hinchcliff, Greenfield, Moldovan, et al., 2013; Melo, 2016; Verma & Moran, 2014).

Accreditation programs, encompassing the continuous quality improvement principle, are noted to have improved the organization of facilities, policies and guidelines, decision making, and safety (Abou Elnour et al., 2014; Davis et al., 2011; Greenfield & Braithwaite, 2008; Hinchcliff, Greenfield, Moldovan, et al., 2013; Melo, 2016; Shaw, 2015; Yan & Kung, 2015). An accreditation program provides a structured framework for engagement and improvement (Abou Elnour et al., 2014; Verma & Moran, 2014). Health care professionals perceived accreditation programs as a strategy for promoting and making transparent quality and collegial decision making. An accreditation program has been shown to stimulate an organization to sustain improvements over the accreditation cycle (Devkaran & O'Farrell, 2015). Similarly, in an acute teaching hospital in Portugal, an accreditation program stimulated improvement though promoting staff reflection on their work, standardization of practices, building upon existing processes, and focusing attention on quality improvement (Melo, 2016). Accredited hospitals formalize, and at times realize, improvements in quality management practices (Braithwaite et al., 2010; Devkaran & O'Farrell, 2015; Hinchcliff, Greenfield, Moldovan, et al., 2013; Jaafaripooyan, 2014; Melo, 2016). In Taiwan, organizational team learning and hospital accreditation awareness was correlated (Yan & Kung, 2015, 2016) and considered to be a viable strategy for improving quality and safety of medical care. Positive correlations were found between accreditation performance and organizational culture and leadership, additionally, a positive trend was noted with clinical performance; however, no link was identified to organizational climate (Braithwaite et al., 2010).

In other studies, however, there are more mixed outcomes. There was no impact on quality outcomes from one program (Almasabi & Thomas, 2016). In another case, the program was seen to bring benefits (e.g., external recognition), as well as drawbacks for individual clinicians (e.g., routinization) (Jaafaripooyan, 2014). Similarly, organizations have undergone improvement processes but failed to reach the standard required by the accreditation program (Lanteigne & Bouchard, 2016).

Accreditation has an undefined impact on patient views or satisfaction reports. A positive effect from accreditation on patient satisfaction has been reported (Alkhenizan & Shaw, 2011) but not identified in other circumstances (Haj-Ali et al., 2014; Mohebbifar et al., 2017). Accredited organizations were perceived by patients as only marginally better than nonaccredited organizations in one study, and the role of accreditation was unclear (Aboshaiqah, Alonazi, & Patalagsa, 2016). Accreditation was unrelated to consumer involvement in another study (Braithwaite et al., 2010). The understanding is that an accreditation program improvement

targets aspects of organizations that are less visible to patients and this mitigates against a relationship between the two issues being identified (Hinchcliff, Greenfield, Moldovan, et al., 2013).

Additionally, there is an ongoing debate about the cost of accreditation programs (Hinchcliff, Greenfield, Moldovan, et al., 2013; Mumford, Forde, Greenfield, Hinchcliff, & Braithwaite, 2013; Mumford, Greenfield, et al., 2013; Mumford, Reeve, et al., 2015). The financial impact for accreditation was reported as proportionally greater for smaller organizations and considered by some to be high overall (Mumford, Greenfield, et al., 2015). However, the argument has been made that the costs incurred are not additional but part of an organization's required investment in quality (Hinchcliff, Greenfield, Moldovan, et al., 2013; Mumford, Forde, et al., 2013; Mumford, Reeve, et al., 2015).

▶ Accreditation Agencies, Standards, and Surveyor Reliability

Accreditation Agencies

Accreditation agencies that assess organizations and services against standards, develop and supervise peer reviewers to maintain a surveyor workforce. Surveyors are a key element of accreditation programs (Teymourzadeh et al., 2016). Accrediting agencies can have surveyor workforces comprised of full-time or part-time surveyors, and they may be on salary, paid a stipend or voluntary. The ongoing support and development of this workforce requires careful management and surveyor workforce sustainability is an ongoing challenge for accreditation agencies. Accrediting agencies need to be able to continually recruit appropriately experienced health professionals as surveyors (Teymourzadeh et al., 2016). However, their regular employment can be incompatible with the time required to participate as a surveyor. Nevertheless, accrediting agencies are continually renewing their workforces. Individuals gain benefits from surveying and it provides value to the institutions in which they are regularly employed (Lancaster, Braithwaite, & Greenfield, 2010; Teymourzadeh et al., 2016). Health professionals who act as volunteer surveyors derive four benefits from doing so, that is, the opportunity to: be exposed to new methods and innovations in health organizations; engage in a unique form of professional development; acquire expertise to enhance quality within the institutions in which they are regularly employed; and contribute to the process of quality improvement and enhance public health in organizations beyond their regular employment.

The status of the accreditation program, whether mandatory or voluntary, shapes the focus of the role and others' perceptions. The surveyor role is a demanding one, including acting as educator, judge, evaluator, regulator, or a combination of these functions (Greenfield, Braithwaite, Pawsey, 2008; Sax & Marx, 2014). A health professional taking on the surveyor role may be comfortable with some part but not others, or with combining the roles. Additionally, potential or perceived conflict of interest issues have been raised when health professionals are surveying colleagues and organizations with which they have ties or with which they may seek to work in the future (Plebani, 2001). Correspondingly, accreditation agencies have instigated policies requiring surveyors to disclose any real or perceived conflicts.

Accreditation agencies, involving many of their stakeholders, have constructed a self-governing system (Greenfield, Pawsey, Naylor, Braithwaite, 2009). It is a system responsive to the conduct and culture of those being regulated; this approach has been labeled "responsive regulation" (Sax & Marx, 2014). The system seeks to influence the attitudes and practices of

those involved, whether they are in the role of accreditation agency personnel, surveyors, or health staff in an organization being accredited (Ingram et al., 2014). Through participation in the development of accreditation programs or the accrediting of health care organizations, a common understanding of standards and shared expectations is constructed. Additionally, participants regulate their own and other colleagues' behaviors to comply with the standards and expectations. The system combines internal assessment, or self-regulation, with self-directed improvement strategies overseen by external peer review. It is a cultural control strategy whose influence is significant on those directly involved (Greenfield et al., 2009; Sax & Marx, 2014). Those health professionals who participate in their organization's accreditation activities generally report improvements to quality and safety.

Accreditation Standards

Government bodies or accrediting agencies can be responsible for the development and revision of standards. It is common for either to develop standards using representatives drawn from the health industry, including combinations of health care experts, researchers, representatives from industry groups, consumers, and governmental agencies; for example, in the United States (The Joint Commission, 2017), Canada (Accreditation Canada, 2016c), France (Haute Autorité de Santé, 2015), and Australia (ACSQHC, 2016), standards are developed through consultation with a wide range of stakeholders. The description, number and status of standards, vary from accreditation program to program. For the accreditation of hospitals, Accreditation Canada has four core standards within its Qmemtum program (Accreditation Canada, 2016d), HAS, the French accreditation agency, has 28 standards and 82 criteria (Haute Autorité de Santé, 2015), and the Australian Commission on Safety and Quality in Health Care program has 10 standards (ACSQHC, 2016). By contrast, the

United States the Public Health Accreditation Board (PHAB) program has 12 domains with multiple standards under each (PHAB, 2014). Accreditation standards cover infrastructure, organizational, service, and continuum of patient care issues (Greenfield & Braithwaite, 2008; Hinchcliff, Greenfield, Moldovan, et al., 2013; Mitchell et al., 2015; Haute Autorité de Santé, 2015). Standards are focused on organizational processes and systems, and the availability of appropriate resources for the organization to deliver the defined services. These types of standards have been termed "process indicators," as they focus on how care is delivered rather than the outcomes of the activity.

Concerns have been raised that when standards do not reflect the outcomes of care, they are not examining all dimensions of quality and safety. Quality indicators are advocated as being more effective measures. However, the use of quality indicators within an accreditation program continues to present many challenges (Hinchcliff, Greenfield, Moldovan, et al., 2013; Mumford, Reeve, et al., 2015). At present, the relationship between accreditation and quality measures—clinical indicators, quality indicators, or clinical performance measures—is not clear (Beatty et al., 2015; Hinchcliff, Greenfield, Moldovan, et al., 2013). Accreditation has been shown to generate improvement in some cases but not in others. The use of quality indicators is likely to remain problematic until the relationship between accreditation and quality indicators is clarified (Hinchcliff, Greenfield, Moldovan, et al., 2013). The question is whether we should expect to find a link between accreditation and different quality measures, given they are developed and implemented separately and not linked. The issue remains unresolved as to whether they examine similar or different aspects of health care performance and quality; the point has been made that they are in fact measuring different aspects of the safety and quality spectrum (Mumford et al., 2014). Nevertheless, concern continues to

be expressed about the lack of a relationship between the two, and the argument persists that this issue needs further investigation (Hinchcliff, Greenfield, Moldovan, et al., 2013; Mumford et al., 2014).

Accrediting agencies are increasingly examining strategies to expand programs or standards to incorporate organizational performance and clinical measures (Accreditation Canada, 2016c; ACHS, 2016; Haute Autorité de Santé, 2015; The Joint Commission, 2016). Accreditation Canada's program Qmentum, uses evidence-based "Required Organizational Practices" "to mitigate risk and contribute to improving the quality and safety of health services" (Accreditation Canada, 2016d). The measures are used to direct surveyors to examine particular parts of an organization requiring close assessment (Mitchell et al., 2015). Alternatively, outcome measures are being reported upon separately to accreditation surveys. Accreditation agencies are producing reports of organizational and clinical compliance with expected guidelines to raise awareness across the industry. For example, in the United States, since 2006, the TJC has tracked and reported upon quality of care measures called "accountability measures" (The Joint Commission, 2016). These items are evidence-based, standardized, national measures that allow comparisons across organizations. In 2016, the TJC reported on 29 measures (down from 45 the previous year with the others retired due to excellent quality performance by TJC accredited hospitals), with data drawn from more than 3,000 accredited hospitals. In particular, the 2016 report documents increased quality performance results in inpatient psychiatric services, venous thromboembolism (VTE) care, stroke care, perinatal care, tobacco use treatment, and substance use care. The report notes that room for improvement exists and there was a decline in the composite accountability score, probably due to the retirement of measures on which many hospitals were performing extremely well.

As these examples demonstrate, the use of quality of care measures in accreditation surveys and the publication of compliance reports are strategies by which accreditation agencies are working with health organizations to assess, measure, and improve their care. Their use forms part of the system of self-governance within and across health organizations. The place of quality indicators within an accreditation program is an important one with which to come to terms. How do organizations use the results from process and quality indicators and accreditation programs? Are they used independently or together? How do we resolve the differences in their findings?

Surveyor Reliability

Reliability is noted as being a critical issue in accreditation, and in health care more broadly. Being able to conduct consistent assessments, interpretations, and judgments, individually and collectively, is a challenge for professionals working in many areas of health care (Greenfield et al., 2009). As such, the challenges of consistency faced by accreditation surveyors are not unique, and surveyors will have encountered them in their normal professional activities. Reliability in accreditation is a concern for accreditation agencies and organizations that have been or are considering going through the accreditation process. Effectively sustaining, developing, and managing a surveyor workforce to maintain and increase the reliability of assessments is a key focus for accrediting agencies (Greenfield, Hogden et al., 2016; Teymourzadeh et al., 2016). When enacting the surveyor role, intra- and inter-rater reliability are issues of note (Greenfield et al., 2009; Greenfield, Hogden et al., 2016; Teymourzadeh et al., 2016). It is important to distinguish between intra- and inter-rater reliability. Intra-rater reliability is high when the assessments made by an individual surveyor or survey team are consistent from case to case. Inter-rater reliability is high when assessments made by different surveyors or survey teams are consistent with one another. Accreditation agencies that use full-time surveyors see this as a strategy that can work toward increasing the mastery of survey techniques and more consistent interpretation of standards. Conversely, part-time surveyors have current knowledge of the health system, management practices, and clinical expectations, but may not be as consistent in surveying as their full-time colleagues.

Accreditation surveying is an activity based on document analysis, observations, and interviews, hence survey findings need to be credible and verifiable (Greenfield, Braithwaite, Pawsey, 2008; Greenfield et al., 2009). Survey teams use these three qualitative data collection methods (document analysis, observations, and interviews) to triangulate their assessments. The results produced through this complex process are not precisely replicable, as human judgments are central to the data collection and analysis process. Nevertheless, striving for rigor in application of standards, individual and team conduct, and transparency in interpretation and decision making is essential (Greenfield, Hogden et al., 2016). Hence the assessment that "Where surveyors and survey teams achieve process consistency and program interpretation from survey to survey, their findings can then be said to be reliable" (Greenfield et al., 2009). In other words, accreditation agencies, rather than focusing on reliability of outcome, need to be encouraged to implement strategies to promote and ensure reliability of process and consistent application of standards (Greenfield et al., 2009; Greenfield, Hogden et al., 2016; Teymourzadeh et al., 2016).

Reliability in surveying has been shown to be promoted or undermined by multiple factors (Greenfield et al., 2009; Greenfield, Hogden et al., 2016; Sax & Marx, 2014). These include: the accreditation program, including documentation requirements for organizations and survey teams; member relationship with the accrediting agency and survey team;

accreditation agency personnel; surveyor workforce renewal; management of the surveyor workforce; performance review of surveyors; and, survey dynamics' effect on the reliability of surveys directly and indirectly. Reliability in the accreditation process is constructed through the interplay of these factors. They realize shared expectations and conduct among stakeholders; together they promote standardized beliefs and actions that become accreditation cultural norms (Greenfield et al., 2009; Greenfield, Hogden et al., 2016; Sax & Marx, 2014). Reliability is an ongoing achievement, to be enacted each and every time a survey team undertakes the task of assessing an organization (Greenfield, Hogden et al., 2016). Two studies developed scenario exercises, using real data, for individual surveyors and survey teams to examine the respective issues. Individual surveyors assessed, at two points in time, scenarios of individual standards relating to a large hospital, and their results were compared. The findings revealed that intra-rater reliability is problematic; that is, individuals struggle to consistently make consistent assessments. A 20% variation in surveyors' individual assessments that potentially could have affected accreditation outcomes was noted (Greenfield et al., 2009). Similarly, scenarios based on real data and comprising written information and a role-play were developed and presented to survey teams. In contrast to the intra-rater findings, the results showed that the examination of the inter-rater reliability of survey teams demonstrated more consistent agreement (Greenfield, Pawsey, Naylor, & Braithwaite, 2008), thus highlighting the mediating effect of teams on individuals.

Differences in how surveyors approach their role can be misinterpreted as a lack of reliability. A typology, using the dimensions of recording (explicit/implicit) and questioning (opportunistic/structured), classifies four accreditation surveyor styles: the discusser, the explorer, the interrogator, and the questioner (Greenfield, Braithwaite,

Pawsey, 2008). In each case the surveyor enacts the role according to their individual preferences, strengths, and interpretation of the survey situation. All have strengths and weakness, depending on the circumstance, no one approach is better than the others. However, each presentation is distinctive to the others and open to misinterpretation, and can be poorly performed, thus affecting reliability. The typology is suggested for use by accreditation agencies in their surveyor training programs, to explore issues of reliability and teamwork, and offers the opportunity to match teams of surveyors with a blend of approaches.

▶ **Public Health Accreditation in the United States**

Public health accreditation programs, specifically in the United States, are now an important driver of improvement (Thielen et al., 2014; Verma & Moran, 2014) and strengthening public health infrastructure (Beatty et al., 2018; Bender et al., 2014; McLees et al., 2014; Singleton et al., 2014); these points are also emphasized in Chapter 11 of this text. Launched in 2011, the Public Health Accreditation Board (PHAB) is leading a voluntary national public health accreditation initiative (Bender et al., 2014; Riley, Bender, & Lownik, 2012) (see the overview section of the Public Health Accreditation Board website). Increasingly more local health departments (LHDs) are seeking PHAB accreditation (Meyerson et al., 2015; Yeager et al., 2016); as of May 2016, 134 LHDs have been awarded accreditation and 176 are undergoing the process (Kronstadt et al., 2016).

The PHAB program has been advocated as a strategy LHDs could use to improve their operations, efficiency, and receive recognition from meeting national industry standards

(Carman, Timsina, & Scutchfield, 2014; Carman & Timsina, 2015). There is recognition of synergies between preparing for PHAB accreditation and the work of other agencies, including: the Centers for Disease Control and Prevention's public health preparedness (Singleton et al., 2014); the Guide to Community Preventive Services (Mercer et al., 2014); collaborating with nonprofit hospitals to conduct community health needs assessments (Singh & Carlton, 2017); and, the Malcolm Baldrige Award for Excellence (Gorenflo et al., 2014). If a LHD would pursue accreditation, or not, has been shown to be determined by the perception as to whether it would impact future funding or performance (Meyerson et al., 2016). Technical assistance was reported as a key initiating factor as well (Meyerson et al., 2015). Prior experience with quality improvement activities has been noted as a contributing factor (Chen et al., 2015; Yeager et al., 2015); conversely, being accredited was seen as strengthening a LHDs quality improvement activities (Madamala et al., 2012). Similarly, if a LHD has completed prerequisites for accreditation and collaborated with other similar bodies then they are orientated to seeking accreditation (Beatty et al., 2015; McLees et al., 2014). Concerns remain, however, for some LHDs who cite the benefits do not match the time, effort, and cost required for accreditation; additionally, some LHDs consider they do not have the capacity to meet the program standards (Beatty et al., 2015; Shah et al., 2015). Rural LHDs, in particular, are identified as being at a disadvantage of lacking staff and resources to do so (Beatty et al., 2018). Accreditation of LHDs in North Carolina is recognized as being amongst the early adopters and best in the United States (Davis et al., 2011; Pestronk et al., 2014; Randolph, Bruckner, & See, 2013). LHDs from across the State conducted activities for improvement, acted on suggestions for improvement and were accredited. They reported improvements in local partnerships as a key benefit from the activity, however many LHDs also identified time and schedule limitations as challenges in the process (Davis et al., 2011). The development of the North Carolina LHD accreditation program is described by Stone and Davis (2012) using a case study format.

▶ Conclusions

Accreditation has been instituted, and has become institutionalized, in health care sectors and jurisdictions around the world. It is a governance strategy that enables health organizations individually and collectively to standardize and self-govern their efforts at improving quality and safety. Accreditation has resulted in improvements and benefits to organization and delivery of care; nevertheless, several significant challenges remain. The sustainability of the current program model and need for further evolution of the component parts, including standards and surveyor workforces, will continue. These are perennial issues inherent in the accreditation, safety, and quality fields. Understanding the role of process and quality indicators within an accreditation program or their relationship to accreditation results is a key one. Differences in findings between them is often associated with unnecessary angst and consternation about the value of accreditation programs. Studies in the field of implementation science are demonstrating how organizational context and human factors matter influence outcomes. It is expected the next few years will shed further light on how and why these variations emerge, and the issue will be reconciled. Clarifying the distinction between the costs associated with implementing safety and quality systems, and those with participation in an accreditation program requires further attention. The difference is confused by many and results in false claims about the cost of accreditation activities. A strength of the field is that accreditation agencies and their partners continue to investigate the organizational and clinical impacts of their programs, and share the knowledge generated.

References

Aboshaiqah, A. E., Alonazi, W. B., & Patalagsa, J. G. (2016). Patients' assessment of quality of care in public tertiary hospitals with and without accreditation: Comparative cross-sectional study. *Journal of Advanced Nursing*, *72*(11), 2750–2761.

Abou Elnour, A., Hernan, A. L., Ford, D., Clark, S., Fuller, J., Johnson, J. K., & Dunbar, J. A. (2014). Surveyors' perceptions of the impact of accreditation on patient safety in general practice. *Medical Journal of Australia*, *201*(3 Suppl), S56–S59.

Accreditation Canada. (2016a). Quality and Safety in Canadian Health Care Organizations: The 2015 Accreditation Canada Report on required organizational practices. Ottawa, Canada: Accreditation Canada.

Accreditation Canada. (2016b). Who we accredit. Retrieved from https://accreditation.ca/who-we-accredit

Accreditation Canada. (2016c). Quality standards. Retrieved from https://accreditation.ca/quality-standards

Accreditation Canada. (2016d). Qmemtum. Retrieved from https://accreditation.ca/qmentum

Agrizzi, D., Agyemang, G., & Jaafaripooyan, E. (2016). Conforming to accreditation in Iranian hospitals. *Accounting Forum*, *40*(2), 106–124.

Alkhenizan, A., & Shaw, C. (2011). Impact of accreditation on the quality of healthcare services: A systematic review of the literature. *Annals of Saudi Medicine*, *31*(4), 407–416.

Almasabi, M., & Thomas, S. (2017). The impact of Saudi hospital accreditation on quality of care: A mixed methods study. *The International Journal of Health Planning and Management*, *32*(4), e261–e278.

Amaral, A., Cuthbertson, B. H. (2016). Balancing quality of care and resource utilisation in acute care hospitals. *BMJ Quality & Safety*, *25*(11), 824.

American Academy of Medical Management. (2018). American Academy of Medical Management: Who we are. Retrieved from http://aammweb.com/about

American Academy of Neurology. (2018). Education offerings. Retrieved from https://www.aan.com

American Academy of Nurse Practitioners. (2018). AANPCB Certification. Retrieved from http://www.aanpcert.org/certs/index

American Association of Tissue Banks. (2018). Accreditation. Retrieved from http://www.aatb.org/?q=content/accreditation-0

American College of Health-System Pharmacists. (2018). ASHP What We Do. Retrieved from http://www.ashp.org/menu/AboutUs/WhatWeDo

American Occupational Therapy Association. (2018). Accreditation. Retrieved from http://www.aota.org/education-careers/accreditation.aspx

Australian Commission on Safety and Quality in Health Care (ACSQHC). Assessment to the NSQHS Standards. Retrieved from https://www.safetyandquality.gov.au

Australian Council on Healthcare Standards (ACHS). (2016). Annual Report 2015/2016. Sydney, Australia: The Australian Council on Healthcare Standards.

Beatty, K. E., Erwin, P. C., Brownson, R. C., Meit, M., & Fey, J. (2018). Public health agency accreditation among rural local health departments: influencers and barriers. *Journal of Public Health Management & Practice*, *24*(1), 49–56.

Beatty, K. E., Mayer, J., Elliott, M., Brownson, R. C., & Wojciehowski, K. (2015). Patterns and predictors of local health department accreditation in Missouri. *Journal of Public Health Management & Practice*, *21*(2), 116–125.

Bender, K. W., Kronstadt, J. L., Wilcox, R., & Tilson, H. H. (2014). Public health accreditation addresses issues facing the public health workforce. *American Journal of Preventive Medicine*, *47*(5 Suppl 3), S346–S351.

Braithwaite, J., Greenfield, D., Westbrook, J., Pawsey, M., Westbrook, M., Gibberd, R., … Lancaster, J. (2010). Health service accreditation as a predictor of clinical and organisational performance: a blinded, random, stratified study. *Quality & Safety in Health Care*, *19*(1), 14–21.

Carman, A. L., & Timsina, L. (2015). Public health accreditation: Rubber stamp or roadmap for improvement. *American Journal of Public Health*, *105*(Suppl 2), S353–S359.

Carman, A. L., Timsina, L. R., & Scutchfield, F. D. (2014). Quality improvement activities of local health departments during the 2008–2010 economic recession. *American Journal of Preventive Medicine*, *46*(2), 171–174.

Chen, L. W., Nguyen, A., Jacobson, J. J., Gupta, N., Bekmuratova, S., & Palm, D. (2015). Relationship between quality improvement implementation and accreditation seeking in local health departments. *American Journal of Public Health*, *105*(Suppl 2), S295–S302.

Commission on Accreditation of Medical Transport Systems. (2018). Welcome to CAMTS. Retrieved from http://www.camts.org/

Council on Podiatric Medical Education. (2018). About the Council. Retrieved from http://www.cpme.org/

Davis, M. V., Cannon, M. M., Stone, D. O., Wood, B. W., Reed, J., & Baker, E. L. (2011). Informing the national public health accreditation movement: Lessons from North Carolina's accredited local health departments. *American Journal of Public Health*, *101*(9), 1543–1548.

Devkaran, S., & O'Farrell, P. (2015). The impact of hospital accreditation on quality measures: An interrupted time series analysis. *BMC Health Services Research*, *15*(1), 137.

Gorenflo, G. G., Klater, D. M., Mason, M., Russo, P., & Rivera, L. (2014). Performance management models for public health: Public Health Accreditation Board

/Baldrige connections, alignment, and distinctions. *Journal of Public Health Management & Practice, 20*(1), 128–134.

Greenfield, D., & Braithwaite, J. (2008). Health sector accreditation research: A systematic review. *International Journal for Quality in Health Care, 20*(3), 172–183.

Greenfield, D., & Braithwaite, J. (2009). Developing the evidence base for accreditation of healthcare organisations: A call for transparency and innovation. *Quality and Safety in Health Care, 18*, 162–163.

Greenfield, D., Braithwaite, J., & Pawsey, M. (2008). Health care accreditation surveyor styles typology. *International Journal of Health Care Quality Assurance, 21*(5), 435–443.

Greenfield, D., Hinchcliff, R., Hogden, A., Mumford, V., Debono, D., Pawsey, M., … Braithwaite, J. (2016). A hybrid health service accreditation program model incorporating mandated standards and continuous improvement: Interview study of multiple stakeholders in Australian health care. *The International Journal of Health Planning and Management, 31*(3), e116–e130.

Greenfield, D., Hinchcliff, R., Pawsey, M., Westbrook, J., & Braithwaite, J. (2013). The public disclosure of accreditation information in Australia: Stakeholder perceptions of opportunities and challenges. *Health Policy, 113*(1–2), 151–159.

Greenfield, D., Hogden A., Hinchcliff R., Mumford V., Pawsey, M., Debono, D., Westbrook, J. I., & Braithwaite, J. (2016). The impact of national accreditation reform on survey reliability: A 2-year investigation of survey coordinators' perspectives. *Journal of Evaluation in Clinical Practice, 22*(5), 662–667.

Greenfield, D., Pawsey, M., & Braithwaite. J. (2012). The role and impact of accreditation on the healthcare revolution [O papel e o impacto da acreditação na revolução da atenção à saúde], *Acreditação, 1*(2), 64–77.

Greenfield, D., Pawsey, M., Naylor, J. M., & Braithwaite, J. (2008). Improving the reliability of an accreditation program: using research to educate and to align practice. In *Conference proceedings: ISQua 2008, twenty-fifth International Safety and Quality Conference: Healthcare quality and safety: Meeting the next challenges,* Copenhagen, Denmark, 19–22 October 2008.

Greenfield, D., Pawsey, M., Naylor, J., & Braithwaite, J. (2009). Are healthcare accreditation surveys reliable? *International Journal of Health Care Quality Assurance, 22*(2), 105–116.

Haj-Ali, W., Bou Karroum, L., Natafgi, N., & Kassak, K. (2014). Exploring the relationship between accreditation and patient satisfaction—the case of selected Lebanese hospitals. *International Journal of Health Policy and Management, 3*(6), 341–346.

Haute Autorité de Santé. (2015). Healthcare organisations accreditation programme in France. Retrieved from http://www.has-sante.fr

Hinchcliff, R., Greenfield, D., Moldovan, M., Westbrook, J. I., Pawsey, M., Mumford, V., & Braithwaite, J. (2013). Narrative synthesis of health service accreditation literature. *BMJ Quality and Safety, 21*(12), 979–991.

Hinchcliff, R., Greenfield D., Westbrook, J. I., Pawsey, M., Mumford, V., & Braithwaite, J. (2013). Stakeholder perspectives on implementing accreditation programs: a qualitative study of enabling factors. *BMC Health Services Research, 13*, 437.

Ingram, R. C., Bender, K., Wilcox, R., & Kronstadt, J. (2014). A consensus-based approach to national public health accreditation. *Journal of Public Health Management & Practice, 20*(1), 9–13.

ISQua. (2018). International Accreditation Programme (IAP) Awards. Retrieved from http://www.isqua.org/accreditation-iap/what-is-the-iap

Jaafaripooyan, E. (2014). Potential benefits and downsides of external healthcare performance evaluation systems: Real-life perspectives on Iranian Hospital Evaluation and Accreditation Program. *International Journal of Health Policy and Management, 3*(4), 191–198.

Kronstadt, J., Meit, M., Siegfried, A., Nicolaus, T., Bender, K., & Corso, L. (2016). Evaluating the impact of National Public Health Department Accreditation—United States, 2016. *MMWR Morbidity & Mortality Weekly Report, 65*(31), 803–806.

Lancaster, J., Braithwaite, J., & Greenfield, D. (2010). Benefits of participating in accreditation surveying. *International Journal for Healthcare Quality Assurance, 23*(2), 141–152.

Lanteigne, G., & Bouchard, C. (2016). Is the introduction of an accreditation program likely to generate organization-wide quality, change and learning? *The International Journal of Health Planning and Management, 31*(3), e175–e191.

Madamala, K., Sellers, K., Beitsch, L. M., Pearsol, J., & Jarris, P. (2012). Quality improvement and accreditation readiness in state public health agencies. *Journal of Public Health Management & Practice, 18*(1), 9–18.

McLees, A. W., Thomas, C. W., Nawaz, S., Young, A. C., Rider, N., & Davis, M. (2014). Advances in public health accreditation readiness and quality improvement: Evaluation findings from the National Public Health Improvement Initiative. *Journal of Public Health Management & Practice, 20*(1), 29–35.

Melo, S. (2016). The impact of accreditation on healthcare quality improvement: A qualitative case study. *Journal of Health Organization and Management, 30*(8), 1242–1258.

Mercer, S. L., Banks, S. M., Verma, P., Fisher, J. S., Corso, L. C., & Carlson, V. (2014). Guiding the way to public health improvement: Exploring the connections between The Community Guide's Evidence-Based Interventions and health department accreditation standards. *Journal of Public Health Management & Practice, 20*(1), 104–110.

Meyerson, B. E., Barnes, P. R., King, J., Degi, L. S., Halverson, P. K., & Polmanski, H. F. (2015). Measuring accreditation activity and progress: Findings from a survey of Indiana local health Departments, 2013. *Public Health Reports, 130*(5), 447–452.

Meyerson, B. E., King, J., Comer, K., Liu, S. S., & Miller, L. (2016). It's not just a yes or no answer: Expressions of local health department accreditation. *Frontiers in Public Health, 4,* 21.

Mitchell, J. I., Izad S., Seyed A., & Kuziemsky, C. (2015). Governance standards: A roadmap for increasing safety at care transitions. *Healthcare Management Forum, 28*(1), 28–33.

Mohebbifar, R., Barnes, P. R., King, J., Degi, L. S., Halverson, P. K., & Polmanski, H. F. (2017). Association between hospital accreditation and patient satisfaction: A survey in the western province of Iran. *Bangladesh Journal of Medical Science, 16*(1), 77–84.

Mumford, V., Forde, K., Greenfield, D., Hinchcliff, R., & Braithwaite, J. (2013). Health services accreditation: What is the evidence that the benefits justify the costs? *International Journal for Quality in Health Care, 25*(5), 606–620.

Mumford, V., Greenfield, D., Hinchcliff, R., Moldovan, M., Forde, K., Westbrook, J. I., & Braithwaite, J. (2013). Economic evaluation of Australian acute care accreditation (ACCREDIT-CBA (Acute)): Study protocol for a mixed-method research project. *BMJ Open, 3*(2).

Mumford, V., Greenfield, D., Hogden, A., Debono, D., Gospodarevskaya, E., Forde, K., Westbrook, J., & Braithwaite, J. (2014). Disentangling quality and safety indicator data: A longitudinal, comparative study of hand hygiene compliance and accreditation outcomes in 96 Australian hospitals. *BMJ Open, 4*(9).

Mumford, V., Greenfield, D., Hogden, A., Forde, K., Westbrook, J., & Braithwaite, J. (2015). Counting the costs of accreditation in acute care: An activity-based costing approach. *BMJ Open, 5*(9).

Mumford, V., Reeve, R., Greenfield, D., Forde, K., Westbrook, J., & Braithwaite, J. (2015). Is accreditation linked to hospital infection rates? A 4-year, data linkage study of Staphylococcus aureus rates and accreditation scores in 77 Australian acute hospitals. *International Journal for Quality in Health Care, 27*(6), 479–485.

Pestronk, R. M., Benjamin, G. C., Bohlen, S. A., Drabczyk, A. L., & Jarris, P. E. (2014). Accreditation: On target. *Journal of Public Health Management and Practice, 20*(1), 152–155.

Plebani, M. (2001). Role of inspectors in external review mechanisms: Criteria for selection, training and appraisal. *Clinica Chimica Acta, 309*(2), 147–154.

Randolph, G. D., Bruckner, J., & See, C. H. (2013). Quality improvement in North Carolina's public health departments. *North Carolina Medical Journal, 74*(2), 137–141.

Riley, W. J., Bender, K., & Lownik, E. (2012). Public health department accreditation implementation: Transforming public health department performance. *American Journal of Public Health, 102*(2), 237–242.

Riley, W. J., Lownik, E. M., Scutchfield, F. D., Mays, G. P., Corso, L. C., & Beitsch, L. M. (2012). Public health department accreditation: Setting the research agenda. *American Journal of Preventive Medicine, 42*(3), 263–271.

Sax, S., & Marx, M. (2014). Local perceptions on factors influencing the introduction of international health-care accreditation in Pakistan. *Health Policy and Planning, 29*(8), 1021–1030.

Shah, G. H., Leep, C. J., Ye, J., Sellers, K., Liss-Levinson, R., & Williams, K. S. (2015). Public Health Agencies' level of engagement in and perceived barriers to PHAB National Voluntary Accreditation. *Journal of Public Health Management & Practice, 21*(2), 107–115.

Shaw, C. (2015). Accreditation is not a stand-alone solution. *Eastern Mediterranean Health Journal, 21*(3), 226–231.

Shearing, C., & Wood, J. (2003). Nodal governance, democracy and the new denizens: Challenging the Westphalian ideal. *Journal of Law and Society, 30,* 400–419.

Singh, S. R., & Carlton, E. L. (2017). Exploring the link between completion of accreditation prerequisites and local health departments' decision to collaborate with tax-exempt hospitals around the community health assessment. *Journal of Public Health Management & Practice, 23*(2), 138–147.

Singleton, C. M., Corso, L., Koester, D., Carlson, V., Bevc, C. A., & Davis, M. V. (2014). Accreditation and emergency preparedness: Linkages and opportunities for leveraging the connections. *Journal of Public Health Management & Practice, 20*(1), 119–124.

Sparrow, M. (2000). *The regulatory craft controlling risks, solving problems, and managing compliance.* Washington, D.C.: Brookings Institute Press.

Stone, D., & Davis, M. V. (2012). North Carolina local health department accreditation program. In C. P. McLaughlin, J. K. Johnson, & W. A. Sollecito, *Implementing continuous quality improvement in health care: A global casebook.* Burlington, MA: Jones & Bartlett Learning.

Teymourzadeh, E., Ramezani, M., Arab, M., Foroushani, A. R., & Sari, A. A. (2016). Surveyor management of hospital accreditation program: A thematic analysis conducted in Iran. *Iranian Red Crescent Medical Journal, 18*(5), e30309.

The Joint Commission. (2016). America's hospitals: Improving quality and safety 2016 annual report. Oakbrook Terrace, IL: Author.

The Joint Commission. (2018). What is accreditation? Retrieved from https://www.jointcommission.org /achievethegoldseal.aspx

Thielen, L., Dauer, E., Burkhardt, D., Lampe, S., & VanRaemdonck, L. (2014). An examination of state laws and policies regarding public health agency accreditation prerequisites. *Journal of Public Health Management & Practice, 20*(1), 111–118.

Triantafillou, P. (2014). Against all odds? Understanding the emergence of accreditation of the Danish hospitals. *Social Science & Medicine, 101,* 78–85.

U.S. Public Health Accreditation Board. PHAB. (2014). Standards and Measures, version 1.5.

Verma, P., & Moran, J. (2014). Sustaining a quality improvement culture in local health departments applying for accreditation. *Journal of Public Health Management & Practice, 20*(1), 43–48.

Yan, Y., & Kung, C. (2015). The impact of hospital accreditation system: Perspective of organizational learning. *Health, 7,* 1081–1089.

Yan, Y., & Kung, C. (2016). Investigation of hospital accreditation awareness and organizational learning promotion from nursing staff perspective. *Arabian Journal of Business Management Review,* S1:007.

Yeager, V. A., Ferdinand, A. O., Beitsch, L. M., & Menachemi, N. (2015). Local public health department characteristics associated with likelihood to participate in national accreditation. *American Journal of Public Health, 105*(8), 1653–1659.

Yeager, V. A., Ye, J., Kronstadt, J., Robin, N., Leep, C. J., & Beitsch, L. M. (2016). National voluntary public health accreditation: Are more local health departments intending to take part? *Journal of Public Health Management & Practice, 22*(2), 149–156.

CHAPTER 13

Quality Improvement in Low- and Middle-Income Countries

Lisa R. Hirschhorn and Rohit Ramaswamy

We need a quality revolution.

—**Precious Matsoso**, Director-General, National Department of Health, South Africa

There has been a growing recognition over the last few decades of the importance of the quality gap in health care and public health programs delivery in many low- and middle-income countries. This gap is critical because poor outcomes are still seen in many conditions (such as maternal and child health, HIV, TB, and noncommunicable chronic diseases), despite significant progress over the past 2 decades in expanding access to these services and work to implement evidence-based interventions known to save lives and increased community access to and utilization of health care (Akachi & Kruk, 2017). This finding of increased access and use with limited benefits is largely due to the quality gap, similar to challenges described in the higher income countries. For example, policies to increase demand for and access to care such as the Janani Suraksha Yojana (JSY) in India that provides cash to women delivering in facilities have been very successful in getting women to facilities, but have failed to reduce maternal and neonatal mortality because of poor quality of care in the facilities (Randive, Diwan, & De Costa, 2013). In this chapter, we discuss some of the growing knowledge and persisting challenges in measuring quality and applying Quality Improvement (QI) methods to solve health problems in low- and middle-income settings, as well as recent successes and areas where more learning is needed.

▶ Variation in Health Outcomes

While multiple factors impact how long individuals live, differences in the quality of the health care delivery system and the care it produces are a major contributor to the variation in life expectancy between countries with similar income levels. Life expectancy and a nation's economic level are not always correlated, partly because of differences in both the level and priorities of funding needed to strengthen the primary care-based

TABLE 13.1 Comparisons of Health Care Spending, Under-five Mortality, and Correct Treatment for Diarrhea in Cambodia and Philippines

Country	Per capita spending on health care (in U.S. dollars)	Percentage of children getting correct diarrhea treatment	Under-five mortality/1,000 live births
Cambodia	30.60	52%	29
Philippines	51.40	53%	28

(Primary Health Care Performance Initiative, n.d.)
Data from Primary Health Care Performance Initiative. (n.d.). Primary Health Care Performance Initiative. Retrieved July 31, 2016, from http://phcperformanceinitiative.org/sites/default/files/PHCPI Two Page Overview.pdf

health care delivery systems that are critical to saving lives. For example, the United States and Chile have about the same life expectancy (78 years), although their populations experience a threefold difference in their average per capita income. The need to ensure effective use of health care funds is also apparent from variations in health outcomes and improvement in countries with similar levels of health care investments. For example, under-five mortality rates and quality of diarrheal care are similar in Cambodia and in the Philippines despite much higher per capita spending on health care in the Philippines (TABLE 13.1). This variability supports the knowledge that simply increasing spending will not bridge the gap between desired outcomes and those achieved.

While the lack of adequate resources do contribute to differential health outcomes between higher- and lower-income countries, the inability of health systems and care delivery processes in facilities and communities to deliver care that meets the six dimensions of quality (safety, effectiveness, patient-centeredness, timeliness, efficiency, and equity) defined by the Institute of Medicine is a greater factor in many countries (Das & Hammer, 2014; Kruk, Chukwuma, & Leslie, 2017; Singh et al., 2016). This has led to the realization that effective and sustainable improvements in population health will require the use of QI methods in health care and public health systems to ensure the delivery of care that meets the needs of individuals and populations now and in the future.

▶ New Challenges and Opportunities for QI

In addition to the need to address gaps in health outcomes and care quality that have persisted for decades, there are a number of emerging challenges that have provided more reasons for increasing the use of QI. First, the epidemiology of global burden of disease is changing—arising from scale-up of effective HIV treatment, reduction of other communicable diseases, rural to urban population shifts, and a rising burden of noncommunicable chronic diseases including diabetes and cardiovascular disease (GBD Collaborators, 2016). This shift has resulted in increased need to build integrated, people-centered health care requiring facilities and systems to establish resilient processes for delivering comprehensive quality health care that meets the evolving range of population health needs including longitudinal care, coordinating referrals to specialists and hospitals as needed, and integrating health promotion and treatment (Bitton et al., 2017). Second, there has been a push toward sharing or shifting tasks, both from specialist to generalist medical staff and from facility-based health providers to community health workers. These changes are designed to increase access by expanding the range of providers, who need to be supported to deliver quality care (Perry, Zulliger, & Rogers, 2014). Third, international goals, such as the health-related sustainable development goal (SDG) "to ensure healthy lives and promote well-being at all ages" (Paule et al., 2017), and the new global HIV targets of 90-90-90 (90% of people with HIV aware of their diagnosis, 90% in care, and 90% with effective treatment defined as viral suppression) are only achievable through systematic improvements in the quality of care. To reach the SDG targets, there is recognition that countries need universal health coverage, which also means universally high-quality care to achieve better outcomes and quality of life regardless of setting. Finally, the Ebola outbreak in 2014 represents another type of challenge because it highlighted the dangers and costs of poor quality of care as well as the often neglected quality domain of safety for patients and their providers (Boozary, Farmer, & Jha, 2014).

▶ QI Frameworks and Methods

There are a number of frameworks and approaches to improve quality that can be implemented in low- and middle-income countries, with a growing evidence base from experiences at the national and local levels in these countries. Over 50 years ago, Donabedian (1988, 2005) developed a model for assessing the quality of health care based on an analysis of the *structure* (i.e., the context in which

health care is delivered and the systems), the *processes* of delivery, and the *outcome*s that are achieved. In 2007, the World Health Organization (WHO) developed a framework designed to help countries strengthen the health systems needed to improve population health. This framework was based on "six pillars" of inputs: health services, information, workforce, commodities, financing, and leadership/governance (WHO, 2007). The WHO framework tracks the link between these important resources through quality to improved population and individual health. Recognizing that simply improving the infrastructure to deliver care does not guarantee the improved quality and quantity of health that are the goals of health care systems (Kruk et al., 2016); more recent frameworks targeting low- and middle-income countries have focused on the processes of delivery of care and systems required to ensure that delivery is people-centered and responsive to the needs and priorities of the communities served (Primary Health Care Performance Initiative, n.d.; WHO, 2015). Only through improving all aspects of the health system—improved delivery of health services, timely availability of the right commodities, adequate financial and human resources, and appropriate leadership and policies—can quality be ensured and health outcomes achieved. This will likely be achieved by a combination of more locally targeted QI, such as value mapping through Lean (see Chapter 5), and supporting supervision combined with broader, national-level system redesign and national policies and strategies to support governance for quality (Ramaswamy et al., 2017; Magge et al., 2014; WHO, 2017b).

QI methods, which emphasize the use of data to inform systematic approaches to reduce variation in the quality of care across varied contexts, are well suited to help advance the work to ensure quality. These methods have been used extensively to strengthen systems in higher-resource settings (Berwick, 1996) and their applicability in strengthening health systems in resource-limited settings is widely recognized (Leatherman et al., 2010). The remarkable improvements in maternal and child health described in Brazil (Macinko, Harris, & Rocha, 2017), Rwanda (Farmer et al., 2013), Costa Rica (Pesec et al., 2017), and a number of other countries (Moucheraud et al., 2016; Ruducha et al., 2017) have been attributed to systems strengthening work both at the macro level (stronger governance and leadership, policies and standards, adequate funding, established processes and protocols for care, supporting expanded access to quality delivery of evidence based interventions known to save lives, etc.) and improving quality at the facility and subnational levels through local QI programs and projects. One clear example is observed by comparing under-five mortality rates in low- and middle-income countries between 1990 and 2016. For example, in Sub-Saharan African countries , under-five mortality rates fell from 183 per 1,000 live births in 1990 to 79 in 2016 (UNICEF, 2018). (Please see UNICEF website that is cited here for annual updates of under-five mortality and other health indices by country and region.) Despite this progress, widespread adoption of QI and accompanying quality assurance and quality control into national policies and governance as well as global and national investments and implementation of improvement efforts at the level of community health systems has been slow. Moreover, the capability to make improvements between countries and within and across income levels has been limited to date.

The most popular QI methods to address process and local system change include those that have been defined and illustrated in a broad range of settings throughout this text, such as the Model for Improvement, Rapid Cycle Change (Plan-Do-Study-Act [PDSA]), Quality Improvement Collaboratives, Lean, and Six Sigma (Chapter 5). The optimal method to use depends on the goals and contextual factors, and there is little evaluation evidence to definitively recommend one method over another. In the sections that follow we briefly describe these methods and provide some examples of their use in low- and middle-income countries.

Quality Improvement Principles

While there is growing work to improve the policies, strategies, and macro-level approaches to improve quality, the fundamental assumption behind the QI approaches highlighted in this chapter is that work in any system is conducted through *processes*. One definition of process is "a collection of activities that takes one or more kinds of input and creates an output that is of value to the customer" (Hammer & Champy, 1993). For example, health care workers at a clinic follow a process of care from registration, to examination, to diagnosis, to treatment, to discharge, and billing. A community-level Ebola eradication effort might involve processes related to case finding, infection control, prevention activities, transport to clinics, and care. These QI methods, are particularly applicable to countries where progress in outcomes has not been seen despite successful investments in building health care facilities to ensure geographic access (Das, 2011; Gage et al., 2017). Transforming a system, regardless of the setting, therefore requires improving processes. Quantitative methods for understanding and improving processes, including the use of process behavior charts, play a central role in QI and were described in Chapter 4.

This focus on processes has three implications:

1. QI often comes about by changing components of or the whole process, not only a single individual step. For example, delays in seeing patients may come from inefficiencies in several interrelated process steps, so addressing just one step is not likely to result in significant

improvement and may even make the problem worse.

2. All processes have a customer targeted to receive their outputs. In the health system context, depending on the process, the customer could be a service provider, the recipient of a service such as a patient, or a community member. Therefore, at the individual or population levels, QI should result in a change that ultimately improves the targeted outcomes for a person or a community. Keeping the focus on the customer helps define the goals of an effective QI effort.

3. The goal of QI is to change the process in a way that adds value to the customer or patient and reduces variation. In QI terminology, *value* is the opposite of *waste*, which refers to process activities that add no benefit to a patient's care or experience. Value can be defined as better health outcomes (including patient-reported outcomes) through higher quality of care, but there are other ways in which value could be measured. Reduced delays, fewer errors, respectful treatment of patients, fewer contact points are all examples of how QI can add value and increase safety. Often adding more people or building more facilities are proposed as improvement solutions. But these kinds of solutions may not always add value because they may just support the workings of a bad process. A commonly quoted aphorism in QI states that "*all improvement is change, but not all change is improvement.*" QI involves changing the process in ways that adds value from the perspective of the targeted customer (see Chapter 14).

Examples of Effective QI Implementation in Low- and Middle-Income Countries

The Model for Improvement, PDSA, and Quality Improvement Collaboratives

The Model for Improvement, developed by the Associates in Process Improvement, helps to structure the thinking and activities that are needed to improve a health care system or specific process (Langley et al., 2009). The model is designed to help teams and organizations determine where to start, what to do, and how to measure change (the three basic questions of the inquiry component). The actual improvement work is then done typically through the application of PDSA cycles (**FIGURE 13.1**). These cycles, which promote the

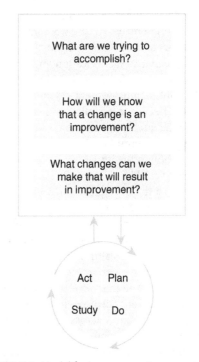

FIGURE 13.1 Model for Improvement

Reproduced from Langley, G.L., Nolan, K.M., Nolan, T.W., Norman, C.L. and Provost, L.P. (2009), The Improvement Guide: A Practical Approach to Enhancing Organizational Performance, 2nd ed., Jossey Bass, San Francisco.

concept of small, iterative tests of change to assess whether they can become part of a larger change package that can be integrated into the system, are core to most process-focused QI.

The model has also been implemented across facilities targeting a common goal using Quality Improvement Collaboratives in a number of low- and middle-income countries. The Collaboratives are organized into "learning sessions" where groups are trained in the basics of the Model for Improvement and share their improvement results and learning. In between these sessions are "action periods," where the groups, supported by individual and group coaching sessions led by QI experts, use PDSA cycles to test improvements in their facilities. For example, in Ghana, Project Fives Alive! was implemented as a series of Collaboratives involving 134 hospitals. By 2014, collaborative participants had collectively achieved a 31% decrease in under-five mortality and a 37% reduction in postneonatal infant mortality. As a result of the learning, a number of new changes to maternal care were introduced across many of the participating facilities, such as early pregnancy identification and immediate postnatal care (Singh et al., 2016).

Quality Improvement Collaboratives have also been successfully implemented to improve the quality of home-based care delivered by community health workers in South Africa, although the impact on quality of care has been variable (Horwood et al., 2015). Horwood and colleagues (2015) described the successful adaptation and implementation of a Learning Collaborative in four QI projects led by local teams and including community-based health workers trained in QI, often supported by facility-based staff. A range of improvements were seen in targeted areas, including effective spread of HIV treatment clubs to expand access to treatment in South Africa. They emphasized the need for initial and ongoing adaptation of the methods to reflect local context and capacity, including simplifying data systems, adjusting QI training methods, and motivation techniques

(see Chapter 14 for further discussion of Quality Improvement Collaboratives).

Lean Management Systems

The Lean paradigm, adapted from manufacturing, is based on the belief that improving a health care system involves the reduction of *waste* in the system (Joosten, Bongers, & Janssen, 2009). (See Chapter 5 for a more detailed description of Lean.) Lean approaches are often used to improve the efficiency of nonclinical processes such as registration, admission, or billing. Although many of these processes may not have a direct impact on patient outcomes, they can improve patient experience and improve facility throughput allowing greater number of patients to be seen when the clinic is open.

One of the simplest and most often used Lean tool is "5S" (standing for "sort, set in order, shine, standardize, and sustain"), which is a systematic approach to clean and organize the workplace and is a common starting point for more advanced Lean projects. 5S has been used in facilities in Brazil, India, Jordan, Senegal, Sri Lanka, Ghana, and Tanzania and has been shown to produce improvements in efficiency (e.g., reduced turnaround time for procedures, or reduction in-patient waiting time), safety (e.g., reduction in postsurgical infections), and patient centeredness (e.g., reduction in time spent on activities other than patient care) (Kanamori et al., 2016). The approach has been adopted as part of national QI strategies in many of these countries. Lean principles were also applied in a hospital in Ghana to improve the admissions process while educating the team about Lean principles (Carter et al., 2012). Overall, the project successfully engaged the team in identifying and working to improve processes. There were also other lessons learned that were important to adaption for further use in similar settings; these included the recognition that implementation required not just training, but, like most QI work, leadership engagement; that tools varied in their feasibility and value; and that the specific type of data required depended on the stage of implementation.

Value chain mapping is another Lean management tool that has also been effectively implemented in a nonprofit-run network of maternal health facilities to map care and identify improvement projects, as well as patient-centered value mapping to improve pediatric HIV care in Togo, although scale-up to national coverage of this approach has not been described (Ramaswamy et al., 2017; Fiori et al., 2016).

Six Sigma

The focus of the Six Sigma QI paradigm is on *eliminating defects and reducing variability* (Trusko et al., 2007). A defect is defined as an outcome that does not meet the requirements of its customers. Six Sigma–based approaches have been used in Ghana as part of an integrated improvement strategy that included clinical skills strengthening, leadership development and to reduce maternal and neonatal mortality in tertiary hospitals (Ramaswamy et al., 2015). The QI approach resulted in a 22.4% reduction in maternal mortality from 2007 to 2011 at one of the largest government hospitals in Ghana, despite a 50% increase in deliveries and a significant increase in mothers admitted with obstetric complications (Srofenyoh et al., 2016). The program was also shown to be highly cost effective (Goodman et al., 2017). Cost effectiveness is another example of QI value and an important component of the triple aim (Berwick, Nolan, & Whittington, 2008) and more recently, the quadruple aim (Bodenheimer & Sinsky, 2014) of health care described in Chapters 1 and 2.

Other Approaches to Improving Care Delivery Quality in Resource-Limited Settings

In addition to the process-focused QI methods described above, there is growing evidence that mentoring or coaching, when done well and integrated into supportive supervision,

can be an important component of improving provider competence to ensure the highest quality of care (Magge et al., 2014; Lazzerini et al., 2017). This has been seen in a range of low- and middle-income settings, including childhood care in Rwanda (Magge et al., 2014), birth practices in India (Marx-Delaney et al., 2017) and management of malaria in Uganda (Mbonye et al., 2014). However, there is significant work needed to understand why it also can be ineffective and how to ensure that individuals providing the supervision follow core principles of supportive supervision and measure the effectiveness of the processes applied (Oursler et al., 2011; Rowe et al., 2005; Leslie et al., 2016). Given the system challenges in many resource-limited settings, one approach that has been recommended is integrating QI coaching with clinical supervision, building capacity for teams to address the systems gaps during more traditional facility and provider support (Mbonye et al., 2014). This approach to coaching also can include working at district levels to build capacity to understand and address higher levels gaps, which require action and leadership at a national or subnational level. One relevant HIV example, is presented by viral load testing; if it is not being done because there is inadequate capacity or stock-out of reagents at the district level, then systems strengthening from the top down is needed, as well as coaching to providers around the timing and performance of viral loads.

Another approach to improve quality used in lower- (and higher-) resourced settings is the use of checklists to improve adherence to protocols (see Chapters 1, 4, and 8). The WHO Safe Childbirth Checklist (SCC) was developed to help birth attendants deliver essential birth practices known to prevent maternal and neonatal harm (Spector et al., 2013). However, as noted in Chapter 4, checklists are tools to be used as part of a larger QI process, and their use alone may not ensure improvement. For example, the Better Birth Program integrated a peer-coaching strategy to support consistent use of the SCC to improve the quality of facility-based delivery in resource-limited settings. Implementation of the program in a number of settings, including India and Namibia, resulted in improvement in delivery of these practices and, in Namibia, in selected outcomes (Kabongo et al., 2017; Marx-Delaney et al., 2017). Similar work has been shown to be effective in improving the safety and outcomes of surgical care across a range of settings (Haynes et al. 2009).

Other interventions have included development of protocols and job aids for common conditions, such as those that are leading causes of childhood, maternal, and neonatal mortality; financial levers such as performance-based financing; quality control; and broader system strengthening (Gergen et al., 2017; Spector et al., 2012; Bryce et al., 2005). These are not within the scope of this chapter but are highly recommended for further study.

Challenges and Proposed Solutions to Scaling Up Effective QI in Low- and Middle-Income Settings

Despite the increase in QI work in recent decades in many resource-constrained settings, the evidence for short term impact and longer term sustainability is variable (Schouten et al., 2008; Franco & Marquez, 2011). There remain a number of challenges at the national and local levels in implementing effective QI programs. These challenges do not suggest the need for completely new QI approaches. Instead what is needed is the adaptation of models that have been successfully implemented in better resourced countries and increasingly in resource-constrained settings to take into consideration the particular contexts, barriers, and constraints of individual countries that prevent delivery of quality care. In a recent review article, Heiby (2014) identified a number of challenges to implementing QI programs in Africa. These include the following:

Focus on inputs and outcomes instead of on processes. While the primary activities of QI methods discussed are focused on making processes better, many health leaders and donors still focus on strengthening the inputs of the health care system and on measuring the resulting outcomes at the health service level (coverage of targeted interventions), the population level (e.g., maternal and under-five mortality, rates of new HIV infections). While inputs are clearly important, large gaps in the performance of systems have been observed even when needed resources are present (Das et al., 2012). For example, in Zambia, researchers found that even when no supplies were needed to deliver quality care to children with fever, the technical quality, defined as following national guidelines for integrated management of childhood illness, was still not delivered (Lunze et al., 2017). A study of delays in the interval between the decision to perform an emergency cesarean section and when the baby was delivered (the "decision-to-delivery interval" or DDI) in a tertiary hospital in Ghana indicated a median DDI of 195 minutes compared to the 30-minute benchmark upheld by most high-resource countries.

Challenges to measurement. Even when greater attention is paid to processes, measuring process quality is often not easy and measuring outcomes valued by customers such as experiential quality and motivation is even more difficult. These measures often require new data collection methods, and the current information systems in many low- and middle-income countries do not provide the necessary infrastructure for routine data collection of needed indicators of quality care (see Chapter 4). For example, measurement of provider competency (e.g., the extent to which providers adhere to recognized protocols of care) is critical but is not routinely captured.

Measurement can use a range of methods including direct observation, chart review, vignettes, patient interviews, simulations, and standardized patients (Das et al., 2012), but many of these are resource intensive and are too complicated to collect, and no global recommendations exist at the time of this publication in 2018. These are also true for measures aligned with Institute of Medicine dimensions, such as timeliness (e.g., waiting time to surgery once the need for an operation has been established). In addition, there is also a rising recognition that transforming care in low- and middle-income countries should involve people-centered health services able to meet the expectations and the needs of individuals and their communities (Bitton et al., 2017; Srivastava et al., 2015; WHO, 2015). There is therefore also a need to measure and improve experiential quality in addition to clinical and operational process measures to ensure the critical quality domain of patient-centeredness. Work to improve routine health management information systems, identify core sets of indicators to measure quality within and across countries beyond inputs, and the growth of field-based mobile data collection systems are promising trends that can improve the quality and ease of collecting process data (Pavluck et al., 2014; WHO, 2017a).

Lack of good guidance on how to implement improvement solutions in a way that fits the context of sites and regions. Even where evidence exists on the evidence-based interventions that can reduce morbidity and mortality and potential solutions to improve critical processes in health or community systems, these are often challenging to implement and sustain. The growing fields of implementation and improvement science (Geng, Peiris, & Kruk, 2017; Marshall, Pronovost, & Dixon-Woods, 2013) offers the tools and frameworks to address these challenges (see Chapter 3), but the field is still emerging in low-resource settings. There is a need for further research on how models and frameworks of implementation science developed and used in high-resource countries translate to low-resource environments, how instruments to measure contexts and barriers and facilitators to implementation apply in these environments and how context-specific implementation guidance can be developed. The need for this work is being recognized more widely, but there is much work still needed to produce the actionable knowledge needed in 2018 and beyond (Ridde, 2016).

Limited documentation of implementation of QI in low-resource settings. Even when effective implementation of QI initiatives takes place, it is often hard to find out what happened because of the lack of available documentation. The Standards for Quality Improvement Reporting Excellence (SQUIRE) guidelines for documenting QI projects were developed in 2008 and updated in 2016 to make them more applicable to practitioners. But there is still a perception that these guidelines are primarily meant for researchers who are publishing QI research and are not widely used to document practice applications, even in high-resource settings. Documentation of the everyday implementation of QI programs at national, state, or local levels—including how QI projects were selected, standard methodologies adapted for use, which stakeholders and leaders were engaged in the process, what changes were tested, and what challenges existed to implementation, scale, and sustainability—are critical for building up a compendium of practice-based evidence of how to make QI work in resource-constrained environments.

Lack of integration of QI into health worker and public health training programs. QI is not only a set of tools and methods; as described in Chapter 1, it also encompasses a QI philosophy, which includes many of the following concepts. Successful QI practitioners have a problem-solving mindset, a willingness to experiment and learn from failure, a passion for bringing about change in organizations and systems, and the ability to engage diverse stakeholders with differing agendas and priorities. The capacity and bandwidth of health care workers, managers and leadership to translate data into action in general represents an ongoing challenge and a need for changing how health workers are trained. A government committed to embedding QI into the health care system, needs to prioritize the development of health care workers and managers to be able to embed QI-trained professionals at all levels and the resources needed to enable them to use these skills. Cadres include senior leaders who can act as champions and drive systemic change while establishing a learning organizational culture; QI professionals who can guide teams through the technical components of the methodologies; front line staff who can be part of QI teams and practice every day, small-scale improvements; and the broader community. Building these capacities will require a number of approaches: preservice training for health care workers, experiential learning that provides them the opportunity to practice and hone their skills, advanced training for improvement coaches, and on-the-job training for leaders and front-line staff. Multilevel training efforts in Kenya and Ghana have been shown to be effective but these programs are rare and have not scaled up to national coverage (Ramaswamy et al., 2015). As online training becomes routine, there is now a possibility to train a larger number of practitioners worldwide,

but building deep QI capability will still initially require coaches on the ground to help translate new theory to meaningful context-relevant practice and this still remains a challenge.

Lack of integration of QI into broader health system strengthening activities. In many resource-limited settings, the challenges faced in implementing QI are no different from the challenges faced by the system in delivering quality services. For example, the weak information systems that make it difficult to collect process data for QI also make it difficult to collect data needed for patient care and effective management. Focusing on strengthening systems for QI alone without integrating with broader health systems strengthening work is unlikely to lead to successful sustainable results. Similarly, health systems strengthening that solely focuses on improving inputs and coverage without measuring and improving quality will also fail to provide the population health gains needed.

Lack of an overall national strategy that ensures learning from and overall coordination of QI to achieve national scale-up of QI. Ultimately, the effectiveness of a national QI program depends on national leadership and a policy and strategy that provides both top-down direction and resources and the ability to innovate and learn from the more local work. This approach is needed to ensure that local improvements that offer promise for broader impact are understood to inform potential scale and work needed to sustain these improvements over time, while ensuring that local efforts reflect national and subnational priorities. Rwanda is an unusual example of a country that has established a culture of quality and learning led by national and local leadership, which has resulted in broadly improved health outcomes (Farmer et al., 2013). In response to the challenges faced by other countries, the WHO recently produced a roadmap for countries to develop these strategies (WHO, 2017b), but this can still be a tough balance to strike. If the projects are not relevant to local staff, then it may be difficult to get buy in. On the other hand, if local priorities are not linked to national strategies and policies, QI teams may spend time and resources on "feel-good projects" that do not bring about changes in critical outcomes. Similarly, some change requires higher level resources and direction to address longer term changes needed to ensure quality such as reorganization of models of care, reform of preservice training and changes in health care funding.

The WHO has been working to develop guidance for national governments to demonstrate how to develop these policies and strategies and other organizations have already been supporting country-led work in a number of low-resource settings (WHO, 2017b). National deployment of any approach will require multilevel capacity building, which, in the absence of commitment of resources from within the country and from partners, is difficult to carry out. Taking lessons from the successes and failures of national quality strategies from high-resource countries and growing work in lower-resourced countries will inform how countries can be more effective in integrating quality and QI into national policies and strategies and improving quality and generate the knowledge needed to accelerate the work within their own borders, the region, and globally.

For a detailed case study of the challenges and lessons learned from a real-world application of QI principles in a resource-limited setting, readers are referred to a case study analysis of a malaria control application in Ghana (Agyepong, Sollecito, & McLaughlin, 2012).

▶ Conclusions

There has been an exciting increase in the focus on quality as core to achieving better and more equitable population health, more efficiently, effectively, and being more responsive to the needs and goals of the communities served. There is a clear recognition that QI methods targeting process changes at the local level are a critical part of the toolkit that resource-limited countries need to facilitate change at the community, facility, and local levels. This can be achieved by adapting lessons learned in higher resourced settings and increasingly from other lower resourced settings. However, this process-focused QI work must be integrated into top-down national level policies and strategies articulating priorities, targeting broader system change and ensuring resources and leadership needed to ensure sustainability of change, resilience of the health system and ultimately meet the ends and goals of their citizens. Only through better understanding gained from integrated research can the global community work and learn together to achieve the important goals of quality care that are effective and affordable for all.

References

Akachi, Y., & Kruk, M. E. (2017). Quality of care: Measuring a neglected driver of improved health. *Bulletin of the World Health Organization, 95*(6), 465–472.

Agyepong, I. A., Sollecito, W. A., & McLaughlin, C. P. (2012). CQI for malaria control in Ghana. In C. P. McLaughlin, J. K. Johnson, & W. A. Sollecito (Eds.), *Implementing continuous quality improvement in health care: a global casebook.* Sudbury, MA: Jones & Bartlett Learning.

Berwick, D. M. (1996). A primer on leading the improvements of systems. *British Medical Journal, 312*, 619–622.

Berwick, D. M., Nolan, T. W., & Whittington, J. (2008). The triple aim: Care, health and cost. *Health Affairs, 27*(3), 759–769.

Bitton, A., Ratcliffe, H. L., Veillard, J. H., Kress, D. H., Barkley, S., Kimball, M., ... Hirschhorn, L. R. (2017). Primary health care as a foundation for strengthening health systems in low- and middle-income countries. *Journal of General Internal Medicine, 32*(5), 566–571.

Bodenheimer, T., & Sinsky, C. (2014). From triple to Quadruple Aim: Care of the patient requires care of the provider. *Annals of Family Medicine, 12*(6), 573–576.

Boozary, A. S., Farmer, P. E., & Jha, A. K. (2014). The Ebola outbreak, fragile health systems, and quality as a cure. *Journal of the American Medical Association, 312*(18), 1859–1860.

Bryce, J., Victoria, C., Habicht, J.-P., Black, R. E., & Scherpbier, R. (2005). Programmatic pathways to child survival: Results of a multi-country evaluation of Integrated Management of Childhood Illness. *Health Policy and Planning, 20*(Suppl 1), i5–i17. https://doi.org/10.1093/heapol/czi055

Carter, P. M., Desmond, J. S., Akanbobnaab, C., Oteng, R. A., Rominski, S. D., Barsan, W. G., & Cunningham, R. M. (2012). Optimizing clinical operations as part of a global emergency medicine initiative in Kumasi, Ghana: Application of lean manufacturing principals to low-resource health systems. *Academic Emergency Medicine, 19*(3), 338–347. https://doi.org/10.1111/j.1553-2712.2012.01311.x

Das, J. (2011). The quality of medical care in low-income countries: From providers to markets. *PLoS Medicine, 8*(4), 4. https://doi.org/10.1371/journal.pmed.1000432

Das, J., & Hammer, J. (2014). Quality of primary care in low-income countries: Facts and economics. *Annual Review of Economics, 6*, 525–553. https://doi.org/10.1146/annurev-economics-080213-041350

Das, J., Holla, A., Das, V., Mohanan, M., Tabak, D., & Chan, B. (2012). In urban and rural India, a standardized patient study showed low levels of provider training and huge quality gaps. *Health Affairs, 31*(12), 2774–2784. https://doi.org/10.1377/hlthaff.2011.1356

Donabedian, A. (1988). The quality of care: How can it be assessed? *Journal of the American Medical Association, 260*(12), 1743–1748.

Donabedian, A. (2005). Evaluating the quality of medical care [reprint of 1966 article]. *The Milbank Quarterly, 83*(4), 691–729. https://doi.org/10.1111/j. 1468-0009.2005.00397.x

Farmer, P. E., Nutt, C. T., Wagner, C. M., Sekabaraga, C., Nuthulaganti, T., Weigel, J. L., … Drobac, P. C. (2013). Reduced premature mortality in Rwanda: Lessons from success. *BMJ Open, 346*(1), f65. https://doi.org/10.1136/bmj.f65

Fiori, J. K., Schechter, J., Dey, M., Braganza, S., Houndenou, S., Gbeleou, C., … Tchangani, E. (2016). Closing the delivery gaps in pediatric HIV care in Togo, West Africa: Using the care delivery value chain framework to direct quality improvement. *AIDS Care, 28*(Suppl 2), 29–33. https://doi.org/10.1080/09540121.2016.1176678

Franco, L. M., & Marquez, L. (2011). Effectiveness of collaborative improvement: evidence from 27 applications in 12 less-developed and middle-income countries. *BMJ Quality & Safety, 20*(8), 658–665. https://doi.org/10.1136/bmjqs.2010.044388

Gage, A. D., Leslie, H. H., Bitton, A., Jerome, J. G., Thermidor, R., Joseph, J. P., & Kruk, M. E. (2017). Assessing the quality of primary care in Haiti. *Bulletin of the World Health Organization, 95*(3), 182–190. https://doi.org/10.2471/BLT.16.179846

GBD Collaborators. (2016). Global, regional, and national life expectancy, all-cause mortality, and cause-specific mortality for 249 causes of death, 1980–2015: A systematic analysis for the Global Burden of Disease Study 2015. *The Lancet, 388*, 1459–1544. https://doi.org/10.1016/S0140-6736(16)31012-1

Geng, E. H., Peiris, D., & Kruk, M. E. (2017). Implementation science: Relevance in the real world without sacrificing rigor. *PLoS Medicine, 14*(4): e1002288. https://doi.org/10.1371/journal.pmed.1002288

Gergen, J., Josephson, E., Coe, M., Ski, S., & Madhavan, S. (2017). Quality of care in performance-based financing: How it is incorporated in 32 programs across 28 countries. *Global Health: Science and Practice, 5*(1), 90–107.

Goodman, D. M., Ramaswamy, R., Jeuland, M., Srofenyoh, E. K., Engmann, C. M., Olufolabi, A. J., & Owen, M. D. (2017). The cost effectiveness of a quality improvement program to reduce maternal and fetal mortality in a regional referral hospital in Accra, Ghana. *PLoS One, 12*(7).

Hammer, M., & Champy, J. (1993). Reengineering the corporation: A manifesto for business revolution. *Business Horizons, 36*(5), 90–91.

Haynes, A. B., Weiser, T. G., Berry, W. R., Lipsitz, S. R., Breizat, A. H., & Dellinger, E. P. (2009). A surgical safety checklist to reduce morbidity and mortality in a global population. *New England Journal of Medicine, 360*, 491–499. https://doi.org/10.1056/NEJMsa0810119

Heiby, J. (2014). The use of modern quality improvement approaches to strengthen African health systems: A 5-year agenda. *International Journal for Quality in Health Care, 26*(2), 117–123.

Horwood, C. M., Youngleson, M. S., Moses, E., Stern, A. F., & Barker, P. M. (2015). Using adapted quality-improvement approaches to strengthen community-based health systems and improve care in high HIV-burden sub-Saharan African countries. *AIDS, 29*, S155–S164. https://doi.org/10.1097/QAD.0000000000000716

Joosten, T., Bongers, I., & Janssen, R. (2009). Application of lean thinking to health care: Issues and observations. *International Journal for Quality in Health Care, 21*(5), 341–347. https://doi.org/10.1093/intqhc/mzp036

Kabongo, L., Gass, J., Kivondo, B., Kara, N., Semrau, K., & Hirschhorn, L. R. (2017). Implementing the WHO Safe Childbirth Checklist: Lessons learnt on a quality improvement initiative to improve mother and newborn care at Gobabis District Hospital, Namibia. *BMJ Open Quality, 6*(2), e000145. https://doi.org/10.1136/bmjoq-2017-000145

Kanamori, S., Castro, M. C., Sow, S., Matsuno, R., Cissokho, A., & Jimba, M. (2016). Impact of the Japanese 5S management method on patients' and caretakers' satisfaction: A quasi-experimental study in Senegal. *Global Health Action, 9*(1), 1–14. https://doi.org/10.3402/GHA.V9.32852

Kruk, M. E., Chukwuma, A., & Leslie, H. H. (2017). Variation in quality of primary-care services in Kenya, Malawi, Namibia, Rwanda, Senegal, Uganda and the United Republic of Tanzania. *Bulletin of the World Health Organization, 95*(6), 408–418.

Kruk, M. E., Leslie, H. H., Verguet, S., Mbaruku, G. M., Adanu, R. M. K., & Langer, A. (2016). Quality of basic maternal care functions in health facilities of five African countries: An analysis of national health system surveys. *The Lancet Global Health, 4*(11), e845–e855. https://doi.org/10.1016/S2214-109X(16)30180-2

Langley, G. L., Moen, R. D., Nolan, K. M., Nolan, T. W., Norman, C. L., & Provost, L. P. (2009). *The improvement guide: A practical approach to enhancing organizational performance.* San Francisco, CA: Jossey-Bass.

Lazzerini, M., Shukurova, V., Davletbaeva, M., Monolbaev, K., Kulichenko, T., Akoev, Y., … Boronbayeva, E. (2017). Improving the quality of hospital care for children by supportive supervision: A cluster randomized trial, Kyrgyzstan. *Bulletin of the World Health Organization, 95*(6), 397–407.

Leatherman, S., Ferris, T. G., Berwick, D., Omaswa, F., & Crisp, N. (2010). The role of quality improvement in strengthening health systems in developing countries. *International Journal for Quality in Health Care, 22*(4), 237–243. https://doi.org/10.1093/intqhc/mzq028

Leslie, H. H., Gage, A., Nsona, H., Hirschhorn, L. R., & Kruk, M. E. (2016). Training and supervision did not meaningfully improve quality of care for pregnant women or sick children in sub-Saharan Africa. *Health Affairs, 35*(9), 1716–1724. https://doi.org/10.1377/hlthaff.2016.0261

Lunze, K., Biemba, G., Lawrence, J. J., Macleod, W. B., Yeboah-antwi, K., Musokotwane, K., … Earle, D. (2017). Clinical management of children with fever: A cross-sectional study of quality of care in rural Zambia. *Bulletin of the World Health Organization, 95*(5), 333–342.

Macinko, J., Harris, M. J., & Rocha, M. G. (2017). Brazil's national Program for Improving Primary Care Access and Quality (PMAQ): Fulfilling the potential of the world's largest payment for performance system in primary care. *The Journal of Ambulatory Care Management, 40*(Suppl 2), S4–S11. https://doi.org/10.1097/JAC.0000000000000189

Magge, H., Anatole, M., Cyamatare, F. R., Mezzacappa, C., Nkikabahizi, F., Niyonzima, S., … Hirschhorn, L. R. (2014). Mentoring and quality improvement strengthen integrated management of childhood illness implementation in rural Rwanda. *Archives of Disease in Childhood, 100*(6), 565–570. https://doi.org/10.1136/archdischild-2013-305863

Marshall, M., Pronovost, P., & Dixon-Woods, M. (2013). Promotion of improvement as a science. *The Lancet, 381*(9864), 419–421. https://doi.org/10.1016/S0140-6736(12)61850-9

Marx-Delaney, M., Saurastri, R., Singh, P., Maji, P., Karlage, A., Hirschhorn, L. R., & Semrau, E. A. (2017). Improving adherence to essential birth practices using the WHO Safe Childbirth Checklist with peer coaching: Experience from 60 public health facilities in Uttar Pradesh, India. *Global Health Science & Practice, 5*(2), 217–231. Erratum: *Global Health Science & Practice, 6*(1), 227.

Mbonye, M. K., Burnett, S. M., Burua, A., Colebunders, R., Crozier, I., Kinoti, S. N., … Weaver, M. R. (2014). Effect of integrated capacity-building interventions on malaria case management by health professionals in Uganda: A mixed design study with pre/post and cluster randomized trial components. *PLoS One, 9*(1), e84945. https://doi.org/10.1371/journal.pone.0084945

Moucheraud, C., Owen, H., Singh, N. S., Ng, C. K., Requejo, J., Lawn, J. E., & Berman, P. (2016). Countdown to 2015 country case studies: What have we learned about processes and progress towards MDGs 4 and 5? *BMC Public Health, 16*(S2), 794. https://doi.org/10.1186/s12889-016-3401-6

Oursler, K. K., Goulet, J. L., Crystal, S., Justice, A. C., Crothers, K., Butt, A. A., … Sorkin, J. D. (2011). Association of age and comorbidity with physical function in HIV-infected and uninfected patients: Results from the Veterans Aging Cohort Study. *AIDS Patient Care and STDs, 25*(1), 13–20. https://doi.org/10.1089/apc.2010.0242

Paule, M., Kieny, M. P., Bekedam, H., Dovlo, D., Habicht, J., Harrison, G., … Travis, P. (2017). Strengthening health systems for universal health coverage and sustainable development. *Bulletin of the World Health Organization, 95*(7), 537–539.

Pavluck, A., Chu, B., Mann Flueckiger, R., & Ottesen, E. (2014). Electronic Data Capture Tools for Global Health Programs. Evolution of LINKS, an Android-, Web-Based System. *PLoS Neglected Tropical Diseases, 8*(4), 8–11. https://doi.org/10.1371/journal.pntd.0002654

Perry, H. B., Zulliger, R., & Rogers, M. M. (2014). Community health workers in low-, middle-, and high-income countries: An overview of their history, recent evolution, and current effectiveness. *Annual Review of Public Health, 35*, 399–421. https://doi.org/10.1146/annurev-publhealth-032013-182354

Pesec, M., Ratcliffe, H. L., Karlage, A., Hirschhorn, L. R., Gawande, A., & Bitton, A. (2017). Primary health care that works: The Costa Rican experience. *Health Affairs (Millwood), 36*(3), 531–538. https://doi.org/10.1377/hlthaff.2016.1319

Primary Health Care Performance Initiative. (n.d.). Primary Health Care Performance Initiative. Retrieved from http://phcperformanceinitiative.org

Ramaswamy, R., Iracane, S., Srofenyoh, E. K., Bryce, F., Floyd, L., Kallam, B., & Owen, M. D. (2015). Transforming maternal and neonatal outcomes in tertiary hospitals in Ghana: An integrated approach for systems change. *Journal of Obstetrics and Gynaecology Canada, 37*(10), 905–914.

Ramaswamy, R., Rothschild, C., Alabi, F., Wachira, E., Muigai, F., & Pearson, N. (2017). Quality in practice using value stream mapping to improve quality of care in low-resource facility settings. *International Journal for Quality in Health Care, 29*(7), 961–965. https://doi.org/10.1093/intqhc/mzx142

Randive, B., Diwan, V., & De Costa, A. (2013). India's conditional cash transfer programme (the JSY) to promote institutional birth: Is there an association between institutional birth proportion and maternal mortality? *PLoS One, 8*(6), e67452. https://doi.org/10.1371/journal.pone.0067452

Ridde, V. (2016). Need for more and better implementation science in global health. *BMJ Global Health, 1*(2), e000115. https://doi.org/10.1136/bmjgh-2016-000115

Rowe, A. K., De Savigny, D., Lanata, C. F., & Victora, C. G. (2005). How can we achieve and maintain high-quality performance of health workers in low-resource settings? *The Lancet, 366*(9490), 1026–1035. https://doi.org/10.1016/S0140-6736(05)67028-6

Ruducha, J., Mann, C., Singh, N. S., Gemebo, T. D., Tessema, N. S., Baschieri, A., ... Zerfu, T. A. (2017). How Ethiopia achieved Millennium Development Goal 4 through multisectoral interventions: A Countdown to 2015 case study. *The Lancet Global Health, 5*(11), e1142–e1151. https://doi.org/10.1016/S2214-109X(17)30331-5

Schouten, L. M. T., Hulscher, M. E. J. L., Everdingen, J. J. E. v., Huijsman, R., & Grol, R. P. T. M. (2008). Evidence for the impact of quality improvement collaboratives: Systematic review. *BMJ, 336*(7659), 1491–1494. https://doi.org/10.1136/bmj.39570.749884.BE

Singh, H., Schiff, G. D., Graber, M. L., Onakpoya, I., & Thompson, M. J. (2016). The global burden of diagnostic errors in primary care. *BMJ Quality & Safety, 26*(6), 484–494. https://doi.org/10.1136/bmjqs-2016-005401

Singh, K., Brodish, P., Speizer, I., Barker, P., Amenga-Etego, I., Dasoberi, I., ... Sodzi-Tettey, S. (2016). Can a quality improvement project impact maternal and child health outcomes at scale in northern Ghana? *Health Research Policy and Systems, 14*(1), 45. https://doi.org/10.1186/s12961-016-0115-2

Spector, J. M., Agrawal, P., Kodkany, B., Lipsitz, S., Lashoher, A., Dziekan, G., ... Gawande, A. (2012). Improving quality of care for maternal and newborn health: prospective pilot study of the WHO safe childbirth checklist program. *PLoS One, 7*(5), e35151. https://doi.org/10.1371/journal.pone.0035151

Spector, J. M., Lashoher, A., Agrawal, P., Lemer, C., Dziekan, G., Bahl, R., ... Gawande, A. A. (2013). Designing the WHO Safe Childbirth Checklist program to improve quality of care at childbirth. *International Journal of Gynaecology and Obstetrics, 122*(2), 164–168. https://doi.org/10.1016/j.ijgo.2013.03.022

Srivastava, A., Avan, B. I., Rajbangshi, P., & Bhattacharyya, S. (2015). Determinants of women's satisfaction with maternal health care: A review of literature from developing countries. *BMC Pregnancy and Childbirth, 15*(1), 97. https://doi.org/10.1186/s12884-015-0525-0

Srofenyoh, E. K., Srofenyoh, N. J., Kassebaum, D. M., Goodman, A. J., & Olufolabi, M. D. O. (2016). Measuring the impact of a quality improvement collaboration to decrease maternal mortality in a Ghanaian regional hospital. *Journal of Gynaecology and Obstetrics, 134*(2), 181–185.

Trusko, B., Pexton, C., Harrington, J., & Gupta, P. (2007). *Improving healthcare quality and cost with six sigma.* Upper Saddle River, NJ: FT Press/Pearson.

UNICEF. (2018, February). UNICEF Data: Monitoring the Situation of Children and Women. Retrieved June 6, 2018, from http://data.unicef.org/topic/child-survival/under-five-mortality/

World Health Organization (WHO). (2007). Everybody's business: Strengthening health systems to improve health outcomes. WHO's Framework for Action. Geneva, Switzerland: WHO. Retrieved from http://www.who.int/healthsystems/strategy/everybodys_business.pdf

World Health Organization (WHO). (2015). WHO global strategy on people-centred and integrated health services. Interim Report. Geneva, Switzerland: WHO. Retrieved from http://apps.who.int/iris/bitstream/10665/155002/1/WHO_HIS_SDS_2015.6_eng.pdf?ua=1&ua=1

World Health Organization (WHO). (2017a). Health Data Collaborative. Retrieved from https://www.healthdatacollaborative.org/

World Health Organization (WHO). (2017b). National quality policy and strategy: Driving change for stronger health. Geneva, Switzerland: WHO. Retrieved from http://www.who.int/servicedeliverysafety/areas/qhc/national-quality-policy-strategy.pdf?ua=1

CHAPTER 14

Future Trends and Challenges for Continuous Quality Improvement in Health Care

Julie K. Johnson and William A. Sollecito

Every system is perfectly designed to get the results it gets.

—**Paul Batalden**

Both the philosophy and processes of continuous quality improvement (CQI) in health care have continued to evolve since the publication of our last edition in 2013. This evolution spans geographical bounds, with ever-widening applications in developing countries; as described in Chapter 13. It also spans health sectors, with probably the best example being the institutionalization of CQI in public health (described in Chapter 11) spurred by external forces such as accreditation (see Chapter 12), as well as internal forces, primarily leadership and cultural influences, encouraging improvement of population health in the most efficient manner. Recent trends in the evolution of CQI have also included broader and more accessible sources of data to carry out CQI, although these are not without some risks, as described in Chapter 4.

Despite the continuing expansion and evolution of CQI in health care, many of the same challenges to quality care and patient safety still persist. These trends are not unlike those that have been seen in other industries and they will not be changed without careful attention to what we have learned in the past coupled with a shared vision across all health care sectors of what we hope to achieve in the future. This leads us to a series of important questions that we can ask here, with answers that we will only know after applying due diligence over the passage of time.

What does the future hold for CQI in health care? What constitutes evidence-based practice across the various *sectors* of health care? How do we implement improvements that have been demonstrated to be effective by evidence-based research? What limits generalizability for evidence-based practices as we attempt to translate them across multiple health care settings? How do we motivate health professionals to engage in improvement activities? How do we put a greater emphasis on adding value as we implement CQI initiatives? Who are the future leaders, where do we find them, and how can we support their development? While to a large extent the future is uncertain, definite trends are under way that we believe will be important themes for the future of CQI. The aim of this chapter is to discuss some of those trends and future challenges, and to create a road map for those who will be leading the transformation of health care.

▶ Setting the Stage for CQI

In patient care settings, we operationalize CQI by asking two separate, but related, questions:

1. How can I improve care for my patients?
2. How can I improve the system of care?

It is generally agreed that the systems we work within are at the root of many of our patient safety and quality problems (IOM, 1999). Quality and safety are both properties of systems, and many of our quality and safety initiatives—the specific changes we put into place to make improvements—belong to the system. Many of these initiatives are described in the recent CQI literature, but not all, since some that have not been successful have suffered the fate of publication bias; that is, they aren't published in peer-reviewed publications and thus are not disseminated, despite their usefulness as mechanisms for learning how to improve our improvement strategies. Many of these initiatives have cross-disciplinary applications, which have been addressed in the preceding chapters, and together these initiatives create a road map for those who wish to lead the future transformation of health care.

The translation of research into practice requires a certain set of skills; similarly, health care professionals will need to be proficient in specialized skills to be able to translate quality improvement concepts into sustained improvements in patient care processes and health outcomes. System-level results do not come from a single initiative or even a series of initiatives when these efforts are not aligned. System improvements require a portfolio of projects that are aligned with strategy to produce and sustain results (Nolan, 2007).

▶ Conceptual Frameworks for Improving Care

Health care has been described as a complex adaptive system (Rouse, 2008; Swensen et al., 2010), and much has been written about both the system itself and solutions that target various levels of the system, so it is not a lack of evidence about system solutions that is holding us back.

FIGURE 14.1 illustrates three fundamental aims of a health system: better patient outcomes, better system performance, and better professional development. A fourth necessary component is the active engagement of

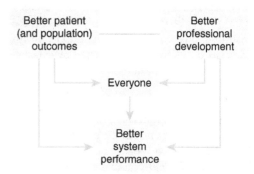

FIGURE 14.1 Fundamental Aims of a Health System
Batalden and Davidoff 2007.

everyone in the health system toward helping to achieve those fundamental aims (Batalden & Davidoff, 2007; Nelson et al., 2008).

We can compare Figure 14.1 to a similar framework, the Institute for Healthcare Improvement (IHI) Triple Aim, which includes improving the patient experience of care, improving the health of populations, and reducing the per capita cost of health care. (Berwick, Nolan, & Whittington, 2008, p. 759). The primary drivers that will make it possible to simultaneously optimize all three aims in the United States are:

1. Measurement that is transparent
2. Public health interventions
3. Design and coordination of care at the patient level
4. Universal access to care
5. A financial management system

A further expansion of these concepts, which recognizes the role of health care providers, adds a fourth aim: improving the work life experience of health care providers, with the specific goals of decreasing burnout, which has been widely reported in recent years, and increasing the intrinsic motivation of providers, a key factor related to the successful implementation of CQI (Deming, 1986). The application of what is now being called the Quadruple Aim, while still a fairly new concept, is expected to have a major impact on achieving the vision of improved safety and quality of care, for individuals and populations (Bodenheimer & Sinsky, 2014; Sikka, Morath, & Leape, 2015).

Derek Feeley, the CEO of the IHI, points out that several institutions have decided to adopt the Quadruple Aim to focus on an additional goal that aligns with their specific organizational vision. He offers some important thoughts on the complementary nature of the Triple and Quadruple Aim with advice for how to incorporate both into a quality health care strategy (Feeley, 2018):

1. *Remember that the Triple Aim is about patients.* Patients are always at the center of what we do.

2. *We haven't finished pursuing the original Triple Aim.* There are still gaps in the health of the populations that we serve. We miss too many opportunities to improve the care experience. We haven't done enough to improve health care quality while reducing costs.

3. *Don't lose focus.* No organization has unlimited resources, so we must deploy what we have in an intentional, purposeful way.

4. *Measure what matters.* Use deliberation and consideration to determine what data you really need, and how to collect and analyze it.

This focus on the individual person is an important reminder for those who wish to lead the future improvement of health care and is highlighted by Don Berwick in *A User's Manual for the IOM's Quality Chasm Report* (Berwick, 2002), in which he suggests that there are four levels of interest:

- Level A: The experience of patients (individuals)
- Level B: The functioning of small units of care delivery (or microsystems)
- Level C: The functioning of the organizations that house or otherwise support microsystems
- Level D: The environment of policy, payment, regulation, accreditation, and other such factors that shape the behavior, interests, and opportunities of the organizations at Level C

"True north," Berwick writes, "lies at Level A: patients [individuals] and their experiences" (Berwick, 2002). The fourth aim of the Quadruple Aim also plays a critical role, albeit at Levels B and C in Berwick's model.

Note that the Triple Aim (improving the experience of care, improving the health of populations, and reducing per capita costs of health care) is slightly different from the fundamental aims shown in Figure 14.1 (better patient outcomes, better system performance, and better professional development). While these aims are not in conflict, better professional development is a key difference in the two models, which aligns very closely with the fourth part of the Quadruple Aim. Educating professionals (including staff) is a critical part of the fourth aim. As described by Bodenheimer and Sinsky (2014), greater training for health care professionals is positive motivation and also a way to foster empowerment. We believe that this aim is necessary in achieving the other aims, and a more detailed discussion about educating professionals to lead quality improvement is presented later in this chapter.

For CQI to add value, have impact, and realize its potential, it will need to be managed at multiple levels. An ecological perspective provides a potential framework for thinking about CQI, because it acknowledges many contextual layers, such as the environment, organization, health care provider, family, and individual patient characteristics, that directly or indirectly influence a range of patient care outcomes. It also provides a model for breaking down the complexity into manageable components and identifying linkages and interdependencies that must be considered when making changes. **FIGURE 14.2** illustrates

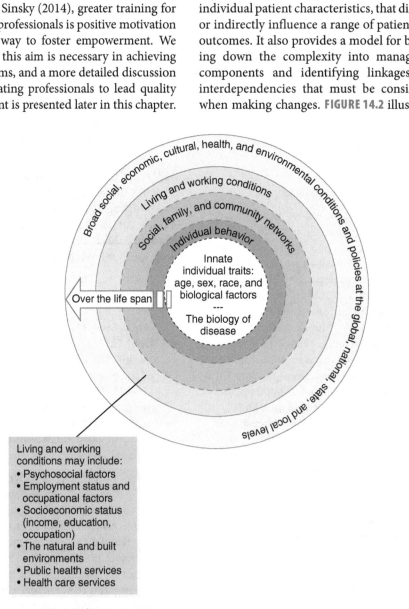

FIGURE 14.2 Ecological Model of Public Health

the ecological perspective in public health; it encompasses the vision that is the critical step in developing constancy of purpose (Deming, 1986) and ultimately developing a culture that embraces improvement (see Chapter 2).

The model shown in Figure 14.2 was developed by the public health profession, which has made great strides in quality improvement (see Chapter 11), spanning education and practice, in recent years and provides another model for accelerating CQI in health care. Much of that progress was initiated with the release of a 2003 Institute of Medicine (IOM) report that "reviews the nation's public health capabilities and presents a comprehensive framework for how the government public health agencies, working with multiple partners from the public and private sectors as an intersectoral public health system, can better assure the health of communities" (IOM, 2003). The extension of this model to other sectors of health requires a conversion of terms, but not concepts; it is another example of cross-disciplinary thinking and interprofessional sharing of ideas.

▶ Road Map for the Future

Every journey begins with a single step.
—**Chinese proverb**

Future trends and challenges related to accelerating CQI in health care, are discussed in the following sections; these are organized into the following sections:

- Education (CQI skills, leadership, teamwork, and collaboration)
- Quality improvement collaboratives (QIC)
- Learning organizations (health systems)
- Value-added health care
- Research and publication

These topics are not listed in order of importance but, taken together, are points of emphasis or priorities for those of us in health care that constitute a starting point for where to go next to ensure a greater focus in the near future on efficient applications of CQI and related concepts such as the Quadruple Aim. These were chosen in part because they are multidisciplinary, and applicable to broad range of health sectors, but are by no means exhaustive.

Education: CQI Skills, Leadership, Teamwork, and Collaboration

We believe that education is the first, and perhaps the most important, step toward accelerating CQI in health care. During the past decade, we have seen an increased focus on educating health professions students to improve the systems they are training to work within by teaching CQI skills and techniques. This has been seen across the continuum of medical education, from students in medical schools to postgraduate residency training programs to initial board certification and maintenance of certification programs. However, further formal efforts are needed—learning from and building upon successful models. The Geisel School of Medicine at Dartmouth has documented its success in incorporating quality improvement into its education using an experiential approach (Adams, 2010); it provides a good model for others to study, including emphasis on the importance of careful evaluation to ensure successful curricular reform (Ogrinc et al., 2011).

While medical education has been criticized because it has not traditionally prepared physicians to work as part of teams, we have seen more efforts to train health professionals to work as part of a team or "microsystem." We have also witnessed an increased focus on quality improvement in public health and nursing education. The Quality and Safety Education for Nurses (QSEN) approach serves as a model for consensus building and, spanning 15 nursing schools, is also an example of how to implement broad levels of change on a national scale (Sherwood and Jones, 2013). It provides for education of students and faculty on the skills needed to practice. (Additional information is available at the website for the QSEN Institute of the Frances Payne Bolton School of Nursing at Case Western Reserve University.) As noted earlier, broader education for staff, nurses, and physicians is an important part of the Quadruple Aim (Bodenheimer & Sinsky, 2014).

One criticism of educational approaches for CQI in medical care is that clinicians, especially physicians, were brought along later, or not at all—sometimes because they were thought to be too busy with the work of caring for patients. Not only did this lead to slow diffusion of CQI in health care, but it sometimes led to frustration or even a sense of failure from frontline clinicians (Ofri, 2010) that could perpetuate a resistance to CQI initiatives (Balestracci, 2009). It is clear now that physicians should be included early on, and their ideas and concerns should be addressed as part of the education process (Berwick & Nolan, 1998). As noted by Solberg and colleagues (2006, p. 298):

> The net result of all of these changes has been to focus attention and pressure on clinicians, especially those in primary care. They are feeling both stressed and unappreciated, as they have to run faster to keep up while being constantly told that what they do isn't good enough. At the same time, it is becoming clearer that if we are to address the cost and quality conundrums we face, clinicians must not only be involved, they must take the lead in making change happen.

In addition to specific CQI skills, there is a need to focus educational efforts on broader areas of leadership and teamwork. They are critical competencies associated with quality improvement and are part of the critical "non-technical skills" (Flin et al., 2008) that will better prepare health care practitioners to shape the quality and safety of health care in the future. As depicted in **FIGURE 14.3**, leadership, teamwork, and CQI skills are the overlapping, complementary foundations of an educational process needed to develop future health care quality improvement leaders. Within those disciplines are specific skill sets that are beneficial to health care in general and CQI specifically.

For everyone to be actively engaged in doing their work and improving their work, there is a basic assumption that everyone will develop a basic understanding of the standards of their own work, as well as the quality improvement skills they need to test changes in that work (Batalden & Davidoff, 2007). As we develop educational programs, an additional consideration for education is that there is a concurrent need to ensure that faculties are both knowledgeable and experienced in the techniques required to implement CQI broadly. It is critical that practitioners learn what to do to improve quality and also become experienced in how it can be done most effectively, using appropriate implementation science techniques to be discussed further later in this chapter. This is described in management science as overcoming the knowing–doing gap (Pfeffer & Sutton, 2000). It is a gap that

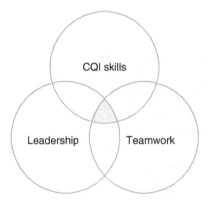

FIGURE 14.3 Educational Components for Future Health Care Leaders

has stalled some very well-intentioned CQI initiatives.

One key to process improvement, which also illustrates overcoming the knowing–doing gap, is statistical thinking. Training in the quantitative sciences is necessary, but not sufficient; statistical thinking must be woven into the culture for all to understand its role in decision making—especially decision making about changes and improvements. In an organization or culture that is dedicated to CQI, "statistical thinking means looking at everything the organization does as a series of processes that have the goal of consistently providing the results your customer desires" (Balestracci, 2009, p. 85). The basics of statistical thinking start with measurement and the ability to learn from the data we have collected (see Chapter 4). We must then take the time to understand what the data tell us, particularly about causes of variation (Deming, 1986), before taking action to make changes. This is a central principle of the application of the Plan, Do, Study, Act (PDSA) cycle.

Leadership

The role of leadership is recognized as fundamental to improving quality and safety because leaders enable connections between the aims (see Figure 14.1 and the preceding discussion of the Quadruple Aim) and the design and testing of those improvements. Leadership has a critical role in setting a vision for change, or constancy of purpose (Deming, 1986) and shaping a culture that embraces quality and safety. Leadership is the first of seven Health Care Criteria for Performance Excellence for the Malcolm Baldrige National Quality Award. According to the Baldrige National Quality Program (2011, p. 49):

An organization's senior leaders (administrative and health care provider leaders) should set directions and create a patient focus, clear and visible values, and high expectations.

. . . Leaders should ensure the creation of strategies, systems, and methods for achieving excellence in health care, stimulating innovation, and building knowledge and capabilities.

Leading an organization that is committed to improving quality and adding value requires creating a "learning organization" that learns from within and formally seeks new ideas from outside as well, which are keys to the diffusion of CQI in health care (Berwick, 2003).

Leadership is not about applying a collection of tools and techniques to those being led; it involves integrating the learning disciplines throughout the organization—vision, values, and purpose; systems thinking; and mental models (Senge, 1990). Successful leaders motivate followers to contribute to the development of a shared vision, that emphasizes the values of CQI, and demonstrate their personal commitment to achieving it. They "inspire" the vision throughout the organization. When defining leadership in the terms of creating a learning organization, the role of the leader is to take responsibility for learning, as a designer of the learning process, a steward of the vision, and a teacher by fostering the learning throughout the organization (Senge, 1990). In so doing, leaders ensure the development of an organizational culture that embraces change and improvement.

Leadership includes not only defining the vision but also living that vision and leading by example. Also important to note is that leadership must occur at all levels within an organization, including scientific leaders, opinion leaders, and those who champion change ideas (Greenhalgh et al., 2005). These individuals may or may not have administrative leadership roles. As discussed earlier, education and training are the critical factors to ensure leadership in the future—and not merely for those at the top levels of an organization. If we want to establish leaders at all levels, then we need leadership training at all levels.

Leadership education is no longer confined to business schools, but is being expanded to the sciences, including medicine, nursing, and public health. This is a trend that must continue. There has also been greater availability of leadership publications that are directed at the unique leadership challenges faced in academic medicine (Houpt, Gilkey, & Ehringhaus, 2015; Viera & Kramer, 2016). Similarly, leadership programs and literature have expanded among other health disciplines that are directly involved in CQI, for example Biostatisticians (LaVange et al., 2012). These are only samples of broader initiatives that need to be replicated to encourage greater leadership development among a wide array of health professionals.

Leadership skills should not be limited to those that are specific to health care challenges but should emphasize those aspects of leadership that are most appropriate for leaders of CQI initiatives in health; for example, an emphasis on transformational leadership and the related broader topic of leading change (Daft, 2015; Kotter, 1996; Rowitz, 2009; Sapienza, 2004). Educational programs should address the predisposing, enabling, and reinforcing factors that lead to higher quality, safer health care, for example, organizational dynamics and diffusion of innovation, and establishing a vision and culture to embrace change.

Teamwork

Closely associated with the role of leadership is the need for teamwork, which is central to CQI initiatives, but is under-represented in health care curriculums. Teamwork, especially in modern health care, is no longer an option but a requirement. Characterized by distribution of responsibilities and leadership at all levels, the use of teams adds value, and improves efficiency, by driving decisions to their lowest competent level. Empowerment of team members and high levels of individual motivation that result are also important in ensuring the development of a culture that is devoted to safety and quality (Daft, 2015; Grove, 1995).

The role of teams in CQI has long been recognized (Deming, 1986); coupled with technology to communicate more effectively, teams are even more important and easier to organize and lead than in earlier years, with more well-defined and well-tested team building and leadership procedures (Daft, 2015; Grove, 1995). However, like many other factors associated with health care CQI, there is an important need to teach practitioners how to be effective members of health care teams, especially CQI teams. (See Chapter 6 for an extensive discussion of health care teams and especially their role in CQI.)

Collaboration

The ability to collaborate, or work across departments, divisions or institutions to improve quality and safety is a clear direction for the future and an important leadership and teamwork skill; it is also described in some leadership textbooks as, boundary spanning leadership (Ernst & Chrobot-Mason, 2010). Improving value can be accomplished through effective collaborations, including acceptance of shared goals among all stakeholders, measurement of process and outcomes, and sharing of best practices. Indeed, outcome improvements and meaningful cost reductions are unachievable without active cooperation among providers committed to functioning as synergistic units. Collaboration is also critical in successful navigation of multidisciplinary efforts that are central to many CQI efforts; collaboration may require spanning departmental boundaries within a health organization or may involve spanning multiple organizations. While collaboration is a particular skill that can be taught, practiced, and refined, Quality Improvement Collaboratives (QICs) are an organizing structure for multiorganizational collaboration that exemplifies the evolution of CQI methods across geographic boundaries and areas of health care. As described in the following sections, QICs are particularly important in both the history and the future of CQI in health care.

Quality Improvement Collaboratives

QICs, also known as Learning Collaboratives, are an example of a broad-based approach with applications that range from primary care to public health. Although some have argued that clear evidence of their effectiveness, in terms of improved outcomes, is lacking, their widespread adoption is well documented (Schouten et al., 2008). QIC implementation requires and ensures practice-based-learning of several skills that are necessary components of successful CQI applications, including teamwork, leadership, and collaboration. Their continued use will be a strong positive force contributing to the spread of CQI in the future. QICs consist of "multidisciplinary teams from various health care departments or organizations that join forces for several months to work in a structured way to improve their provision of care" (Schouten et al., 2008, p. 1491). They have been described as temporary learning organizations. (Ovretveit et al., 2002). Greenhalgh et al., (2005), in their comprehensive review of the literature on diffusion of innovation in health service organizations, describe the goal of QICs as "spread of ideas":

> Participants in a quality collaborative work together over a number of months, sharing ideas and knowledge, setting specific goals, measuring progress, sharing techniques for organizational change and implementing rapid-cycle, iterative tests of change. Learning sessions are the major events of a Collaborative; these are 2-day events where members of the multi-disciplinary project teams from each health care organization gather to share experiences and learn from clinical and change experts and their colleagues. The time between learning sessions is called an action period in which participants work within their own organizations towards major,

"breakthrough" improvement, focusing on their internal organizational agenda and priorities for changes and improvements whilst remaining in continuous contact with other Collaborative participants. (p.163)

Introduced initially in the United States in the mid-1980s, QICs are now used in many countries with varying health care financing systems, including Canada, Australia, and European countries, where several national health authorities support nationwide quality programs based on this strategy. One of the first uses of QICs was The Northern New England Cardiovascular Disease Study Group in 1986. A similar approach has been used in the United Kingdom through its National Health Service Modernization Agency; it is called the Beacon Model and focuses on transfer of best practices, derived from Beacon organizations "that have achieved a high standard of service delivery and are regarded as centers of best practice" (Greenhalgh et al., 2005, p. 168). Recently, QICs have also been successful in low- and middle-income countries (see Chapter 13).

QICs were initially developed and are still used in primary care; for example, see Solberg's description of the DIAMOND QIC, which has a goal of improving care and outcomes for adult patients with depression in primary care clinics (2013). They have now evolved to a broader number of settings, and their widespread adoption in the United States has led to the formation of a national organization, the Network for Regional Healthcare Improvement (Network for Regional Healthcare Improvement, 2018).

QICs have become particularly prevalent in surgical care, especially at the state level (Dellinger et al., 2005; Campbell et al., 2009; Guillamondegui et al., 2012; SCOAP Collaborative et al., 2012). A recent example of a large scale surgical QIC is the Illinois Surgical Quality Improvement Collaborative (ISQIC), which was developed in late 2014. ISQIC is a payer-funded initiative and includes

57 diverse Illinois hospitals that agreed to adopt the widely recognized American College of Surgeons (ACS) National Surgical Quality Improvement Program (NSQIP) as the common data sharing platform. In addition, ISQIC includes 21 components, organized into five domains, to facilitate quality improvement that target the hospital, the surgical QI team, and the perioperative microsystem: guided implementation (e.g., mentors, coaches, statewide QI projects), education (e.g., process improvement curriculum), hospital- and surgeon-level comparative performance reports (e.g., process, outcomes, costs), networking (e.g., forums to share QI experiences and best practices), and funding (e.g., for the overall program, pilot grants, and bonus payments for improvement) (Nadeem et al., 2013; Nembhard, 2009; Hall, Hamilton et al., 2009; Hall, Richards, Ingraham, & Ko, 2009).

There are many other examples of successful QICs in CQI (de Vries et al., 2010; Haynes et al., 2009), such as the National Cancer Institute's Community Clinical Oncology Program (Minasian et al., 2010) and the National Community Cancer Centers Program (Clauser et al., 2009; Johnson et al., 2011) developed to provide access to state-of-the-art cancer care in community settings. An exciting example of the future of collaboratives can be seen with the Collaborative Improvement and Innovation Networks (CoIINs), which are multidisciplinary teams of federal, state, and local leaders working together to tackle a common problem. Using technology to remove geographic barriers, participants with a collective vision share ideas, best practices, and lessons learned, and track their progress toward similar benchmarks and shared goals. CoIIN provides a way for participants to self-organize, forge partnerships, and take coordinated action to address complex issues through structured collaborative learning, quality improvement, and innovative activities (HRSA, 2018).

The success and widespread adoption of QICs are directly related to the exchange and application of best practices by experts and peers to carry out improvement initiatives. Referring to the work of Ovretveit et al. (2002), the reasons for the success of QICs can be grouped into four general categories: topics chosen for improvement, participant and team characteristics, skills of facilitator and expert advisers, and ensuring ways to maximize spread of ideas. Greenhalgh et al. (2005, p. 167) explain that these success factors result from:

1. Clearly focused important topics that address clear gaps between current and best practice.
2. Highly motivated participants who clearly understand individual and corporate goals in a supportive organizational culture.
3. Effective teams and team leadership whose goals are in alignment with those of the organization.
4. Facilitation by credible experts, who provide adequate support outside as well as through the learning events.
5. Maximizing the spread of ideas through networking between teams and other mechanisms.

Based on their systematic review of the literature, these authors conclude that QICs have been demonstrated to be successful and popular ways of implementing improvements in health service delivery. However, they also point out two major criticisms—they are expensive, and gains from them have been difficult to measure. Indeed, creating and maintaining a collaborative is resource intensive, requiring significant financial and labor support. Therefore, it is critical to evaluate the most effective way to learn and engage front line clinicians in the QIC process.

This key point about engaging frontline clinicians in the QIC process cannot be over-emphasized and is an underlying factor that helps explain the attraction and success of using QICs in health care. For example, this principle is also noted in a description of the success of the Michigan ICU program for decreasing central venous catheter blood-stream infections (CVC-BSIs). Dixon-Woods and colleagues provide an in-depth analysis of the success of this program, including the fact that in addition to being founded on evidence-based, consensus driven interventions and other well defined scientific factors, it also succeeded because of evidence drawn from social science about physician behavior (Dixon-Woods et al., 2011, p. 186):

> Clinicians' behavior is not only influenced by abstract knowledge and formal bodies of evidence but also by trusted peers ... people are more likely to change their behaviors when they see liked and trusted peers doing the same ... Critical to the Michigan's ability to create a professional community focused on reducing CVC-BSIs and to secure legitimacy within the community was its use of leaders who were ICU "insiders" with whom members of the community could identify.

This is an important factor that must be emphasized on its own, to help define the road map for the future success of CQI in health care, and it is also an underlying feature of QICs that help to guarantee their continued role in that future.

Learning Organizations (Health Systems)

To succeed in a rapidly changing environment, including improving quality and safety in the future, health care organizations/systems need to smoothly manage the transformation process and take on the challenge of becoming what Peter Senge (1990, p. 3) described as "learning organizations," places where "people continually expand their capacity to create the results they truly desire, where new and expansive patterns of thinking are nurtured, where collective aspiration is set free and where people are continually learning to learn together."

As presented in TABLE 14.1, health care has experienced and must continue to strive for a process of transitioning from a professional model characterized by individual responsibility, professional autonomy, and accountability to a transformational model characterized by shared responsibility and collaborative decision making, continuous innovation, and

TABLE 14.1 Emergence of Transformational Models for Organizational Performance

Professional	CQI	Transformational
<ul><li>Individual responsibility</li><li>Professional leadership</li><li>Autonomy</li><li>Administrative authority</li><li>Professional authority</li><li>Goal expectations</li><li>Rigid planning</li><li>Responses to complaints</li><li>Retrospective performance appraisal</li><li>Quality assurance</li></ul>	<ul><li>Collective responsibility</li><li>Managerial leadership</li><li>Accountability</li><li>Participation</li><li>Performance and process expectations</li><li>Flexible planning</li><li>Benchmarking</li><li>Concurrent performance appraisal</li><li>Continuous improvement</li></ul>	<ul><li>Leaders and employees share overall responsibility, as well as take individual responsibility</li><li>People at multiple levels assume leadership</li><li>Outcome and value driven</li><li>Shared decision making</li><li>Continuous planning</li><li>Future orientation</li><li>Performance enhancement appraisals</li><li>Continuous innovation</li></ul>

learning (Upshaw, Steffen, and McLaughlin 2013). Traditional CQI provides important skills needed to make the transition, but transformational models provide organizations the opportunity to ensure that both incremental and radical learning occur in order to meet the challenges of an uncertain and complex environment. Through organizational learning, health care organizations can better face the reality of managing costs, providing high-quality services, and improving outcomes while accommodating individual needs through case management, patient education, and support of patient decision making.

Table 14.1 presents the following distinguishing characteristics of the transformational model that are fundamental to CQI.

Shared and Individual Responsibility by Leaders and Employees

Operating under transformational models, health care managers and clinical leaders share responsibility for accomplishing the organizational mission with other personnel. Everyone understands that they are important to the success of the organization, and they know what role they play in that success. Individuals, teams, units, and departments are committed to carrying out their responsibilities.

Leadership by People at Multiple Levels

Leadership roles for making decisions and guiding change must be afforded to people working in managerial or clinical roles, line staff, and field positions. Changes and decisions designed by people in offices apart from where the work is performed usually have limited effect. Their role should be limited to determining and communicating the broader environmental context in which local decision making takes place. For real innovation and improved performance, people working directly with

problems and systems need to be empowered to be fully involved in designing and deciding how to improve processes and quality. These are the people on the sharp end of processes, who will experience intrinsic motivation to lead the transformations that are needed, including innovation and improvement.

Outcome- and Value-Driven Process

People throughout transformative health care organizations demonstrate commitment to achieving outcomes, improving quality, and adding value. Employees, providers, and managers recognize that improving outcomes means that individual expectations for quality and clinical services, such as disease treatment and management, meet and exceed standards.

Shared Decision Making

It is critically important that people understand the core business, values, and mission of the organization so that they can participate in the decisions that affect them. Straight talk about what is occurring in the environment, how the organization is positioned to respond, and what people need to do to make necessary changes must be modeled and supported by managers and leaders. People need to understand their roles in helping the organization succeed, but they also need to define their roles and how they will contribute.

Continuous Planning

People must be motivated to make change and able to participate meaningfully in the change process. In general, participation will be more effective when the issues and changes are not routine (Schwarz, 1989). Transformational change in organizations prepares people to participate in planning and anticipating next steps in an evolutionary change process. When the organization is undergoing regular and dynamic change, people from across the organization must be informed and involved in deciding what changes should be made, in what order, and by what methods. Through functional and cross-functional teams, providers and managers can involve others in mapping strategies and preparing for new challenges (Carroll & Edmondson, 2002).

Future Orientation

Unlike what has come before, health care organizations and systems must be defining what the future will be and setting their sights on how they will make that happen. A potential danger for the transformative organization is that it might achieve its objectives for the immediate future and turn its attention to categorizing its accomplishments. Such a retrospective orientation will slow the organization and reduce people's motivation to stay ahead of the trends in the ever-changing health care sector. Transformational leadership continually brings forward the vision of the future organization and indicates how the organization can get from where it is in the present to where it wants to be in the future.

Performance Enhancement Appraisals

In addition to rewarding and assessing performance improvements for individual employees and teams, transformational organizations need to commit real resources and support structures to recognizing creativity and innovation. We need to look beyond improving how we get things done and begin to question and explore new ways of doing what needs to be done. Employees need to know that they will be rewarded for going outside the traditional structures to redesign and recreate the organization. Such changes will improve more than employee performance; they will increase employee dedication and contributions to the organization's future success. Commitment is greater in organizations that are actively managing change, obviously uncomfortable with

the status quo, and creating a new standard for performance (McNeese-Smith, 1996; Pascale et al., 1997).

Some of that uneasiness could be mitigated by training staff to understand that health care has two types of processes side by side, ranging from evidence-based to discovery (Bohmer 2009) and exhibiting a continuum of complexity and uncertainty (Green et al., 2001).

Continuous Innovation

To excel in the future, health care organizations will need to establish systems that reward people for good work to recognize efforts that surpass expectations. Transformative models provide support for people to demonstrate creativity and innovation that extend beyond standard performance. Clear systems for highlighting outstanding performance and contributions of providers, administrators, and employees can energize others and provide standards against which to assess poor performance (Pascale et al., 1997).

A Focus on Value-Added Health Care

Clearly a trend that must continue is the focus on improving the "value" of the health care service contribution to better health. Value, as a framework for efficiently improving outcomes, is a concept that all stakeholders—patients, providers, payers, and policy makers—can embrace (Lee, 2010). This is critical for all health care systems, including those in low- and middle-income countries since they are dealing with limited resources for access and services as well as for CQI initiatives. But how is value achieved? Value has been defined as "a function of three elements: its design (the right treatment for the right patient at the right time), its execution (reliably doing it right every time to achieve the best outcomes), and its cost over time" (Swensen et al., 2010). More simply, value can be defined as "health outcome achieved per dollar spent" (Porter, 2010). This definition implies that value is created around the patient, for the patient (Porter, 2010). If value improves, patients, payers, providers, and suppliers all benefit since the economic sustainability of the health care system increases.

The CQI evolution has emphasized many fundamental concepts of health improvement and change including health care services as a system and process; system leadership; measurement of outcome; unwanted variation; system failure and unreliability; organization-wide contributions to better health; making improvement part of everyone's job; and accountability for better performance. To some extent we have de-emphasized the focus on value. Moving forward, value has reemerged as a key concept for the future of healthcare and its roots go back many years to Philip Crosby (Crosby, 1980) and others. Crosby does not talk about the business case for quality, but his idea that "quality is free" is at the heart of this concept, in that the cost of poor quality is the expense of not doing things correctly the first time, which directly relates to the value proposition; the costs of a quality program are more than offset by the value produced, and avoidance of costs of rework and the loss of customers as well (Crosby, 1980).

Clinicians and patients coproduce health care services. Good health outcomes, experience, and value are created by bringing the right people together with the right information, the right technology, in the right way, and at the right time, in response to a patient's needs (Batalden, 2016). The conversation about value needs to address value to patients, internal customers, and suppliers, as well as the overall population. The focus on internal as well as external customers has been discussed for many years as a basic tenet of CQI (Crosby, 1980; Deming, 1986) and is also consistent with the new thinking on provider well-being that is incorporated in the Quadruple Aim. Individual physicians are not necessarily compelled to change when faced with data on their own patients; data must be given with the context of an organizational culture that is dedicated to quality and safety,

as illustrated by the Intermountain Healthcare example (Savitz, 2012). Fjeldstadt suggests a "value model," which is an organizational architecture for health care service that builds on three complementary and interdependent value-creating building blocks: the value shop, the value chain, and the value network (Stabell & Fjeldstad, 1998). The *value shop* has been the predominant way of creating value in health care. It enables highly customized responses to individual problems. It is based on one-to-one patient–professional relationships where there is a predictable cycle of steps, including case acquisition, developing a diagnosis, selecting a customized treatment, and testing of the proposed solution. This model was formed in the mid-20th century (Kaba & Soorikumaran, 2007), when the complexity of medical care was far more limited. The main tradeoff in the value shop is between breadth (the number and diversity of conditions that can be managed) and depth (the level of expertise that can be provided). As the number of diagnostic and therapeutic interventions has increased, medical knowledge expanded, and expectancies for longer and better life increased, the "shop" has changed. The tradeoff has been managed by moving from work done by *individual professionals* who knew what was needed and acted accordingly, to work done by multiple professionals from multiple disciplines in *organizational systems* supported by information systems and greatly increasing contributions by patients (Batalden, Ogrinc, & Batalden, 2006).

The *value chain* represents another way of creating value (Porter, 1985). It consists of repeatable, standardized treatment processes that professionals and patients use to produce the desired outcome. In product manufacturing, value chains have enabled gains in efficiency linking processes and standardization. For those products and activities in health care service systems that are similar, this mental model may be very helpful. For example, adopting a chain model for total hip and knee repair may result in efficiency of the linked processes, improved outcomes, and lower costs. Two key tradeoffs in the value chain architecture are between cost and differentiation. Very efficient chains (e.g., those with the fewest, most standardized processes) are less able to address a diversity of needs. This is why some attempts to "install" the chain model widely in health care service systems have been frustrating. The challenge is that only a modest percentage of health care service really fits this product–chain framework. Indeed, patients with complex medical problems might resent being treated to standardized solutions and experts who advertise that they are less expensive. When something major is wrong, patients want the most customized care possible.

The *value network* represents a third way of creating value. A *value network* is a set of activities that facilitates interaction among people, places, and things (e.g., patients, clinicians, researchers, organizational entities, and databases). Learning Health Systems, in which science, informatics, incentives, and culture are aligned for continuous improvement and innovation, with best practices seamlessly embedded in the delivery process and new knowledge captured as an integral by-product of the delivery experience (IOM, 2013), is an example of a value network. There is a vast literature from economics, computer science, business, mathematics and evolutionary biology that provides the scientific basis for how networks function and create value (Benkler, 2006; Wilson, Ostrom, & Cox, 2013). In other industries, combinations of platforms and personnel facilitate networks to increase the efficiency and effectiveness of interaction and exchange.

Research into Improvement Science and Implementation Science

In health care, and especially medical care, evidence-based practice is defined by rigorous research methods. At times, quality improvement research has been criticized because it does not always require the rigor that is expected of more traditional biomedical studies. As a consequence, the results of important CQI initiatives may not be disseminated in the literature because they do not meet publication standards regarding clarity of the study population, interventions, outcome measurements, and procedures for data collection (Pronovost & Wachter, 2006). As CQI continues to evolve into a broader range of health applications—and there is an increased focus on benefits, costs, and the value of health care—there will be increased demand for rigorous CQI studies, which will lead to better education of health professions students as well as better education in research methods for individuals working in the field. Furthermore, there will be more widespread adoption of guidelines for publishing quality improvement initiatives, such as the Standards for QUality Improvement Reporting Excellence (SQUIRE) initiative (Davidoff et al., 2008). The SQUIRE guidelines help authors write peer-reviewed, usable articles about quality improvement in health care so that findings may be easily discovered and widely disseminated.

It is important to clarify that rigor does not always require large-scale randomized, controlled clinical trials (RCTs). In fact, RCT designs can sometimes be at cross-purposes with quality improvement studies (Balestracci, 2009). Similarly, as described in Chapter 4, the use of judgment sampling instead of scientific random sampling to select cases for study is often preferable in CQI initiatives (Perla, Provost, & Murray, 2013). Instead, rigorous studies should emphasize careful design, careful selection of representative patients for study, and analyses appropriate for the design chosen and the decision to be made; that is, in some cases a descriptive analysis may be most appropriate. Most important, rigor implies the use of the scientific method and appropriate attention to patient rights and privacy.

Research methods play an important role but should not serve as an impediment to application of CQI innovations; rather, our research perspective should be broadened to use a wider array of methods to achieve our ultimate goal, which is to make the correct decisions about the application of new CQI ideas. In many cases, the most cost-effective approach is best; to reach the correct decision, we may be better served by implementing a number of repetitive small-scale trials, using a PDSA approach, by which we learn and adapt from each cycle.

Many decisions can be made by simple analyses of properly collected data, perhaps substituting control charts for complex statistical inference models. In some cases, the use of complex design and analysis strategies has produced strong evidence in favor of change, and the widespread adoption of a new approach or CQI tool has met resistance for reasons other than scientific conclusions. Value considerations also enter into this discussion, as the use of RCTs may be unduly expensive and may not always be required and in some cases may not be appropriate, since they may not include the decision-making dimensions that are relevant and will continue to be relevant in the future, such as clinical experience and patient preference. This argument is especially pertinent for CQI decisions as CQI continues to evolve beyond medical care to other health sectors. To address this multidisciplinary perspective, it has been proposed that a transdisciplinary model of evidence-based practice be developed for application to a wide array of disciplines, including nursing, psychology, social work and public health, in addition to medicine. Such a model can be grounded in an ecological framework, such as that presented earlier in Figure 14.1, and can include an emphasis on shared decision making, an increasing demand in health care as well as other health disciplines (Satterfield et al., 2009).

Where more complex methods are required to make decisions, a broader array of research tools that have been proven to be effective should be considered, spanning both traditional experimental designs and observational studies using quasi-experimental designs (Shadish, Cook, & Campbell, 2002). Likewise, consideration should be given to qualitative research methods, as they offer unique tools and perhaps more in-depth probing to help understand the needs of patients, providers, and administrators while complementing and providing context to traditional quantitative methods. Qualitative research has an important role in that it can provide insights into both the quality and safety of care. More importantly, it can provide insight into what may be required to improve care because improvement work requires contextual data about health care settings—specifically the people, processes, and patterns that make up the daily work of providing health care.

Implementation science, introduced and described in substantial detail in Chapter 3, will be critical to ensuring that best practices for clinical care, research, and quality improvement are well implemented. Multiple implementation frameworks and models exist, but perhaps most importantly is the focus on understanding the context in which a CQI initiative was developed and how and where it is adapted for use in other practice settings. Context is critical to understanding why some CQI initiatives are very successful in one setting but do not translate well to other settings; from a design perspective, this can be considered an issue of poor generalizability (i.e., limited external validity) (Shadish, Cook, & Campbell, 2002; Speroff et al., 2004).

One of the key issues that we have faced in the past and that could limit CQI use in the future is failure of a CQI initiative that has been successful on a small scale (e.g., a specific project) to be scalable. The challenge is how to demonstrate improvement on a larger scale, or in other settings with value added to the organizations in which it is applied. This has been attributed to a variety of factors, including lack of fidelity in its application and failure to explain and understand the context in which the initiative was carried out (Dixon-Woods & Martin, 2016). For example, a 2016 systematic review of Lean interventions indicated only limited process improvement impact, and there was evidence of negative impacts in regard to value, as indicated by high financial costs and poor worker satisfaction (Moraros, Lemstra, & Nwankwo, 2016).

What is the context where our improvement work takes place? Clinical process improvement takes place at the front line of care, where providers and patients meet. This can be a clinic, an operating room, an emergency department, a community health center, etc.

Context can be defined as: "Understanding how and why programs work—not simply whether they work" (Dixon-Woods et al., 2011, p. 167). The use of evidence-based methods directly influences the internal validity of a CQI process, but it is external validity that must be considered as well when we intend to generalize a successful implementation to another setting, time or place; this requires careful attention to context. "Knowing how the contextual features compare to one's own circumstances is key to determining the generalizability and relevance of results. The context of individual, group, organization, and system characteristics that surround and interact with the quality improvement initiative may explain critical conditions or barriers to replication" (Speroff et al., 2004, p. 35).

Understanding and carefully evaluating context of successful CQI methods plays a significant role in generalizability of the CQI implementation to other settings. Care must be taken avoid what some authors call "looking for the magic bullet" without careful attention to fidelity and context of successful approaches that we adopt, especially from other industries; this helps to explain some of the controversy about the wholesale use of checklists; for example, see Ramaswamy et al. (2018) and Bosk et al. (2009). Dixon-Woods and Martin (2016) provide a very good description of steps that should be taken to "improve the quality of quality improvement," including greater attention to context and fidelity and the need to focus on organizational and larger program (vs. project) issues when scaling CQI initiatives. Similarly, guidelines have been developed for the appraisal of PDSA methodology

that appears in the literature, before accepting individual study findings and generalizing them to other settings (Speroff et al., 2004).

The Salzburg Global Seminar Session 565 brought together improvement leaders from 22 countries and included researchers, evaluators, and improvers. The primary conclusion that resulted from the session was the need for evaluation to be embedded as an integral part of the improvement (Massoud et al., 2018). Evaluation can take many forms, but for improvement work, Ramaswamy et al. call for "unpacking the black box" of improvement, where the black box is actually the complex relationship between improvement and context (Ramaswamy et al., 2018).

▶ Conclusions

Our vision for this edition of *Continuous Quality Improvement in Health Care* was to provide a foundation for those interested in learning about CQI—the history of the field as well as some of the most relevant topics in improving quality and safety. But at the same time an important goal was to identify what has changed since the last edition and what we have learned in health care about CQI; new methods and new applications (e.g., from other fields) that have become part of the latest wave of the evolution of CQI from industry to health care. Probably the most important new application to have evolved into health care CQI has been implementation science, addressing the critical issue of how to put into practice the innovations and improvements that we have developed through the CQI methodology described here and elsewhere. Another important new idea is the expansion of the Triple Aim (an important concept that has helped to increase the use of CQI methods) by introducing a fourth aim directed at improving provider well-being via the Quadruple Aim. A new, but old concept that has re-emerged is the need for a greater focus on value in health care. In parallel with new ideas and applications has been a further broadening of CQI to other sectors of health and to other geographic locations that have institutionalized CQI as a way ensuring quality, safety and continuous innovation. The interprofessional learning and adaption from medicine to nursing to public health and from developed countries to an increasing number of developing regions is illustrative of the growth that has occurred.

While great progress has been made we are sobered by the realization that much more needs to be done. As with health care itself wider adoption of new scientific methods have led to a new vision of what can be achieved, and through an ongoing learning process we recognize how to achieve that vision, but also realize that some mistakes have been made along the way, which can only be corrected by applying the scientific method, through ongoing education about what we have done right and what we have done wrong. We have learned that more is not necessarily better. For example, electronic medical records are important and useful, but not always optimal to achieve the specificity needed to carry out CQI initiatives, which rely detailed measurement of change over time. Thus, we have also evaluated what works well, what doesn't, and how to close that gap. For example, the successes achieved by a focus on the Triple Aim have been shown to be important but also in need of further improvement, giving rise to the Quadruple Aim.

We have illustrated that broader applications of CQI in multiple health care arenas have led to improved quality and safety, but have also provided lessons for what is missing in the methodology of CQI and the understanding of how to apply these powerful methods correctly and efficiently.

At the same time, we have reiterated some of the constants regarding what must be done to bring value to the patient experience as we continue our improvement work. We have reinforced the importance of understanding variation, teamwork and leadership to foster organizational learning and create a culture of safety and quality throughout all health sectors, locally and globally.

The other important growth trend that has continued since our last edition has been within health delivery. The goal in health care should be to treat not one condition at a time but the total patient—as the patient progresses through the many phases of care, across diverse care settings, with different teams of providers caring for the patient's multiple overlapping conditions. The future will surely bring linkages aided by technology for collaboration across health care sectors and will lead to a new, broader goal for CQI to break out of our silos.

Finally, we recognize the challenges of ongoing CQI growth, including the need for the greatest rigor in CQI research and the need to emphasize value—not only in the large health care systems of the industrialized world but perhaps especially in low- and middle-income countries where health challenges are enormous, and funding is in short supply.

We find it fitting to conclude this chapter with words from Avedis Donabedian, one of the most well-recognized forefathers of quality in health care (Best & Neuhauser, 2004):

Systems awareness and systems design are important for health professionals, but they are not enough. They are enabling mechanisms only. It is the ethical dimensions of individuals that are essential to a system's success. Ultimately, the secret of quality is love. You have to love your patient, you have to love your profession, you have to love your God. If you have love, you can then work backward to monitor and improve the system. (p. 472)

With Donabedian's words in mind, and with the future growth of CQI not an option but a necessity, we close this discussion with one further question, "Who are the future leaders in health care, and where are they from?" The answer is easy: They will come from us, our students, and our children.

References

Adams, R. (2010). Leading health care organizations announce collaborative effort to improve care, lower costs. (Dartmouth-Hitchcock Medical Center press release.) Retrieved from http://www.dhmc.org

Baldrige National Quality Program. (2011). *2011–2012 Health care criteria for performance excellence.* Gaithersburg, MD: National Institute of Standards and Technology.

Balestracci, D. (2009). *Data sanity: A quantum leap to unprecedented results.* Englewood, CO: Medical Group Management Association.

Batalden, M., Batalden, P., Margolis, P., Seid, M., Armstrong, G., Opipari-Arrigan, L., & Hartung, H. (2016). Coproduction of healthcare service. *BMJ Quality & Safety, 25,* 509–517.

Batalden, P. B., & Davidoff, F. (2007). What is "quality improvement" and how can it transform healthcare? *Quality & Safety in Health Care, 16*(1), 2–3.

Batalden, P., Ogrinc, G., & Batalden, M. (2006). From one to many. *Journal of Interprofessional Care, 20,* 549–551.

Benkler, Y. (2006). *The wealth of networks: How social production transforms markets and freedom.* New Haven, CT: Yale University Press.

Berwick, D. (2002). A user's manual for the IOM's Quality Chasm report. *Health Affairs (Millwood), 21*(3), 80–90.

Berwick, D. M. (2003). Disseminating innovations in health care. *Journal of the American Medical Association, 289,* 1969–1975.

Berwick, D., & Nolan, T. (1998). Physicians as leaders in improving health care. *Annals of Internal Medicine, 128,* 289–292.

Berwick, D. M., Nolan, T. W., & Whittington, J. (2008). The triple aim: Care, health, and cost. *Health Affairs (Millwood), 27*(3), 759–769.

Best, M., & Neuhauser, D. (2004). Avedis Donabedian: Father of quality assurance and poet. *Quality & Safety in Health Care, 13*(6), 472–473.

Bodenheimer, T., & Sinsky, C. (2014). From triple to quadruple aim: Care of the patient requires care of the provider. *Annals of Family Medicine, 12*(6), 573–576.

Bosk, C. L., Dixon-Woods, M., Goeschel, C. A., & Pronovost, P. J. (2009). The art of medicine—Reality check for checklists. *The Lancet, 374,* 444–445.

Byrne, J. A. (1993, February 8). The virtual corporation. *Business Week,* 98–103.

Campbell, D. A., Jr., Kubus, J. J., Henke, P. K., Hutton, M., & Englesbe, M. J. (2009). The Michigan Surgical Quality Collaborative: A legacy of Shukri Khuri. *American Journal of Surgery, 198*(5 Suppl), S49–S55.

Classen, D. C., Resar, R., Friffen, F., Federico, F., Frankel, T., Kimmel, N., ... James, B. C. (2011). 'Global Trigger Tool' shows that adverse events in hospitals may be ten times greater than previously measured. *Health Affairs (Millwood), 30,* 581–589. https://doi.org/10.1377/hlthaff.2011.0190

Clauser, S. M., Johnson, D., O'Brien, J., Beveridge, J. M., Fennell, M. L., & Kaluzny, A. D. (2009). A new approach to improving clinical research and cancer care delivery in community settings: Evaluating the NCI Community Cancer Centers Program. *Implementation Science, 4,* 63. https://doi.org/10.1186/1748-5908-4-63

Crosby, P. (1980). *Quality is free: The art of making quality certain.* New York, NY: Penguin Group.

Daft, R. L. (2015). *The leadership experience* (6th ed.). Mason, OH: Cengage Learning.

Davidoff, F., Batalden, P., Stevens, D., Ogrinc, G., Mooney, S., Standards for QUality Improvement Reporting Excellence Development Group. (2008). Publication guidelines for quality improvement in health care: Evolution of the SQUIRE project. *Quality & Safety in Health Care, 17*(Suppl 1), i3–i9.

de Vries, E. N., Prins, H. A., Crolla, R. M., den Outer, A. J., van Andel, G., van Helden, S. H., ... SURPASS Collaborative Group. (2010). Effect of a comprehensive surgical safety system on patient outcomes. *The New England Journal of Medicine, 363*(20), 1928–1937.

de Vries, E., Ramrattan, M., Smorenburg, S. M., Gouma, D. J., & Boermeester, M. A. (2008). The incidence and nature of in-hospital adverse events: A systematic review. *Quality & Safety in Health Care, 17,* 216–223.

Dellinger, E. P., Hausmann, S. M., Bratzler, D. W., Johnson, R. M., Daniel, D. M., Bunt, K. M., ... Sugarman, J. R. (2005). Hospitals collaborate to decrease surgical site infections. *American Journal of Surgery, 190*(1), 9–15.

Deming, W. (1986). *Out of crises.* Cambridge, MA: Massachusetts Institute of Technology Center for Advanced Engineering Study.

Dixon-Woods, M., Bosk, C. L., Aveling, E. L., Goeschel, C. A., & Pronovost, P. J. (2011). Explaining Michigan: Developing an ex post facto theory of a quality improvement program. *Millbank Quarterly, 89*(2), 167–205.

Dixon-Woods, M., & Martin, G. P. (2016). Does quality improvement improve quality? *Future Hospital Journal, 3*(3), 191–194.

Ernst, C., & Chrobot-Mason, D. (2010). *Boundary spanning leadership—Six practices for solving problems, driving innovation and transforming organizations.* New York, NY: McGraw-Hill.

Feeley, D. (2018). The Triple Aim or the Quadruple Aim? Four points to help set your strategy. IHI Improvement Blog. Retrieved from http://www.ihi.org

Flin, R., O'Connor, P., & Crichton, M. (2008). *Safety at the sharp end: A guide to non-technical skills.* Aldershot, UK: Ashgate.

Grady, D. (2010, November 10). Study finds no progress in safety at hospitals. *New York Times.* Retrieved from www.nytimes.com

Greenhalgh, T., Robert, G., Bate, P., Macfarlane, F., & Kyriakidou, O. (2005). *Diffusion of Innovations in Health Service Organisations: A Systematic Literature Review*. Oxford, UK: Blackwell Publishing.

Grove, A. (1995). *High output management*. New York, NY: Random House.

Guillamondegui, O. D., Gunter, O. L., Hines, L., Martin, B. J., Gibson, W., Clarke, P. C., ... Cofer J. B. (2012). Using the National Surgical Quality Improvement Program and the Tennessee Surgical Quality Collaborative to improve surgical outcomes. *Journal of the American College of Surgeons, 214*(4), 709–714; discussion 714–706.

Hall, B., Hamilton, B., Richards, K., Bilimoria, K., Cohen, M., & Ko, C. (2009). Does surgical quality improve in the American College of Surgeons National Surgical Quality Improvement Program: An evaluation of all participating hospitals. *Annals of Surgery, 250,* 363–376.

Hall, B., Richards, K., Ingraham, A., & Ko, C. (2009). New approaches to the National Surgical Quality Improvement Program: The American College of Surgeons experience. *American Journal of Surgery, 198,* S56–S62.

Haynes, A. B., Weiser, T. G., Berry, W. R., Lipsitz, S. R., Breizat, A. H., Dellinger, E. P., ... Safe Surgery Saves Lives Study Group. (2009). A surgical safety checklist to reduce morbidity and mortality in a global population. *The New England Journal of Medicine, 360,* 491–499.

Health Resources & Services Administration (HRSA). (2018). Collaborative Improvement & Innovation Networks (CoIINs). Retrieved from https://mchb .hrsa.gov

Houpt, J. L., Gilkey, R. W., & Ehringhaus, S. H. (2015). *Learning to lead in the academic medical center—A practical guide*. New York, NY: Springer.

Hussey, P. S., Anderson, G. F., Osborn, R., Feek, C., McLaughlin, V., Millar, J., & Epstein, A. (2004). How does the quality of care compare in five countries? *Journal of Health Affairs, 23*(3), 89–99.

Institute of Medicine (IOM). (1988). *The future of public health*. Washington, D.C.: National Academies Press.

Institute of Medicine (IOM). (1999). *To err is human: Building a safer health system*. Washington, D.C.: National Academies Press.

Institute of Medicine (IOM). (2001). *Crossing the quality chasm: A new health system for the 21st century*. Washington, D.C.: National Academies Press.

Institute of Medicine (IOM). (2003). *The future of the public's health in the 21st century*. Washington, D.C.: National Academies Press. Retrieved from http:// www.nationalacademies.org

Johnson, M., Clauser, S., O'Brien, D., Beveridge, J., & Kaluzny, A. (2011). Improving community cancer care and expanding research in community hospitals. *Oncology Issues, 26*(1), 26–28.

Kaba, R., Soorikumaran, P. (2007). The evolution of the doctor-patient relationship. *International Journal of Surgery, 5,* 57e65.

Kotter, J. P. (1996). *Leading change*. Boston, MA: Harvard Business School Press.

Landrigan, C. P., Parry, G. J., Bones, C. B., Hackbarth, A. D., Goldmann, D. A., & Sharek, P. J. (2010). Temporal trends in rates of patient harm resulting from medical care. *The New England Journal of Medicine, 363*(22), 2124–2134.

LaVange, L., Sollecito, W., Steffen, D., Evarts, L., & Kosorok, M. (2012, February). Preparing biostatisticians for leadership opportunities. *Amstat News,* 5–6. Retrieved from http://magazine.amstat.org

Leape, L., & Berwick, D. (2005). Five years after "To Err Is Human": What have we learned? *Journal of the American Medical Association, 293*(19), 2384–2390.

Lee, T. H. (2010). Putting the value framework to work. *The New England Journal of Medicine, 363*(26), 2481–2483.

Massoud, M. R., Kimble, L. E., Goldmann, D., Ovretveit, J., & Dixon, N. (2018). Salzburg Global Seminar Session 565—'Better Health Care: How do we learn about improvement?' *International Journal of Quality in Health Care, 30*(Suppl 1), 1–4.

McGlynn, E. A., Asch, S. M., Adams, J., Keesey, J., Hicks, J., DeCristofaro, A., & Kerr, E. A. (2003). The quality of health care delivered to adults in the United States. *The New England Journal of Medicine, 348*(26), 2635–2645.

McLaughlin, C. P., Johnson, J. K., & Sollecito, W. A. (Eds.). (2012). *Implementing continuous quality improvement in health care: A global casebook*. Sudbury, MA: Jones & Bartlett Learning.

McLaughlin, C. P., & Kaluzny, A. D. (Eds.). (2006). *Continuous quality improvement in health care: Theory, implementations, and applications* (3rd ed.). Sudbury, MA: Jones and Bartlett Publishers.

Millenson, M. (2002). Pushing the profession: How the news media turned patient safety into a priority. *Quality & Safety in Health Care, 11,* 57–63.

Minasian, L. M., Carpenter, W., Weiner, B., Anderson, D. E., McCaskill-Stevens, W., Nelson, S., Whitman, C., ... Kaluzny, A. D. (2010). Translating research into evidence-based practice: The National Cancer Institute's Community Clinical Oncology Program. *Cancer, 116*(19), 4440–4449.

Moraros, J., Lemstra, M., & Nwankwo, C. (2016). Lean interventions in healthcare: do they actually work? A systematic literature review. *International Journal of Quality in Health Care, 28,* 150–165.

Nadeem, E., Olin, S. S., Hill, L. C., Hoagwood, K. E., & Horwitz, S. M. (2013). Understanding the components of quality improvement collaboratives: A systematic literature review. *The Millbank Quarterly, 91*(2), 354–394.

Nelson, E., Godfrey, M., Batalden, P. B., Berry, S. A., Bothe, A. E., Jr., McKinley, K. E., … Nolan, T. W. (2008). Clinical microsystems, part 1. The building blocks of health systems. *The Joint Commission Journal of Quality Patient Safety, 34*(7), 367–378.

Nembhard, I. M. (2009). Learning and improving in quality improvement collaboratives: Which collaborative features do participants value most? *Health Services Research, 44*(2 Pt 1), 359–378.

Network for Regional Healthcare Improvement. (2018). [Website home page]. Retrieved from http://www.nrhi.org/

Nolan, T. (2007). Execution of strategic improvement initiatives to produce system-level results. [IHI Innovation Series white paper]. Cambridge, MA: Institute for Healthcare Improvement.

Ofri, D. (2010). Quality measures and the individual physician. *The New England Journal of Medicine, 363*(7), 606–607.

Ogrinc, G., Mooney, S. E., Estrada, C., Foster, T., Goldmann, D., Hall, L. W., … Watts, B. (2008). The SQUIRE (Standards for QUality Improvement Reporting Excellence) guidelines for quality improvement reporting: Explanation and elaboration. *Quality & Safety in Health Care, 17*(Suppl 1), i13–i32.

Ogrinc, G., Nierenberg, D. W., & Batalden, P. B. (2011). Building experiential learning about quality improvement into a medical school curriculum: The Dartmouth Experience. *Health Affairs (Millwood), 30,* 716–722. https://doi.org/10.1377/hlthaff.2011.0072

Perla, R. J., Provost, L. P., & Murray, S. K. (2013). Sampling considerations for health care improvement. *Quality Management in Health Care, 22*(1), 36–47.

Pfeffer, J., & Sutton, R. (2000). *The Knowing–Doing Gap: How Smart Companies Turn Knowledge into Action.* Boston, MA: Harvard Business School Press.

Porter, M. (1985). *Competitive Advantage.* New York, NY: Free Press

Porter, M. E. (2010). What is value in health care? *The New England Journal of Medicine, 363*(26), 2477–2481.

Pronovost, P., & Wachter, R. (2006). Proposed standards for quality improvement research and publication: One step forward and two steps back. *Quality & Safety in Health Care, 15*(3), 152–153.

Ramaswamy, R., Reed, J., Livesley, N., Boguslavsky, V., Ellorio, E., Sax, S., Houleymata, D., Kimble, L., & Parry, G. (2018). Unpacking the black box of improvement. *International Journal for Quality in Health Care, 30*(Suppl 1), 15–19.

Rouse, W. (2008). Health care as a complex adaptive system. *Bridge, 38*(1), 17–25.

Rowitz, L. (2009). *Public health leadership—Putting principles into practice* (2nd ed.) Gaithersburg, MD: Aspen Publishers, Inc.

Sapienza, A. M. (2004). *Managing scientists—Leadership strategies in scientific research* (2nd ed.). Hoboken, NJ: Wiley-Liss, Inc.

Satterfield, J. M., Spring, B., Brownson, R. C., Mullen, E. J., Newhouse, R. P., Walker, B. B., & Whitlock, E. P. (2009). Toward a transdisciplinary model of evidence based practice. *The Millbank Quarterly, 87,* 2.

Savitz, L. (2012). The Intermountain way to positively impact costs and quality. In C. P. McLaughlin, J. K. Johnson, & W. A. Sollecito. *Implementing continuous quality improvement in health care: A global casebook.* Sudbury, MA: Jones & Bartlett Learning.

SCOAP Collaborative, Writing Group for the SCOAP Collaborative, Kwon, S., Florence, M., Grigas, P., Horton, M., … Flum, D. R. (2012). Creating a learning healthcare system in surgery: Washington State's Surgical Care and Outcomes Assessment Program (SCOAP) at 5 years. *Surgery, 151*(2), 146–152.

Senge, P. (1990). *The fifth discipline.* New York, NY: Doubleday.

Shadish, W., Cook, T., & Campbell, D. T. (2002). Experimental and Quasi-Experimental Designs for Generalized Causal Inference. Boston, MA: Houghton Mifflin.

Sherwood, G., & Jones, C. B. (2013). Quality Improvement in Nursing. In W. A. Sollecito & J. K. Johnson (Eds.), *Continuous quality improvement in health care,* 4th ed. Sudbury, MA: Jones & Bartlett Learning.

Sikka, R., Morath, J. M., & Leape, L. (2015). The Quadruple Aim: Care, health, cost and meaning in work. Retrieved from http://qualitysafety.bmj.com/content/24/10/608

Solberg, L. (2013). The role of organizations, systems, and collaboratives. In W. A. Sollecito and J. K. Johnson (Eds.), *McLaughlin and Kaluzny's Continuous Quality Improvement in Health Care* (4th ed.). Burlington, MA: Jones & Bartlett Learning.

Solberg, L., Kottke, T., & Brekke, M. L. (2006). Quality improvement in primary care. In C. McLaughlin & A. Kaluzny. (Eds.), *Continuous quality improvement in health care: Theory, implementations, and applications* (3rd ed.). Sudbury, MA: Jones and Bartlett Publishers.

Speroff, T., James, B. C., Nelson, E. C., Headrick, L. A., & Brommels, M. (2004). Guidelines for appraisal and publication of PDSA quality improvement. *Quality Management in Health Care, 13*(1), 33–39.

Stabell, C., & Fjeldstad, Ø. (1998). Configuring value for competitive advantage: on chains, shops, and networks. *Strategic Management Journal, 19,* 413–437.

Swensen, S. J., Meyer, G. S., Nelson, E. C., Hunt, G. C., Pryor, D. B., Weissburg, J. I., … Berwick, D. M. (2010). Cottage industry to postindustrial care—The revolution in health care delivery. *The New England Journal of Medicine, 362*(5), e(12)1–e(12)4.

Upshaw, V. M., Steffen, D. P., & McLaughlin, C. P. (2013). CQI, transformation and the "learning" organization. In W. A. Sollecito & J. K. Johnson (Eds.), *McLaughlin and Kaluzny's continuous quality improvement in health care*, 4th ed. Sudbury, MA: Jones & Bartlett Learning.

Viera, A. J., & Kramer, R. (2016). *Management and leadership skills for medical faculty—A practical handbook*. New York, NY: Springer.

Wachter, R. M. (2004). The end of the beginning: Patient safety five years after To Err Is Human. *Health Affairs (Millwood)*, Suppl Web Exclusives, 534–545.

Wachter, R. M. (2010). Patient safety at ten: Unmistakable progress, troubling gaps. *Health Affairs (Millwood)*, *29*(1), 165–173.

Wilson, D. S., Ostrom, E., & Cox, M. E. (2013). Generalizing the core design principles for the efficacy of groups. *Journal of Economic Behavior & Organization, 90*, S21–S32.

Index

Page numbers followed by *f*, *t*, and *b* indicate figures, tables and boxes, respectively.

W

X